ATLAS OF
Clinical
Gynecology

SERIES EDITOR

Morton A. Stenchever, MD

Professor, Chairman Emeritus
Department of Obstetrics and Gynecology
University of Washington Medical Center
Seattle, Washington

Volume **III**

Reproductive
Endocrinology

VOLUME EDITOR

Daniel R. Mishell, Jr., MD

Lyle G. McNeile Professor and Chairman
Department of Obstetrics and Gynecology
University of Southern California School of Medicine
Los Angeles, California

With 30 contributors

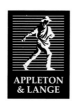

Developed by Current Medicine, Inc.
Philadelphia

010152

Current Medicine, Inc.

400 Market Street
Suite 700
Philadelphia, PA 19106

Director, Product Devlopment	*Lori J. Bainbridge*
Senior Development Editor	*Susan L. Hunsberger*
Editorial Assistant	*Charlene A. French*
Art Director	*Paul Fennessy*
Design	*Robert LeBrun*
Layout	*Christopher Allan, Christine Keller-Quirk, Robert LeBrun*
Illustration Director	*Ann Saydlowski*
Illustrators	*Nicole Mock, Wendy Jackelow, Ann Saydlowski, Beth Starkey, Debbie Wertz*
Production Manager	*Lori Holland*
Production Associate	*Amy Watts*
Indexer	*Dorothy Hoffman*

Reproductive endocrinology / volume editor, Daniel R. Mishell;
   with 20 contributors.
    p. cm. — (Atlas of clinical gynecology ; v. 3)
    1. Endocrine gynecology—Atlases. 2. Human reproduction—
Endocrine aspects—Atlases. 3. Infertility—Atlases. I. Mishell,
Daniel R.II. Series.
    [DNLM: 1. Gonadal Disorders—diagnosis atlases. 2. Menstruation
Disorders—diagnosis atlases. 3. Infertility—diagnosis atlases.
    4. Reproduction Techniques atlases.WP 17 A8806 1997 v.3]
RG79.A88 1998 vol. 3
[RG159]
618.1'0022'2 s—dc21
[618.1]
DNLM/DLC
for Library of Congress   98-9640
ISBN: 0-8385-0319-5   CIP

Although every effort has been made to ensure that drug doses and other information are presented accurately in this publication, the ultimate responsibility rests with the prescribing physician. Neither the publishers nor the authors can be held responsible for errors or for any consequences arising from the use of information contained herein. Products mentioned in this publication should be used in accordance with the prescribing information prepared by the manufacturers. No claims or endorsements are made for any drug or compound at present under clinical investigation.

©Copyright 1999 by Current Medicine, Inc. All rights reserved. No part of this publication may be reproduced, stored in a retrieval system or transmitted in any form by any means electronic, mechanical, photocopying, recording, or otherwise, without prior written consent of the publisher.

Printed in Singapore by Imago Productions (FE) Pte Ltd.

10 9 8 7 6 5 4 3 2 1

Series Preface

The *Atlas of Clinical Gynecology* is an ambitious 5-volume series covering the field of gynecology. Volume topics include pediatric and adolescent gynecology, oncology, pathology, reproductive endocrinology, urogynecology, and reparative surgery. Each volume contains more than 500 images. The images in this collection include not only traditional photographs, but also charts, tables, algorithms, and diagrams, making this collection much more than an atlas in the conventional sense.

The atlas series serves as an excellent teaching tool and resource. In the past few decades, individual learning styles have changed dramatically. In the past, the printed work in book and journal was the primary way in which information was transferred and learning accomplished. In recent decades, however, education has been greatly enhanced by the addition of audio and visual technology. More recently, the advent of personal computers has further enriched the types of learning modalities available.

The *Atlas of Clinical Gynecology* series is designed to use the printed word and visual modalities. The series is available in atlas format as well as in slide sets and on CD-ROM. The information can be used by individual students and by those who teach physicians, medical students, and other health care professionals. The atlas may also serve as a valuable patient education tool.

The series is comprehensive and includes topics that may be neglected in the literature or absent from some training programs. Often practitioners do not see enough patients with a given condition to develop expertise in diagnosis and management. The series is designed to expose the clinician to the unfamiliar as well as to update information on more common gynecologic problems.

I wish to thank the volume editors for their expertise and dedication—Alvin Goldfarb, Barbara Goff, Daniel Mishell, Benjamin Greer, and J. Thomas Benson. We hope that physicians, health care professionals, and the educators who train them find the quality and format of this series useful in the diagnosis and treatment of women of all ages. They deserve the best care available.

Morton A. Stenchever, MD

Volume Preface

A great amount of new information in the field of reproductive endocrinology is being accumulated at a rapid rate. Busy clinicians and resident physicians who encounter women with reproductive endocrine disorders and infertility have difficulty synthesizing all the new information in the field. This volume was developed in order to provide clinicians with an easily understood means of summarizing current knowledge in the area. It provides the reader with a means to use current information in order to diagnose and treat reproductive endocrinologic disorders and infertility. All 15 chapters have been written by individuals who are recognized as experts in the particular area of reproductive endocrinology about which they have written. The chapters are written in a succinct, easily read format that will provide the clinician and student a way to retain and utilize the information with a minimum of effort. The atlas format also allows an easy means of referral when the clinician needs to make a decision about diagnosis or treatment of an individual patient.

As editor of this atlas, I would like to thank each of the authors who contributed a great amount of time and effort in order to prepare this volume. I would also like to thank the staff of Current Medicine, particularly Susan Hunsberger, for her expert assistance in the preparation of this volume.

Daniel R. Mishell, Jr., MD

Contributors

Eli Y. Adashi, MD
Professor and Chair
Department of Obstetrics, Gynecology
    and Pediatrics
University of Utah Health Sciences Center
Salt Lake City, Utah

Sandra M. Bello, MD
Fellow
Division of Reproductive Endocrinology
    and Infertility
Department of Obstetrics and Gynecology
University of Southern California School
    of Medicine
Los Angeles, California

Sarah L. Berga, MD
Associate Professor
Division of Reproductive Endocrinology
Departments of Obstetrics, Gynecology,
    and Reproductive Sciences and Psychiatry
University of Pittsburgh School of Medicine
Attending Physician
Magee-Women's Hospital
Pittsburgh, Pennsylvania

Paul F. Brenner, MD
Professor and Vice Chairman
Department of Obstetrics and Gynecology
University of Southern California
    Medical School
Los Angeles, California

John E. Buster, MD
Professor
Department of Obstetrics and Gynecology
Baylor College of Medicine
Houston, Texas

Bruce R. Carr, MD
Paul C. MacDonald Professor of Obstetrics
    and Gynecology
Department of Obstetrics and Gynecology
University of Texas
Southwestern Medical Center
Dallas, Texas

Peter L. Chang, MD
Assistant Professor
Department of Obstetrics and Gynecology
College of Physicians and Surgeons of
    Columbia University
New York City, New York

John Collins, MD
Professor
Department of Obstetrics and Gynecology
McMaster University
Hamilton, Ontario, Canada

Tammy L. Daniels
Research Associate
Magee-Women's Research Hospital
Pittsburgh, Pennsylvania

Michael P. Federle, MD
Professor
Department of Radiology
University of Pittsburgh School of Medicine
Pittsburgh, Pennsylvania

Lyndon M. Hill, MD
Professor and Medical Director
Department of Obstetrics, Gynecology, and
    Reproductive Sciences
University of Pittsburgh School of Medicine
Pittsburgh, Pennsylvania

Gloria E. Hoffman, PhD
Professor
Department of Anatomy and Neurobiology
University of Maryland School of Medicine
Baltimore, Maryland

Robert Israel, MD
Professor
Department of Obstetrics and Gynecology
University of Southern California
Los Angeles, California

Howard S. Jacobs, MD, FRCP, FRCOG
Professor
UCL Medical School
The Middlesex Hospital
London, England

Brinda N. Kalro, MD
Fellow
Department of Obstetrics, Gynecology, and
    Reproductive Sciences
Magee-Women's Hospital
Pittsburgh, Pennsylvania

Charles M. March, MD
Professor
Department of Obstetrics and Gynecology
University of Southern California
Women's and Children's Hospital
Los Angeles, California

Kenneth S. McCarty, Jr., MD, PhD
Professor
Departments of Pathology and Internal
    Medicine
University of Pittsburgh School of Medicine
Pittsburgh, Pennsylvania

Monica McKinnon, MD
Resident
Department of Obstetrics and Gynecology
University of Massachusetts Medical Center
Worcester, Massachusetts

Veronica Ravnikar, MD
Professor
Director of Reproductive Endocrinology
Department of Obstetrics and Gynecology
University of Massachusetts Medical Center
Worcester, Massachusetts

Robert W. Rebar, MD
Professor and Director
Department of Obstetrics and Gynecology
University of Cincinnati
Cincinnati, Ohio

Mark V. Sauer, MD
Instructor
Department of Obstetrics and Gynecology
College of Physicians and Surgeons of
    Columbia University
New York City, New York

Michael D. Scheiber, MD
Instructor
Department of Obstetrics and Gynecology
University of Cincinnati
Cincinnati, Ohio

Donna Shoupe, MD
Professor
Department of Obstetrics and Gynecology
University of Southern California
Women's and Children's Hospital
Los Angeles, California

Rebecca Z. Sokol, MD
Professor
Department of Obstetrics and Gynecology
University of Southern California
Women's and Children's Hospital
Los Angeles, California

Patricia J. Sulak, MD
Associate Professor
Department of Obstetrics and Gynecology
Texas A&M Health Science Center
Temple, Texas

Jules Sumkin, DO
Associate Professor
Department of Radiology
University of Pittsburgh School of Medicine
Pittsburgh, Pennsylvania

Melvin H. Thornton, MD
Clinical Assistant Professor
Department of Obstetrics and Gynecology
University of Southern California School
    of Medicine
Los Angeles, California

Laurence C. Udoff, MD
Assistant Professor
Department of Obstetrics and Gynecology
University of Utah
Salt Lake City, Utah

Kenneth H.H. Wong, MD
Clinical Fellow
Department of Obstetrics and Gynecology
University of Utah
Salt Lake City, Utah

Paul M. Yandell, MD
Assistant Professor
Department of Obstetrics and Gynecology
Texas A&M Health Science Center
Temple, Texas

Contents

Primary Amenorrhea

Paul F. Brenner

Indications of malfunction of the reproductive axis include the absence of spontaneous menstruation by the age of 16.5 years, the failure of secondary sex characteristics (breast development) to appear by age 14, and the appearance of secondary sex characteristics that is not followed by menarche within 2 years. The presence of the clinical manifestations of Turner syndrome at any age is predictive of the absence of ovarian follicles and the apparatus to synthesize estrogen. Primary amenorrhea is defined as the absence of spontaneous uterine bleeding (menarche) by the age of 16.5 years. The cause can be physiologic (pregnancy), endocrinologic (failure of the reproductive axis to attain full maturity) or anatomic (obstruction of the lower reproductive tract including the cervix, vagina, or hymen that blocks the egress of the desquamated endometrial tissue and blood). Individuals with ambiguous external genitalia should be evaluated as soon after birth as is feasible to establish the correct diagnosis and formulate a plan of management. The phenomenon of ambiguous external genitalia is not considered in this chapter.

HORMONES AND PUBERTY

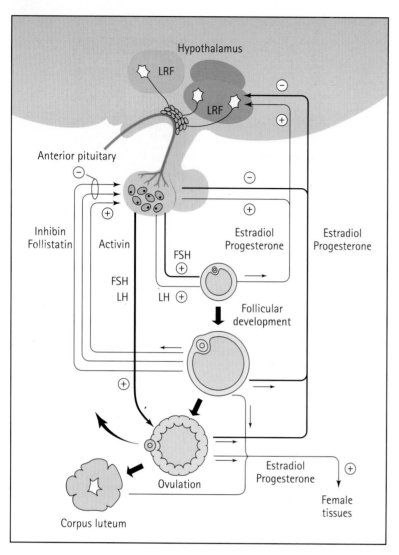

FIGURE 1-1.

Hormonal control of ovarian function. The hypothalamus produces a gonadotropin-releasing hormone factor (GnRH), which acts on the pituitary cells to secrete follicle-stimulating hormone (FSH) and luteinizing hormone (LH). A secretion of FSH together with tonic LH stimulates the follicular development. The developed follicles secrete estradiol, progesterone, inhibins, activins, and follistatins. Estradiol and progesterone, at different concentrations or ratios, either positively or negatively feed back to the hypothalamic hypophysial axis in regulating the secretion of FSH and LH. Inhibins and follistatins specifically suppress, whereas activin and transforming growth factor-β enhance the secretion of FSH by the pituitary.

Menarche requires a patent outflow tract, a hormonally responsive endometrium, ovarian sex steroidogenesis and follicular development, anterior pituitary hormaonal signals of FSH and LH, and release from the hypothalamus of GnRH. The normal function of the reproductive axis involves negative and positive feedback signals of ovarian estrogen, progesterone, activin, inhibin and follistatin on the hypothalamus and the anterior pituitary gland as well as properly timed pulses of GnRH and the cyclicity of the production and release of the pituitary gonadotropins. (*Adapted from* Ying [1]; with permission.)

MEAN AGES OF US GIRLS AT THE ONSET OF PUBERTAL EVENTS

Event	Mean age ± SD, y
Initiation of breast development	10.8 ± 1.10
Appearance of pubic hair	11.0 ± 1.21
Menarche	12.9 ± 1.20

FIGURE 1-2.

Mean ages of US girls at the onset of pubertal events. Menarche is only one of the clinical events that are a part of normal female puberty. Menarche is preceded by breast budding and development, changes in the contour of the pelvis, appearance of pubic and axillary hair, and acceleration of the rate of increase in height (peak height velocity). Breast budding is considered one of the earliest events of puberty, and the first spontaneous menstrual period is one of the latest events of puberty. These morphologic pubertal changes occur in response to the endocrinologic changes in estrogen and androgen secretion. The definition of primary amenorrhea assumes that menarche occurs with a normal frequency distribution and is statistically derived based on multiples of the SD above the mean. The definition used in this discussion of primary amenorrhea is based on the mean age at menarche in US women as 12.9 years SD, 1.2 years). Three SDs above the mean age at menarche is 16.5 years. The incidence of primary amenorrhea is less that 0.1% of the female population. (*Adapted from* Frisch and Revelle [2].)

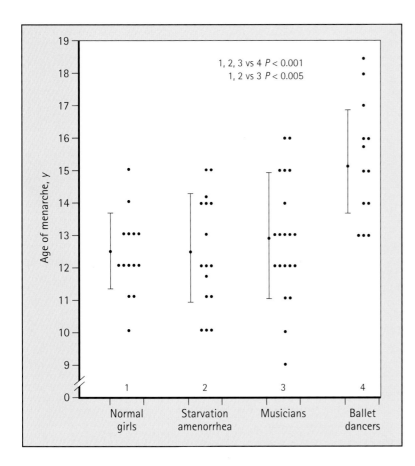

FIGURE 1-3.

The age of menarche in normal girls compared with that of girls with starvation amenorrhea, musicians, and ballet dancers. The age at menarche is influenced by many factors. Onset of menstruation has a positive correlation with the age of maternal menarche. If the mothers had relatively late menarche, their daughters are likely to experience their menarche at a later age; if the mothers had a relatively early menarche, their daughters tend to experience an early menarche. Blind women tend to have menarche earlier than do women with unimpaired vision. Women with diabetes mellitus have a later menarche than do women with normal carbohydrate metabolism. Menarche is related to both body weight as well as body composition. Compared with girls of normal body weight, those whose body weight exceeds the ideal by 20% to 30% have an earlier menarche and those whose body weight exceeds the ideal by more than 30% have a delayed menarche. Rigorous exercise programs, rural living, colder climate, and higher altitude are also associated with a later onset of menstruation. It is suggested that a percent body fat between 17% and 22% is usually required for menstruation. Ballet dancers and individuals who participate in strenuous exercise programs before menarche have a reduced ratio of fat to lean body weight and often experience a delay in menarche. *T bars* indicate mean ± SD. (*Adapted from* Warren [3].)

MEAN INTERVALS BETWEEN BREAST BUDDING AND OTHER PUBERTAL CHANGES

Pubertal events	Interval between pubertal events, y ± SD
Breast budding to peak height velocity	1.0 ± 0.77
Breast budding to menarche	2.3 ± 1.03
Breast budding to last stage pubic hair growth	3.1 ± 1.04
Breast budding to last stage breast development	4.5 ± 2.04

FIGURE 1-4.

Mean intervals between breast budding and other pubertal changes. Once the mean age for the onset of the clinical landmarks that comprise normal female puberty are determined, the mean intervals between the stages of these events are easily calculated. The mean interval for US girls between the initial breast budding and menarche is 2.3 years (SD, 1.03). The interval obviously varies, with some individuals progressing from breast budding to menarche in 1.5 years and as long as 5 years in others. Primary amenorrhea is defined as the absence of spontaneous menstruation by age 16.5 years. An evaluation of sexual infantilism or the absence of secondary sex characteristics should be initiated for a woman 14 years of age or older who presents with the absence of breast budding. Because the mean interval from breast budding to menarche is 2.3 years with an SD of approximately 1 year, it is unlikely that these individuals will menstruate in the next 2 years. (*Adapted from* Frisch and Revelle [2].)

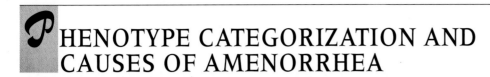

PHENOTYPE CATEGORIZATION AND CAUSES OF AMENORRHEA

CATEGORIZATION OF PHENOTYPES OF INDIVIDUALS WITH PRIMARY AMENORRHEA

Group	Breasts	Uterus
I	Absent	Present
II	Present	Absent
III	Absent	Absent
IV	Present	Present

FIGURE 1-5.

Categorization of phenotypes of individuals with primary amen-orrhea. This classification is based on the presence or absence of breast and uterine development. Individuals with primary amen-orrhea for whom an anatomic disorder and pregnancy have been excluded can be categorized into four phenotypic groups. Presence or absence of uterus is determined by palpation, which may be performed as a vaginal-abdominal or a rectal-abdominal exami-nation. The breast is the most estrogen-sensitive human tissue; therefore, the use of exogenous estrogen, depending on dose and duration of administration, may stimulate breast development and confuse this classification. Classifications based on positive and negative clinical findings reduces the need for adjunctive diagnostic aids.

Group I women (breasts absent, uterus present) were never exposed to normal estrogen production by the ovary. Because the normal development of pelvic organs derived from the müllerian system results in the presence of the uterus, women with group I primary amenorrhea never had normal estrogen production by

the ovaries but did have the normal development of the stuctures that are part of the müllerian system.

Women with group II primary amenorrhea (breasts present but no uterus) will have either a congenital absence of the uterus or androgen-insensitivity (testicular feminization) syndrome. Congenital absence of the uterus is a separate, non-inherited event that results in failure of development of the müllerian system. Androgen-insensitivity syndrome is a genetic inherited disorder.

Group III primary amenorrhea (breasts and uterus absent) is very rare. These patients have a male karyotype (46,XY), elevated gonadotropin levels, and serum testosterous levels that are within or below the normal female range. Women with group III primary amenorrhea include those with 17,20-desmolase deficiency, agonadism, and 17α-hydroxylase deficiency. Patients with a 46,XY karyotype differ from those with gonadal failure in that they lack a uterus, whereas those with gonadal failure have a uterus present. These patients differ from those with androgen-insensitivity syndrome in that they do not have breast develop-ment and their circulating testosterone levels are in the normal female range, whereas those with androgen-insensitivity syndrome have breast development and their circulating testosterone levels are in the normal male range.

Group IV primary amenorrhea comprises those women who have both spontaneous breast development and the presence of the uterus. The presence of spontaneous breast development indi-cates that the female reproductive axis had attained sufficient maturity to produce enough endogenous estrogen for a sufficient length of time to stimulate the growth and development of breast tissue as an early puberal event. Some time after puberty had been initiated and before the later events of puberty (such as menarche) could be completed, the hypothalamic-pituitary-ovarian axis failed to function normally.

CLASSIFICATION OF CAUSES OF PRIMARY AMENORRHEA

Group I primary amenorrhea (breasts absent, uterus present)

  Gonadal failure

    45,X (Turner syndrome)

    46,X, abnormal X (eg, short- or long-arm deletion)

    Mosaicism (eg, X/XX, X/XX/XXX)

    46,XX or 46,XY pure gonadal dysgenesis

    17 α-Hydroxylase deficiency with 46,XY karyotype

  Hypothalamic failure secondary to inadequate GnRH release

    Insufficient GnRH secretion due to neurotransmitter defect

    Inadequate GnRH synthesis

    Congenital anatomic defect in central nervous system

  Pituitary failure

    Isolated gonadotropin insufficiency

    Chromophobe adenoma

    Mumps, encephalitis

    Newborn kernicterus

    Prepubertal hypothyroidism

Group II primary amenorrhea (breasts present, uterus absent)

    Androgen insensitivity (testicular feminization)

    Congenital absence of the uterus

Group III primary amneorrhea (breasts and uterus absent)

    17,20-Desmolase deficiency

    Agonadism

    17α-Hydroxylase deficiency with 46,XY karyotype

Group IV primary amenorrhea (breasts and uterus present)

    Hypothalamic

    Pituitary

    Ovary

    Uterine

FIGURE 1-6.

Classification of causes of primary amenorrhea. The various causes of primary amenorrhea have been classified in several different ways. The most common classification relates to the anatomic site in the reproductive axis that is involved (hypothalamus, pituitary, ovary, uterus, vagina) and malfunctioning. Mashchak *et al.* [4] proposed a phenotypic classification based on the presence or absence of the breast and uterus. Using this system, individuals can be placed in one of four groups in descending order of frequency. The groups are individuals with absent breast development and a uterus present, individuals with both breast development and a uterus present, individuals with breast development present and an absent uterus, and the least common group of individuals without breast development and without a uterus present.

 # ROUP I: BREASTS ABSENT, UTERUS PRESENT

FAILURE OF OVARIAN ESTROGEN PRODUCTION (HYPOGONADISM)

Anatomic site	Gonadotropins
Hypothalamus-pituitary	Low or normal hypogonadotropic
Ovary	Elevated hypergonadotropic

FIGURE 1-7.

Failure of ovarian estrogen production in group I primary amenorrhea. A failure of ovarian estrogen production is caused by either a hypothalamic-pituitary disorder or ovarian failure. A central nervous system disorder results in diminished gonadotropin output by the hypothalamic-pituitary unit to the ovary. The ovary has the potential for normal estrogen production, but the pituitary stimulus is not delivered to the ovary (hypogonadotropic hypogonadism). Ovarian follicles are the site of estrogen and inhibin production. As a consequence of the ovary's inability to produce estrogen and inhibin, the negative feedback of estrogen and inhibin on the hypothalamus and pituitary is absent. In the absence of any inhibition of gonadotropin, the levels of follicle-stimulating hormone and luteininzing hormone become elevated in women with ovarian failure (hypergonadotropic hypogonadism).

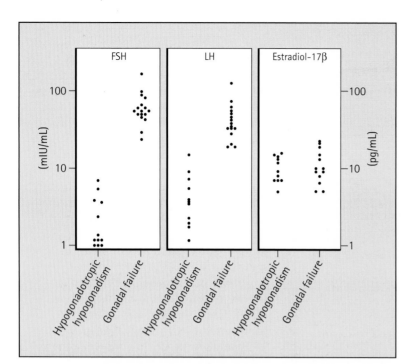

FIGURE 1-8.

Serum levels of follicle-stimulating hormone (FSH) luteinizing hormone (LH), and estradiol in women with hypogonadotropic hypgonadism and gonadal failure. Individuals who lack primordial follicles to make estrogen or have an enzyme deficiency in the sex steroid biosynthetic pathway so that they are unable to synthesize estrogen will lack the negative feedback of estrogen and inhibin or estrogen alone on the hypothalamus and pituitary. Without the negative feedback of estrogen and inhibin on the hypothalamic-pituitary axis, gonadotropin levels increase. Therefore, measurement of gonadotropin levels can be used to differentiate hypogonadtropic hypogonadism and gonadal failure.

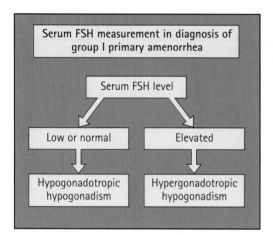

FIGURE 1-9.

Measurement of serum follicle-stimulating hormone (FSH) in diagnosis of group I primary amenorrhea. Prior to the maturity of the reporductive axis, FSH basal levels are greater than LH basal levels. During the reproductive years, basal LH concentrations are higher than basal FSH concentrations; postmenopausally, the reverse occurs. Both FSH and LH concentrations rise in women with gonadal failure. The increase is FSH is more pronounced than the increase in LH levels in women with ovarian failure, and serum FSH concentrations are the preferred marker to distinguish this disorder from hypothalamic-pituitary disorders in women with group I primary amenorrhea. (*Adapted from* Mashchak *et al.* [4].)

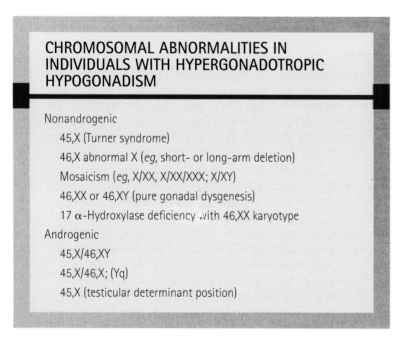

FIGURE 1-10.

The most common chromosomal abnormalities in women with hypergonadotropic hypogonadism. All individuals have elevated follicle-stimulating hormone and luteinizing levels and low estradiol levels. Two X sex chromosomes that are normal in number and structure are required for the normal development of the ovary. Genetic disorders are the most common cause of primary amenorrhea. Approximately 30% of individuals with primary amenorrhea have a genetic disorder. Women with ovarian failure due to a genetic cause usually have a deletion of all or part of one X chromosome. Sometimes even if two normal X chromosomes are present, ovarian failure can occur, indicating a genetic and not a chromosomal disorder. The most common chromosomal abnormalities associated with hypergonadotropic hygonadism include 45,X karyotype (Turner syndrome), structurally abnormal X chromosome, mosaicism, pure gonadal dysgenesis (46,XX and 46,XY with streak gonads), and 17 α-hydroxylase deficiency with a 46,XX karyotype.

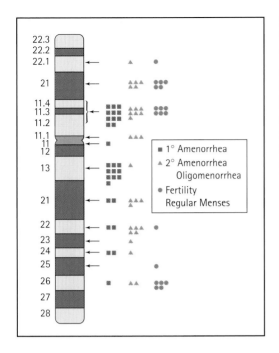

FIGURE 1-11.

The X chromosome, including the effects of deletions in different parts of the chromosome. The most common chromosomal abnormality that results in gonadal failure is the complete absence of the X chromosome. The absence of an entire X chromosome results in a karyotype of 45,X, or Turner syndrome. The principal features of Turner syndrome include sexual infantilism, short stature, and streak gonads. Approximately 98% of pregnancies in which the fetus has one X chromosome end in spontaneous abortion. The remaining 2% of such pregnancies accounts for an incidence of Turner syndrome that is between one in 2000 and one in 7000 births. The diagnosis is usually made in neonatal period because of the unique somatic characteristics of individuals with this disorder. (*Adapted from* Simpson [5]; with permission.)

■ 1° Amenorrhea
▲ 2° Amenorrhea
    Oligomenorrhea
● Fertility
    Regular Menses

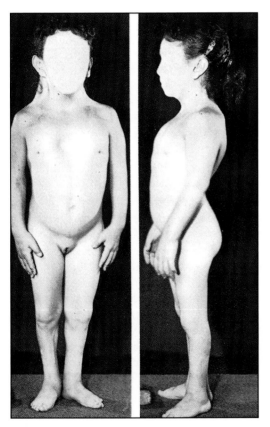

FIGURE 1-12.

Physical characteristics of gonadal dysgenesis. Note the short stature (final height, 42 in), webbing of the neck, multiple nevi, low-set hairline and ears, lack of secondary sex characteristics, wide-spaced nipples, and edema of the feet and hands. Other somatic abnormalities that are usually part of Turner syndrome include a short, thick and webbed neck, low posterior hairline, congenital lymphedema, broad shield-like chest, hypoplastic or inverted nipples, cubitus valgus, short fourth metacarpal bones, multiple pigmented nevi, tendency to keloid formation, and recurrent otitis media. A variety of cardiovascular anomalies are associated with Turner syndrome, including bicuspid aortic valve, coarctation of the aorta, mitral valve prolapse, and aortic aneurysms. Renal anomalies associated with Turner syndrome include a horseshoe kidney, unilateral pelvic kidney, rotational anomalies, and partial or complete duplication of the collecting system. Hashimoto's thyroiditis, Addison's disease, alopecia, and vitiligo are autoimmune disorders associated with this syndrome. In addition, individuals with Turner syndrome may have mild insulin resistance, hearing loss, and osteoporosis. Patients with Turner syndrome have normal intelligence. (*From* Federman [6]; with permission.)

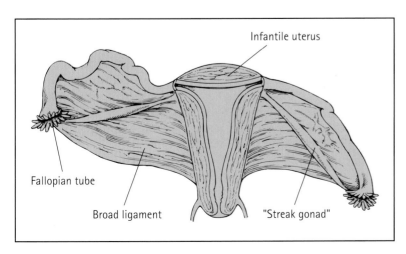

FIGURE 1-13.

The internal genitalia of a patient with Turner syndrome, featuring a normal but infantile uterus, normal fallopian tubes, and pale glistening streak gonads (*ie*, fibrous tissue without follicles) in both broad ligaments. The only indications for surgical removal of the streak gonads are the presence of a Y chromosome in the karyotype of the peripheral blood leukocytes or clinical evidence of excess androgen production without the presence of a Y chromosome. In the absence of these two conditions it is not necessary to surgically extirpate the streak gonads, because malignant transformation is extremely rare.

Infantile uterus

Fallopian tube

Broad ligament

"Streak gonad"

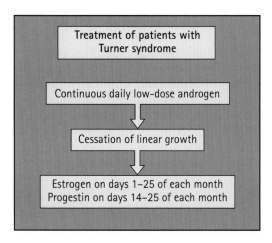

FIGURE 1-14.

Treatment of patients with Turner syndrome. Treatment aims are to maximize the patient's final height, initiate breast development, and prevent osteoporosis. The diagnosis of Turner syndrome is usually based on the presence of the clinical features of this syndrome coupled with an elevated serum follicle-stimulating hormone value. The diagnosis is confirmed by a 45,X karyotype. Individuals with Turner syndrome require hormonal replacement therapy. The administration of estrogen will stimulate breast development and prevent osteoporosis. Progestins should also be given to reduce the risk of developing endometrial hyperplasia and adenocarcinoma. To maximize the individual's final height, low-dose androgens should be administered before or during estrogen replacement therapy [ERT]. One regimen uses continuous fluoxymesterone, 2.5 mg/d, until there is a cessation of linear growth over a 3-month interval. Another regimen uses a testosterone analogue, oxandrolone (0.1 mg/kg/body weight daily). Once the patient demonstrates no further increase in height, ERT is initiated.

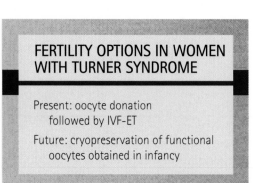

FIGURE 1-15.

Fertility options in women with Turner syndrome. Individuals with Turner syndrome 45,X have ovarian failure. Oocyte donation followed by *in vitro* fertilization–embryo transfer (IVF-ET) is the only successful treatment for those patients with Turner syndrome who desire fertility. Estradiol is administered first to prepare the endometrium to receive the embryo. The endometrium response to exogenous estrogen is monitored with transmaginal ultrasonography. When the endometrium achieves a thickness that is considered favorable for receiving the embryo, the oocytes are aspirated from the donor, progesterone administration is begun, and the oocytes are fertilized *in vitro*. On the third day of progesterone administration, the embryo transfer is performed. Following embryo transfer, daily doses of estrogen and progesterone are given to the recipient until 9 to 12 weeks of gestation, when placental production of steroids is sufficient to maintain a pregnancy. Shortly after birth, functional ovarian follicles may be present in individuals with Turner syndrome. Currently, ovarian cryopreservation is rarely successful; however, in the future, women with Turner syndrome may be able to have their functional oocytes aspirated early in infancy and cryopreserved until a time in their reproductive years when fertility is desired.

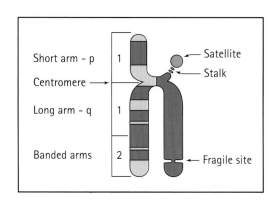

FIGURE 1-16.

An idealized "composite" chromosome demonstrating various features of chromosomes. Women with gonadal failure due to a structurally abnormal X chromosome disorder have a 46,XX karyotype, but genetic information is missing from one of the X chromosomes. The clinical manifestations of the stucturally incomplete chromosome varies depending on the amount of genetic material that has been lost and the specific site on the stucturally abnormal X chromosome from which the genetic material was deleted. Individuals who have a deletion of the long arm of the X chromosome (Xq) have streak gonads, sexual infantilism, and usually (but not always) normal stature and an absence of the somatic abnormalities. Individuals who have deletion of the short arm of the X chromosome (Xp) have streak gonads, sexual infantilism, short stature, and the clinical signs of Turner syndrome. Individuals with isochromosome of the long arm of the X chromosome also manifest many of the clinical features of Turner syndrome. Occasionally an individual with structurally abnormal X chromosome may have a few ovarian follicles that allow the production of sufficient estrogen to initiate breast development, experience a few spontaneous menses, and even become pregnant. (*Adapted from* Mishell *et al.* [7]; with permission.)

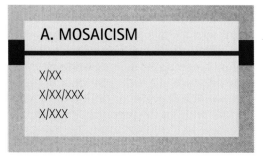

FIGURE 1-17.

Karyotypes of various disorders causing primary amenorrhea. **A**, Mosaicism. Individuals with a mosaic karyotype have a wide spectrum of phenotypes. The most common mosaic karyotype associated with ovarian failure is X/XX. In general, individuals with the X/XX karyotype are taller and have fewer anomalies than individuals with 45,X karotype. They are usually shorter than individuals with a normal female karyotype. Two thirds of individuals with X/XX mosaicism have some anomaly and one fifth have spontaneous menstruation and very rarely do they ovulate spontaneously, conceive, and deliver a normal infant. Estrogen production depends on the number of follicles present in the gonadal tissue as well as the funcitonal capacity of the follicles. The clinical presentation of individuals with X/XXX and X/XX/XXX karyotypes is similar to those individuals with X/XX mosaicism.**B**, Pure Gonadal dysgenesis. Individuals with a normal karyotype may still have their ovaries fail to develop.Individuals with pure

(*Continued on next page*)

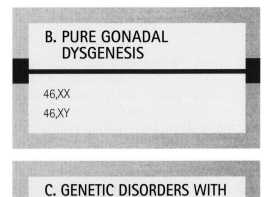

B. PURE GONADAL DYSGENESIS

46,XX

46,XY

C. GENETIC DISORDERS WITH HYPERANDROGENISM

45,X/46,XY

45,X/46,Xi (Yq)

45,X (testicular determinate position)

FIGURE 1–17. *(Continued)*
gonadal dysgenesis have streak gonads, sexual infantilism, and primary amenorrhea, but they lack the other morphologic features found in individuals with Turner syndrome and a 45,X karyotype. Patients are normal in stature and do not have the clinical signs of Turner syndrome. Breast development usually does not occur in individuals with pure gonadal dysgenesis. A few of these patients have been reported to have breast development and a few episodes of spontaneous menses, which is most likely caused by a few ovarian follicles that have persisted until puberty and then, in response to gonadotropin stimulation, synthesize estrogen. **C**, Gonadal dysgenesis and hyperandrogenism. Approximately one tenth of patients with gonadal dysgenesis have a genetic disorder that is associated with hyperandrogenism. Most often these individuals with gonadal dysgenesis have a karyotype that includes a Y chromosome or a fragment of a Y chromosome. Less often, some of these individuals may only have a DNA fragment that contains the testis-determining gene (probably *SRY*). Screening for testis-determining genes, including the Y chromosome *SRY* gene, will eventually become part of the evaluation of all individuals with gonadal dysgenesis, but it is not the standard at this time. Gonadal neoplasms frequently occur in individuals with gonadal dysgenesis who have a Y chromosome in at least one cell line of their karyotype. These individuals should have their gonads removed as soon as the Y chromosome is identified. Individuals with gonadal dysgenesis who are also hirsute or have clinical evidence of virilization should also have their gonads surgically extirpated for the same reason, even if a Y chromosome has not been identified in the karyotype.

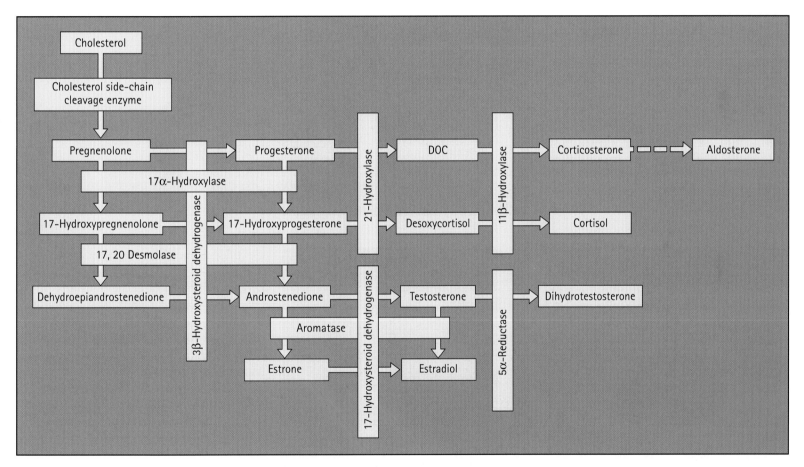

FIGURE 1–18.

The steroid biosynthetic pathway. A few women have been reported to have gonadal failure due to an enzyme defect in the biosynthetic pathway. These individuals have primary amenorrhea group I, normal female external genitalia, and 17α-hydroxylase deficiency. 17α-hydroxylase is essential for the conversion of pregnenolone to 17-hydroxypregnenolone and progesterone to 17-hydroxyprogesterone. 17-Hydroxypregnenolone and 17-hydroxyprogesterone are precursors in the biosynthetic pathway to androgens and estrogens. Women with 17α-hydroxylase deficiency are unable to produce sex steroids, resulting in low serum estrogen concentrations, the absence of the negative feedback of estrogen on the hypothalamus and pituitary, and the elevation of gonadotropin levels. Although control of cortisol and adrenal androgens are adrenocorticotropic dependent, aldosterone is not. Aldosterone is regulated by the renin-angiotensin system and plasma sodium concentration. 17α-Hydroxylase deficiency results in an elevation of deoxycorticosteroid (DOC) and corticosteroid. The increase in DOC and corticosterone concentrations leads to sodium retention, which lowers serum aldosterone levels. Women with 17α-hydroxylase deficiency manifest sodium retention, hypokalemia, and hypertension caused by the increase in mineralocortioid precursors in the aldosterone pathway. 17α-Hydroxylase deficiency is a potentially life-threatening disease. The treatment of this disorder includes not only estrogen and progestin replacement therapy, but also cortisone administration. Successful pregnancies have been achieved in women with 17α-hydroxylase deficiency using *in vitro* fertilization–embryo transfer technology.

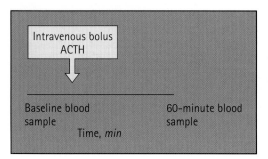

FIGURE 1-19.

Adrenocorticotropic hormone (ACTH) sitmulation test. The diagnosis of 17α-hydroxylase deficiency can be made by demonstrating an elevation in the immediate precursors and a decrease in the immediate product involved in the enzymatic pathway. Serum levels of progesterone exceeding 3 ng/mL (precursor) and 17α-hydroxyprogesterone levels less than 0.2 ng/mL (product) are very suggestive of the diagnosis of 17α-hydroxylase deficiency. An ACTH stimulation test confirms the diagnosis. Between 8:00 and 9:00 AM following overnight fasting, 0.25 mg of cosyntropin is given intraveously over a 30- to 60-s interval. Blood samples are obtained just prior to the administration of ACTH (baseline) and 60 minutes after ACTH in injected. Patients with 17α-hydryoxylase deficiency will demonstrate a marked increase in serum progesterone concentrations and little or no change in 17α-hydroxyprogesterone levels.

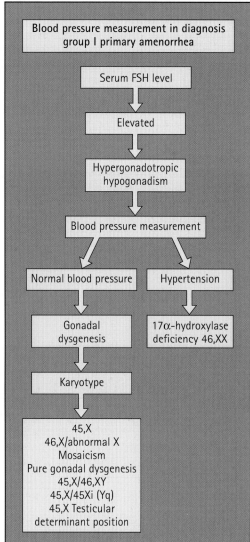

FIGURE 1-20.

Blood pressure measurement in diagnosis of group I primary amenorrhea. Patients with hypergonadotropic hypogonadism as determined by serum follicle-stimulating hormone (FSH) level can be categorized into two groups. Those with 17α-hydroxylase deficiency will have an elevated blood pressure. The diagnosis is established by the measurement of serum progesterone and 17α-hydroxyprogesterone levels and confirmed by an adrenocorticotropic hormone challenge test. In the absence of hypertension a karyotype is necessary to establish the precise diagnosis.

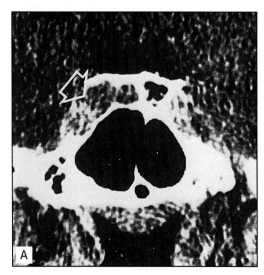

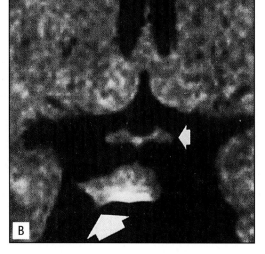

FIGURE 1-21.

Anatomic defects causing gonadotropin-releasing hormone (GnRH) failure. Such defects are rare. One woman was found to have anterior encephalocele and no sellar floor. Another had stenosis of the aqeduct with dilated ventricles. Central nervous system neoplasms that impinge on the hypothalamic-pituitary region, such as a craniopharyngioma, may also rarely cause hypogonadotropic hypogonadism. Pituitary tumors are rarely identified as the cause of primary amenorrhea associated with hypogonadotropic hypogonadism. Most of these tumors secrete prolactin. A computed tomography (CT) scan or magnetic resonance imaging (MRI) study of the sella turcica should be performed in all individuals with hypogonadotropic hypogonadism.

These images were selected to demonstrate pathology, and do not exactly correspond in level of section through the sella. A, CT scan (coronal section) showing bony erosion of right sella turcica (arrow) with possible soft tissue extension into the right cavernous sinus. Height of pituitary gland (not shown) is 9 mm. B, MRI (coronal section) showing a soft tissue mass extending into the right cavernous sinus near the carotid artery (small arrow). Height of the pituitary gland is 9 mm. A normal optic chiasm is seen (small arrow). (From Stein et al. [8]; with permission.)

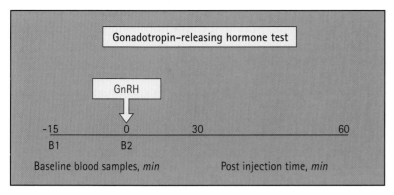

FIGURE 1-22.

Gonadotropin-releasing hormone (GnRH) test. Most individuals with hypogonadotropic hypogonadism will demonstrate a positive result to this test. The pituitary is primed with daily intramuscular administration of 100 µg GnRH for 1 week before the test. Two baseline blood samples are obtained 15 minutes apart on the day of the test. A single intravenous bolus of 100 µg GnRH is then administered over a 30 second interval. Blood samples are obtained 30 and 60 minutes after the GnRH is administered. The peak response of luteinizing hormone occurs 30 minutes after the GnRH injec-

tion, and the peak response of follicle-stimulating hormone (FSH) occurs 60 minutes after the injection. In response to a single bolus of GnRH there is an increase in LH and a greater increase in FSH when pituitary gonadotropin function is intact. Once the pituitary has been sufficiently primed, a significantly response of FSH and LH to a single bolus of GnRH indicates that the defect is in the hypothalamus. GnRH synthesis or GnRH secretion is usually found to be insufficient in individuals with hypogonadotropic hypogonadism. Some women with hypothalamic hypogonadotropic hypogonadism also have anosmia (Kallmann syndrome). All individuals with group I primary amenorrhea and hypogonadotropic hypogonadism should have testing for olfaction. Coffee, orange, cocoa, and tobacco are appropriate substances to be included in a qualitative test of olfactory function. Anosmia indicates an impaired development of the rhinencephalic brain structure.

Failure to demonstrate an increase in serum gonadotropin levels after a GnRH stimulation test indicates pituitary hypogonadotropic hypogonadism. These patients usually have associated disorders such as thalassemia major or retinitis pigmentosa. Other very rare causes of hypogonadotropic hypogonadism due to pituitary failure include prepubertal hypothyroidism, newborn kernicterus, and mumps encephalitis.

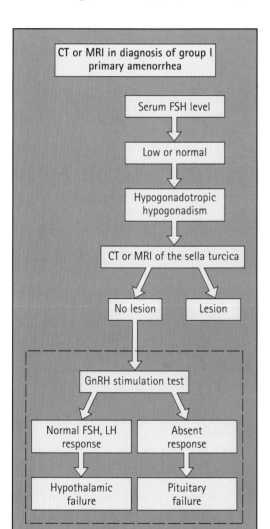

FIGURE 1-23.

Use of computed tomography (CT) or magnetic resonance imaging (MRI) in diagnosis of group I primary amenorrhea. Patients with hypogonadotropic hypogonadism as determined by serum follicle-stimulating hormone (FSH) level should have a CT or MRI study, which can identify any lesions impinging on the hypothalamic-pituitary region or a pituitary adenoma. For women who do not have a lesion, the gonadotropin-releasing hormone (GnRH) stimulation test will distinguish those individuals with hypothalamic hypogonadotropic hypogonadism from those with pituitary hypogonadotropic hypogonadism. This distinction is of academic importance and has little clinical relevance because the management of both groups is the same. Therefore, the GnRH stimulation test is an optional diagnostic test. LH—luteinizing hormone.

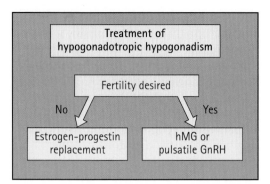

FIGURE 1-24.

Treatment of disorders causing hypogonadotropic hypogonadism. All women with group I primary amenorrhea and hypogonadotropic hypogonadism are estrogen deficient. Despite that gonadotropin deficiency usually has a hypothalamic cause, it is not practical to offer these women long-term gonadotropin-releasing hormone (GnRH) administration. These women should receive an estrogen or progestin replacement regimen (either cyclic or continuous). Estrogen administration will initiate breast development and protect the skeletal system. There may be other benefits to estrogen replacement therapy, including protection from cardiovascular disease, reduction in Alzheimer's disease, a decrease in colon cancer, and even less age-related macular degeneration. These latter benefits are not universally acknowledged as clinical advantages related to estrogen-replacement therapy. A progestin is recommended as part of the regimen to protect the endometrium from the hyperstimulation of unopposed estrogen. If pregnancy is desired, either human menopausal gonadotropins (hMGs) or pulsatile GnRH can be used to successfully induce ovulation. Clomiphene citrate is not effective in the induction of ovulation in hypoestrogenic individuals.

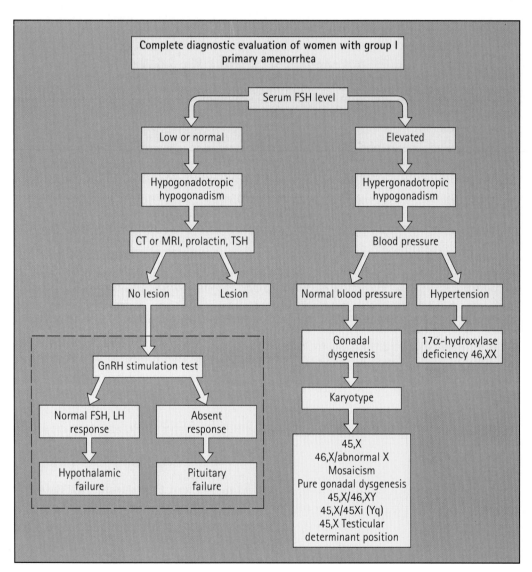

FIGURE 1-25.

Complete diagnostic evaluation of women with group I primary amenorrhea. The first step in the evaluation is to determine if the patient is hyper- or hypogonadotropic. An elevated follicle-stimulating hormone (FSH) level indicates hypergonadotropic hypogonadism. A low or normal FSH level indicates hypogonadotropic hypogonadism. Patients with hypergonadotropic hypogonadism and hypertension most likely have a 17α-hydroxylase deficiency in the steroid biosynthetic pathway. An elevated serum progesterone level and a low 17-hydroxyprogesterone level is indicative of this diagnosis, and an adrenocorticotropic hormone stimulation test confirms the diagnosis. Patients with hypergonadotropic hypogonadism who are normotensive have gonadal dysgenesis, thus a karyotype is required.

Individuals with hypogonadotripic hypogonadism should have a computed tomography (CT) or magnetic resonance imaging (MRI) study to identify those patients with a lesion impinging on the hypothalamic-pituitary region. In the absence of a lesion, a gonadotropin-releasing hormone (GnRH) stimulation test will differentiate those individuals who have a normal response in gonadotropin levels, indicating hypothalamic failure, from those who have no gonadotropin response to GnRH stimulation, which indicates pituitary failure. The *dashed lines* indicate that the GnRH stimulation test is optional: the test distinguishes pituitary from hypothalamic casues of hypogonadatropic hypogonadism, but the clinical management is the same for both groups. PrL—prolactin; TSH—thyroid-stimulating hormone.

ROUP II: BREASTS PRESENT, UTERUS ABSENT

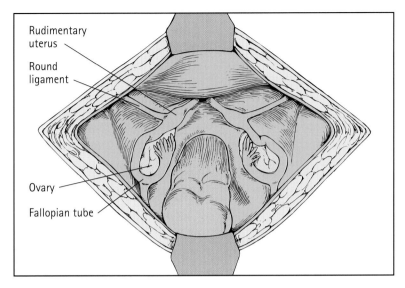

FIGURE 1–26.

Congenital absence of the vagina. Laparotomy revealed a rudimentary uterus that showed evidence of failure of fusion of müllerian ducts. That this finding is common in this condition indicates that the disorder is more extensive than a simple anomaly of the vagina. Complete uterine agenesis is second only to genetic abnormalities as the most common cause of primary amenorrhea. The incidence of uterine agenesis is one in 4000 to 5000 female births, and 15% of individuals with primary amenorrhea have a congenital absence of the uterus. individuals with complete uterine agenesis have a normally functioning hypothalamic-pituitary-ovarian axis. With the obvious exception of menarche, all other pubertal events are normal. Breast development and axillary and pubic hair growth are normal in women with a congenital absence of the uterus. Absence of the vagina in addition to absence of the uterus is referred to as Mayer-Rokitansky-Kuster-Hauser syndrome.

Women with congenital absence of the uterus with or without a vagina also have an increase in the presence of other associated congenital anomalies. Congenital anomalies of the renal system occur in one third or more of these individuals. Absence of a kidney has been reported in approximately 15% of woman and a double-collecting system in as many as 40% of women with congenital absence of the uterus. An intravenous pyelogram should be part of the diagnostic evaluation of any woman with uterine agenesis. Skeletal abnormalities occur in 5% to 10% of women with the congenital absence of the uterus. Congenital fusion of cervical vertebrae, one of the most common of these anomalies, is clinically relevant should the patient require general anesthesia. The rigidity of the neck hampers attempts at successful endotracheal intubation.

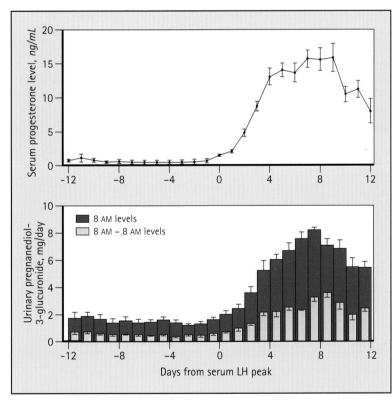

FIGURE 1–27.

Mean and standard errors of daily 8:00 AM serum progesterone concentrations and 24-hour (8:00 AM to 8:00 AM) and overnight urinary excretion of radioimmunoassayable pregnanediol 3-glucuronide in seven women during an entire menstrual cycle. The data obtained in individual subjects were grouped according to the day of the midcycle luteinizing hormone (LH) peak and averaged.

Women with uterovaginal agenesis have an otherwise normal female reproductive axis. The reproductive function of the hypothalamus-pituitary-ovarain axis is entirely normal, which results in ovulation and normal steroidogenesis. The levels and patterns of estradiol and progesterone are consistent with those found in normal ovulatory women who have a uterus. Clinically these women notice breast and mood changes one would normally associate with ovulation. Ovarian follicles can be identified with ultrasonography of the pelvis. Indirect parameters of ovulation such as once-a-week measurement of progesterone serum concentration that exceeds 3 ng/mL indicates ovulation. The documentation of ovulation in an individual with group II primary amenorrhea excludes the diagnosis of androgen insensitivity.

Women of reproductive age with congenital absence of the uterus can be expected to have normal ovarian estrogen production and excretion. The complement of ovarian follicles is normal in these women and they will experience menopause at the same time as ovulatory women with a uterus. Early hormonal replacement is not necessary. Because women with a congenital absence of the uterus have normal complement of ovarian follicles, normal ovarian steroidogenesis, and normal ovulation, these women may donate their own eggs to a surrogate mother and have their own genetic children. Women with congenital absence of the uterus who also have an absent vagina can use a series of progressively larger dilators or a vaginoplasty to create a vaginal vault. (*Adapted from* Stanczyk *et al.* [9]; with permission.)

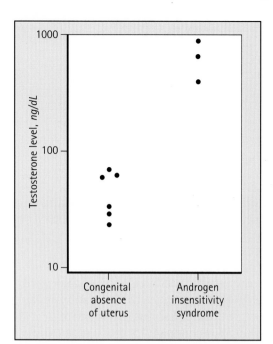

FIGURE 1-28.
Serum testosterone levels in women with group II primary amenorrhea. Determination of serum concentrations of testosterone can be used in a diagnostic algorithm to distinguish between women with congenital absence of the uterus and androgen insensitivity syndrome. Women with uterovaginal agenesis have normal ovarian steroidogenesis of both estrogens and androgens. These women with congenital absence of the uterus have testosterone levels in the normal female range (20 to 85 ng/dL). Individuals with androgen insensitivity syndrome have testes and normal testicular steroidogenesis. Their serum testosterone concentrations are in the normal male range (> 300 ng/mL). Serum testosterone determination is a specific, relatively rapid and inexpensive method to distinguish between the two disorders (uterovaginal agenesis and androgen insensitivity syndrome), both of which cause group II primary amenorrhea with or without vaginal atresia. Individuals with congenital absence of the uterus have normal pubic and axillary hair growth. Individuals with androgen insensitivity syndrome have absent or very sparse pubic and axillary hair growth.

CAUSES OF GROUP II PRIMARY AMENORRHEA

Congenital absence of uterus (uterovaginal anenesis)

Androgen insensitivity syndrome (testicular feminization)

FIGURE 1-29.
Causes of group II primary amenorrhea. An individual with androgen insensitivity syndrome may have a complete or, less commonly, incomplete forum. The complete forum is clinically characterized by an absence of or decreased axillary and pubic hair, normal breast development, and a blind vaginal pouch. Androgen insensitivity is a genetically inherited disorder that is either X-linked recessive or X-linked dominant, with incomplete penetrance. This disorder can be present in several members of the family. thus the family pedigree is an integral part of the investigation.

The basic defect is either the lack of or abnormal function of the androgen receptor. More specifically, the defect appears to be in androgen-receptor binding. The clinical result is the failure of the gonadal and genetic male fetus to masculinize *in utero* or at puberty, because testosterone and dihydrotestosterone are necessary to stimulate growth of internal and external male genitalia. The testis secretes müllerian inhibiting substance, which does not require the presence of androgen receptors and the uterus and oviducts do not develop. The presence of the Y chromosome and the genes that control stature usually results in a tall, slender individual.

Incomplete androgen insensitivity is far less common than the complete form. There may be partial fusion of the labioscrotal folds and some degree of clitoromegaly at birth. At puberty there is pubic hair growth and growth of the clitoris as well as breast development. The breast development is not as great in the incomplete forms of androgen insensitivity as in the complete forms.

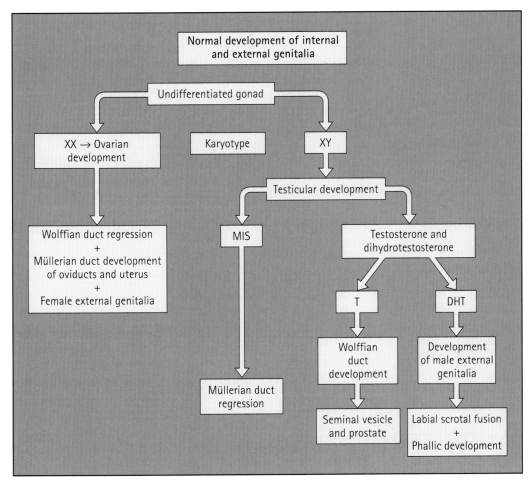

FIGURE 1-30.

Normal development of internal and external genitalia. Individuals with androgen-insensitivity sydrome are phenotypically and psychologically female, but genetic (46,XY) and gonadal (testes) males. They have normal testicular determining factor genes. The testes produce normal amounts of male androgens and müllerian-inhibiting substance (MIS). The MIS accounts for the failure of development of müllerian duct–derived structures, particularly the uterus and oviducts. The testes produce testosterone and estradiol levels that are in the normal male range, but testosterone does not stimulate development of internal and external male genitalia due to the absence of receptors. Normal hypothalamic-pituitary feedback mechanisms result in normal gonadotropin levels. Normal breast development occurs with low estradiol levels (30 pg/mL) becuase of the lack of inhibition by androgens. The breast tissue that is present in individuals with

androgen-insensitivity syndrome has more adipose than glandular tissue.

The testes appear grossly normal but spermatogenesis is incomplete or absent. The testes may be found in an intra-abdominal, inguinal, or labioscrotal location. The incidence of testicular neoplasia in individuals with androgen-insensitivity syndrome varies from 2% to 22% if the testes are left *in situ* following puberty. These tumors are usually dysgerminomas or gonadoblastomas, and they nearly always occur after age 20. Because normal breast development and epiphyseal closure occurs from endogenous estrogen produced by the testes, the testes are usually left in place until puberty is completed, especially if the testes are intra-abdominal in location. Testes in an inguinal or labioscrotal location are more likely to develop tumors and should be removed at the time of diagnosis. Once the testes are surgically extirpated, unopposed estrogen replacement therapy should be initiated to prevent osteoporosis. Progestins are unnecessary as there is no endometrial tissue to be stimulated.

If the vaginal pouch is inadequate for coitus, progressive vaginal dilation or vaginoplasty should be performed. A vaginoplast should not be considered until the individual is sexually active and capable of maintaining the patency of the enlarged vagina.

The counseling of individuals with androgen insensitivity syndrome takes a great deal of sensitivity. They can be told they have an abnormal gonad and abnormal sex chromosome, but the terms *testes* and *Y chromosome* are to be avoided. They must be advised that they are unable to become pregnant.

FIGURE 1-31.

Variations in clinical and laboratory parameters in women with group II primary amenorrhea. Women with congenital absence of the uterus are gonadal (ovaries) and genetic (46,XX) females. They have normal female pubic hair growth at puberty. Testosterone concentrations in the peripheral circulation are in the normal female range. These individuals have normal function of the hypothalamic-pituitary-ovarian axis and are ovulatory. Indirect evidence of ovulation, biphasic basal body temperature, and ovulatory level of progesterone are present.

Patients with androgen-insensitivity syndrome are gonadal (testes) and genetic (46,XY) males. They have absent or sparse hair growth at puberty. Testosterone concentrations in the peripheral circulation are in the normal male range. These individuals do not have any evidence of ovulation.

VARIATIONS IN CLINICAL AND LABORATORY PARAMETERS IN WOMEN WITH GROUP II PRIMARY AMENORRHEA

Parameter	Congenital absence of the uterus	Androgen-insensitivity syndrome
Gonad	Ovary	Testes
Karyotype	46,XX	46,XY
Pubic hair	Present	Absent, sparse
Testosterone	Female range	Male range
Weekly progesterone level	Ovulation	No ovulation
Vagina	Present, small pouch, or absent	Present, small pouch, or absent

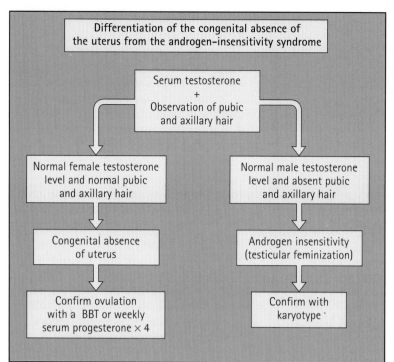

FIGURE 1-32.

Differentiation of the congenital absence of the uterus from the androgen-insensitivity syndrome. There are only two possible diagnoses for women with group II primary amenorrhea: congenital absence of the uterus or androgen-insensitivity syndrome. The presence or absence of pubic and axillary hair and the determination of serum testosterone level will differentiate between the two possibilities. A testosterone level in the normal female range and normal pubic and axillary hair growth indicates congenital absence of the uterus. Indirect evidence of ovulation and 46,XX karyotype confirms the diagnosis. A testosterone level in the normal male range and absent or sparse pubic and axillary hair indicates the individual has androgen-insensitivity syndrome. A 46,XY karyotype confirms the diagnosis.

ROUP III: BREASTS AND UTERUS ABSENT

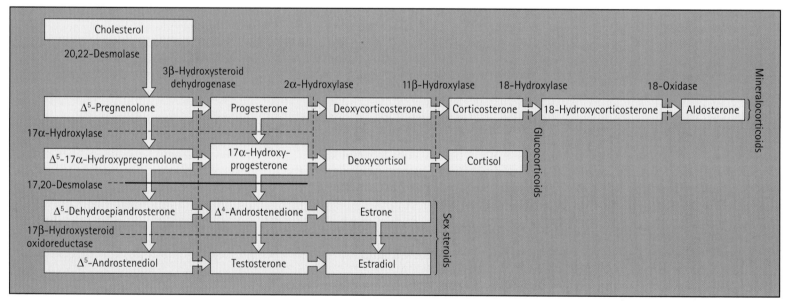

FIGURE 1-33.

The steroid biosynthetic pathway of a patient with 17,20-desmolase deficiency. The *solid line* denotes the block in the pathway. Individuals with the deficiency of the enzyme 17,20-desmolase are unable to convert 17α-hydroxypregnenolone to dehydroepiandrosterone and are unable to convert 17α-hydroxyprogesterone to androstenedione. A complete enzyme deficiency of 17,20-desmolase results in the inability to synthesize all sex steroids. The cortisol synthetic pathway is not affected by this specific enzyme deficiency. These rare cases of 17,20-desmolase deficiency have a 46,XY karyotype and testes. When the diagnosis is confirmed, the testes should be surgically extirpated. (*Adapted from* Goebelsmann *et al.* [10]; with permission.)

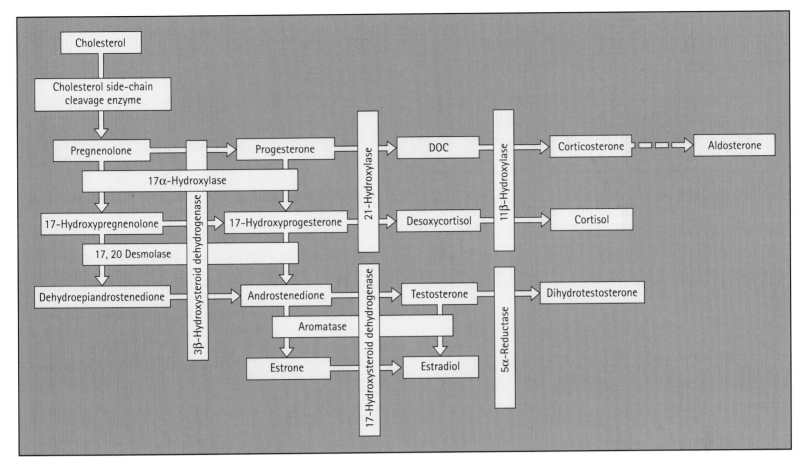

FIGURE 1-34.

Individuals with the deficiency of the enzyme 17 α-hyroxylase are unable to convert pregnenolone to 17 α-hydroxypregnenolone and progesterone to 17 α-hydroxyprogesterone. A complete enzyme deficiency of 17 α-hydroxylase also results in the inability to synthesize sex steroids. These individuals with a 17-hydroxylase deficiency have a constellation of findings which include absence of the uterus, primary amenorrhea, absence of secondary sex characteristics and hypertension. Individuals with 17 α-hydroxylase deficiency with a 46, XY karyotype do not have a uterus as distiguished from idividuals with 17 α-hydroxylase deficiency with a 46, XX karyotype who do have a uterus. The lack of breast development distinguishes individuals with a 17 α-hydroxylase deficiency from those with androgen insensitivity syndrome. The diagnosis and management of individuals with 17 α-hydroxylase deficiency with a XY karyotype is the same as it is for individuals with the same enzyme deficiency and an XX karyotype. They require estrogen replacement therapy as well as cortisol.

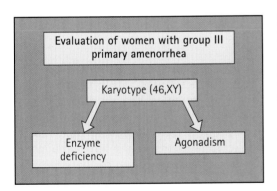

FIGURE 1-35.

Evaluation of women with group III primary amenorrhea. Another cause of this phenotype, in addition to enzyme deficiency, is testicular agonadism. It is theorized that patients with agonadism had testicular tissue present early enough in embryonic development to suppress the müllerian system, after which this testicular tissue disappeared. This syndrome is also known as the "vanishing testes syndrome." If the enzymatic deficiencies of 17,20-desmolase and 17α-hydroxylase are excluded in patients with group III primary amenorrhea, then a presumptive diagnosis of agonadism is made.

GROUP IV: BREAST AND UTERUS PRESENT

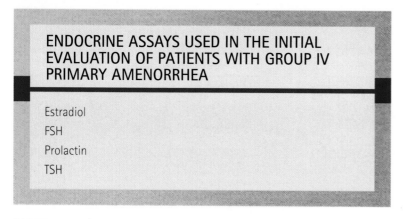

ENDOCRINE ASSAYS USED IN THE INITIAL EVALUATION OF PATIENTS WITH GROUP IV PRIMARY AMENORRHEA

Estradiol

FSH

Prolactin

TSH

FGIURE 1-36.

Endocrine assays used in the initial evaluation of patients with group IV primary amenorrhea. The evaluation of individuals with group IV primary amenorrhea is very similar to the diagnostic evaluation of women with secondary amenorrhea. The history should include details pertaining to strenuous exercise, marked weight loss, severe stress, diet, breast discharge and symptoms of hypothyroidism. Before any other evaluation of women with group IV primary amenorrhea is undertaken, pregnancy and obstruction of the lower reproductive tract should be excluded. This initial phase of laboratory screening includes measurement of prolactin, thyroid-stimulating hormone (TSH), estradiol, and follicle-stimulating hormone (FSH) levels in serum.

The progesterone challenge test has been used in the past as an *in vivo* assay of estrogen. If the endometrium has been primed with sufficient estrogen, the administration of an intramuscular injection of progesterone or oral progestins would result in vaginal bleeding when the progesterone or progestin influence had dissipated. A positive progesterone challenge test indicates levels of endogenous estradiol$_2$ greater than 40 pg/mL, a reactive endometrium and a patent outflow tract. If the endometrium had not been primed with sufficient estrogen, then the administration of progesterone or progestins would not result in bleeding when the circulating levels of exogenous steroids begin to fall. Estradiol concentrations of 40 pg/mL or greater usually results in bleeding and a positive progesterone challenge test. The use of serum estradiol determinations are more precise and accurate and have progesterone or pregestin challenge test in the diagnostic evaluation of patients with amenorrhea.

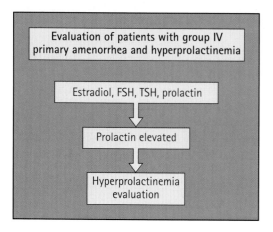

FIGURE 1-37.

Evaluation of patients with group IV primary amenorrhea and hyperprolactinemia. Approximately one fourth of the women with group IV primary amenorrhea have elevated serum prolactin levels. Serum prolactin level should be measured whether galactorrhea is present or absent. If hyperprolactinemia is found, then the further evaluation is focused on determining the cause (*eg*, pituitary macroadenomas, which can cause blindness).

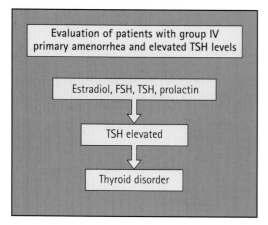

FIGURE 1-38.

Evaluation of patients with group IV primary amenorrhea and elevated thyroid-stimulating hormone (TSH)-levels. A sensitive assay is used to determine TSH levels in the peripheral circulation. This assay is useful in identifying patients with subtle, asymptomatic thyroid disorders. TSH measurements to assess the presence of thyroid gland hypofunction are also part of the evolution of women with group IV amenorrhea and hyperprolactinemia, those who are under the age of 35 years of age and have premature ovarian failure and may have multiple endocrine gland involvement, and in women with hypothalamic-pituitary failure.

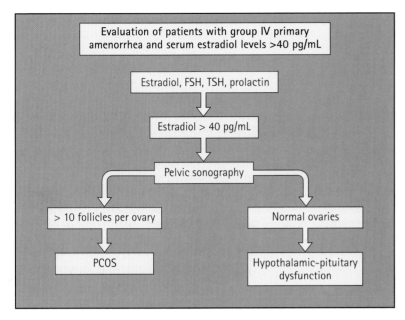

FIGURE 1-39.

Evaluation of patients with group IV primary amenorrhea and serum estradiol levels greater than 40 pg/mL. These patients will have polycystic ovary syndrome (PCOS), hypothalamic-pituitary dysfunction, moderate stress amenorrhea, or exercise weight loss amenorrhea. A pelvic ultrasound finding of 10 or more follicles in each ovary confirms the diagnosis of PCOS. Hyperandrogenism is often an integral part of PCOS, and all women with PCOS should have their serum testosterone and serum dehydroepiandrosterone sulfate levels determined. When the pelvic ultrasound examination fails to confirm the diagnosis of PCOS in women with group IV primary amenorrhea and serum estradiol levels greater than 40 pg/mL, then the diagnosis is hypothalamic-pituitary dysfunction. To determine the cause of hypothalamic-pituitary dysfunction, a history should be taken to determine if drug ingestion, severe stress, marked weight loss, or strenuous exercise is the cause. In the absence of any of these causes, idiopathic hypotalamic pituitary dysfunction is present. Hypothalamic-pituitary dysfunction is usally a self-limiting disorder that does not adversely affect the patient's general health. Fertility is usally feasible with the assistance of agents that induce ovulation.

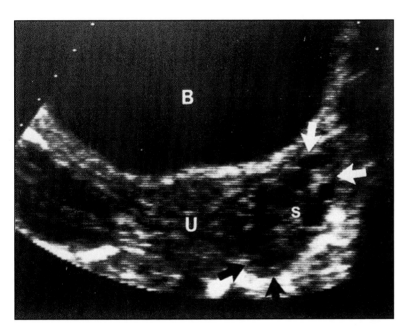

FIGURE 1-40.

Polycystic ovaries shown an transverse ultrasonographic scan of the pelvis. Enlarged ovaries containing more than 10 peripherally distributed multiple cysts (*arrows*) with increased stroma can be seen. Diagnosis of polycystic ovary syndrome (PCOS) in women with group IV primary amenorrhea is confirmed by a pelvic ultrasound examination demonstrating 10 to more follicles in each ovary. Polycystic ovaries are described as enlarged ovaries containing an increased number of follicles that are located peripherally underneath the capsule in the increased ovarian stroma. The scale shows 1-cm markers. B—bladder; S—stroma; U—uterus. (*From* Frank *et al.* [11]; with permission.)

FIGURE 1-41.

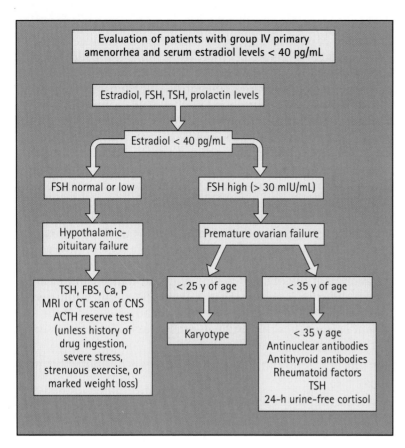

```
┌─────────────────────────────────────────┐
│ Evaluation of patients with group IV primary │
│ amenorrhea and serum estradiol levels < 40 pg/mL │
└─────────────────────────────────────────┘
                    │
                    ▼
        ┌─────────────────────────────┐
        │ Estradiol, FSH, TSH, prolactin levels │
        └─────────────────────────────┘
                    │
                    ▼
            ┌──────────────────┐
            │ Estradiol < 40 pg/mL │
            └──────────────────┘
             │                    │
             ▼                    ▼
   ┌──────────────────┐   ┌──────────────────────┐
   │ FSH normal or low │   │ FSH high (> 30 mIU/mL) │
   └──────────────────┘   └──────────────────────┘
             │                    │
             ▼                    ▼
   ┌──────────────────┐   ┌──────────────────────┐
   │ Hypothalamic-     │   │ Premature ovarian failure │
   │ pituitary failure │   └──────────────────────┘
   └──────────────────┘        │              │
             │                 ▼              ▼
             ▼          ┌────────────┐  ┌────────────┐
   ┌──────────────────┐ │ < 25 y of age │ │ < 35 y of age │
   │ TSH, FBS, Ca, P   │ └────────────┘  └────────────┘
   │ MRI or CT scan of CNS │    │              │
   │ ACTH reserve test │      ▼              ▼
   │ (unless history of │ ┌──────────┐  ┌──────────────────────┐
   │ drug ingestion,   │ │ Karyotype │  │ < 35 y age            │
   │ severe stress,    │ └──────────┘  │ Antinuclear antibodies │
   │ strenuous exercise, or │          │ Antithyroid antibodies │
   │ marked weight loss) │            │ Rheumatoid factors     │
   └──────────────────┘              │ TSH                    │
                                     │ 24-h urine-free cortisol │
                                     └──────────────────────┘
```

FIGURE 1-41.

Evaluation of patients with group IV primary amenorrhea and serum estradiol levels less than 40 pg/mL. These women have a failure of the reproductive axis to maintain physiologic levels of estrogen. This failure in estrogen steroidogenesis may be the result of hypothalamic-pituitary disorders, which include pituitary tumors, marked weight loss or anorexia nervosa, strenuous exercise, severe stress, or other rare hypthalamic-pituitary lesions. The failure in estrogen production may also be caused by premature ovarian failure. Hypothalamic-pituitary failure may be distinguished from premature ovarian failure by the measurement of serum follicle-stimulating hormone (FSH). Women with estradiol levels less than 40 pg/mL and normal or low FSH levels have hypothalamic-pituitary failure, and women with estradiol levels less than 40 pg/ml and elevated FSH levels (>30 mIU/ml) have premature ovarian failure.

A woman with hypothalamic-pituitary failure whose history is negative for severe stress, marked weight loss, or strenuous exercise should have a radiologic imaging study of this region of the central nervous system to rule out a space-occupying lesion. Either a computed tomography (CT) scan or magnetic resonance imaging (MRI) study of the hypothalamus-pituitary area is indicated, irrespective of the prolactin level. If a lesion is visualized, a test of adrenocarticotropic hormone (ACTH) reserve is mandatory. An insulin tolerance test is used to determine ACTH function. Hypoglycemia is induced and the cortisol response is determined 120 minutes later. In a normal test of ACTH reserve, the cortisol level will increase 6 µg/100 mL above baseline. If a lesion is not identified by a central nervous system (CNS) imaging study, the diagnosis of functional hypothalamic-pituitary failure is made. Some women with this diagnosis will have the spontaneous return of normal ovarian function as they grow older. FSB—fasting blood suger; TSH—thyroid-stimulating hormone.

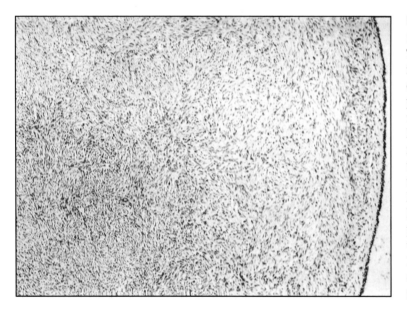

FIGURE 1-42.

Section of ovary from a woman with premature ovarian failure. The cortex the ovary is devoid of follicles. A patient with ovarian failure who is under the age of 35 years, and for whom no cause of ovarian destruction can be identified, should be tested for the presence of autoimmune disease, which produces failure of follicular development owing to antibodies to follicle-stimulating hormone (insensitive ovary syndrome). Other endocrine organs may also be involved. The autoimmune disease may involve the thyroid gland, adrenal glands, and parathyroid glands as well as the ovaries. Antithyroid antibodies, antinuclear antibodies, a 24-hour urine-free cortisol level, rheumatoid factors, thyroid-stimulating hormone, fasting blood sugar, and serum calcium, phosphorus, and thyroxine concentrations should be determined. A women with premature ovarian failure who is under the age of 25 years should also have a karyotype to rule out presence of a chromosomal abnormality and determine whether a Y chromosome is present. (*From* Tulandi and Kinch [12]; with permission.)

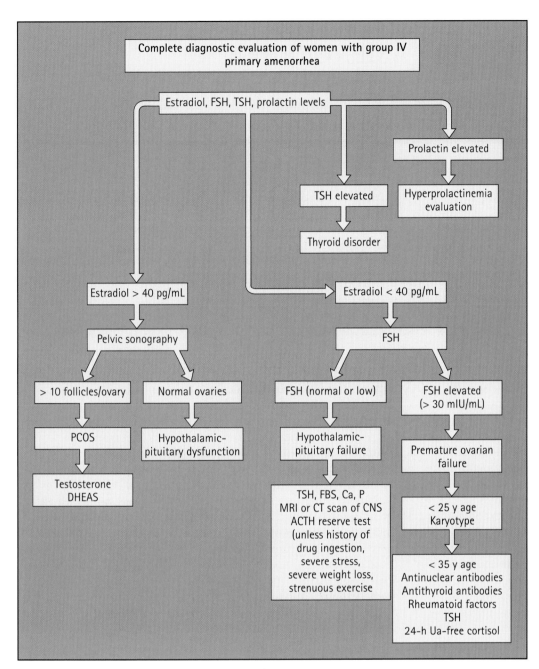

FIGURE 1–43.

Complete diagnostic evaluation of women with group IV primary amenorrhea (breasts and uterus present). Based on serum estradiol, follicle-stimulating hormone (FSH), thyroid-stimulating hormone (TSH), and prolactin levels, these women may be categorized as having hyperprolactinemia, hypothyroidism, hypoestrogenism, or estrogen levels equal to or greater than 40 pg/mL. Women with hyperprolactinemia require a work-up specific for this endocrinopathy. Those women with estradiol levels less than 40 pg/mL have either premature ovarian failure or hypothalamic-pituitary failure. The former will have elevated FSH and the latter will have normal or low FSH levels. Those women with estradiol levels greater than 40 pg/mL have either polycystic ovary syndrome (PCOS) or hypothalamic-pituitary dysfunction. The former have more than 10 follicles per ovary as demonstrated by pelvic ultrasonography, whereas the latter have normal-appearing ovaries. ACTH—adrenocorticotropic hormone; CNS—central nervous system; CT—computed tomography; DHEAS—dehydroepiandrosterone sulfate; FBS—fasting blood sugar; MRI—magnetic resonance imaging.

MANAGEMENT OF PRIMARY AMENORRHEA

TREATMENT OF PRIMARY AMENORRHEA WITH BREAST AND UTERUS PRESENT

| | Serum estradiol level | | |
| | | <40 pg/mL | |
Conception	>40 pg/mL	FSH ↓	FSH ↑
Desired	Clomid	hMG or GnRH	Donor eggs
Not desired	Progesterone 12d/mo	HRT	HRT
	or	or	or
	Ocs	Ocs	Ocs

FIGURE 1-44.

Breast and uterus present. The management of individuals with primary amenorrhea who have breast development and an uterus presnet depends on whether they desire conception or not, and their circulating estradiol levels. Women in this group who desire conception and whose serum estradiol concentrations are greater than 40 pg/ml have their own ovarian follicles. Clomiphene citrate is the agent of choice for the induction of ovulation is those women. Women in this group whose serum estradiol levels are less than 40 pg/ml have either hypogonadotropic hypogonadism, or hypergonadotropic hypogonadism. Individuals with hypogonadotropic hypogonadism, low or normal FSH, have their own ovarian follicles. These women rarely respond to clomid and the choices for the induction of ovulation include human menopausal gonadotropin or gonadotropin releasing hormone. Women with hypergonadotropic hypogonadism have ovarian failure and depletion of their complement of ovarian follicles. Their only option for conception requires the use of donor oocytes.

Women in this group who do not desire conception and whose estradiol levels exceed 40 pg/ml require progestin administration to prevent the hyperstimulation of the endometrium. One regimen is to administer medroxyprogesterone acetate orally 5 mg each day for the first twelve days each month. Another option for those women is the use of combination oral contraceptives. Women in the group who do not desire conception and whose serum estradiol levels are less than 40 pg/ml are managed with hormone replacement therapy. There are many hormonal regimens available to provide phsiologic estrogen replacement. For these women combination oral contraceptives are also an option. FSH—follicle-stimulating hormone; hMG—human menopausal gonadotropin; GnRH—gonadotropin releasing hormone; HRT—hormone replacement therapy; OCs—oral contraceptives.

REFERENCES

1. Ying S-Y: Inhibins, activins and follistatins: gonadal proteins modulating the secretion of follicle-stimulating hormone. *Endocr Rev* 1988, 9:267-293.

2. Frisch RE, Revelle R: Height and weight at menarche and a hypothesis of menarche. *Arch Dis Child* 1971, 46:695-701.

3. Warren MP: The effects of exercise on pubertal progression and reproductive function in girls. *J Clin Endocrinol Metab* 1980, 51:1150-1157.

4. Mashchak CA, Kletzky OA, Davajan V, *et al*.: Clinical and laboratory evaluation of patients with primary amenorrhea. *Obstet Gynecol* 1981, 57:715-721.

5. Simspon JL: Phenotypic-karyotypic correlations of gonadal determinants: current status and relationship to molecular studies. *Hum Genet* 1987, 224–232.

6. Federman DD: Abnormal Sexual Development: A Genetic and Endocrine Approach to Differential Diagnosis. Philadelphia: WB Saunders; 1967:48.

7. Mischell DR Jr, Davajan V, Lobo RA (eds.): *Infertility, Contraception and Reproductive Endocrinology*, edn 3. Cambridge, MA: Blackwell Scientific Publications; 1991:S47.

8. Stein A, Levenik MN, Kletzky OA: Computed tomography versus magnetic resonance imaging for the evaluation of suspected pituitary adenomas. *Obstet Gynecol* 1989, 73:996-999.

9. Stanczyk FZ, Miyakawa I, Goebelsmann U: Direct radioimmunoassay of urinary estrogen and pregranediol glucuronides during the menstrual cycle. *Am J Obstet Gynecol* 1980, 137:443-450.

10. Goebelsmann U, Zachmann M, Davajan V, *et al*.: Male pseudohermaphroditism consistent with 17,20-desmolase deficiency. *Gynecol Invest* 1976, 7:138-156.

11. Frank S, Adams J, Mason H, *et al*.: Ovulatory disorders in women with polycystic ovary syndrome. *Clin Obstet Gynecol* 1985, 12:605-632.

12. Tulandi T, Kinch RAH: Premature ovarian failure. *Obstet Gynecol Surv* 1981, 36:521-527.

Secondary Amenorrhea

Sarah L. Berga, Tammy L. Daniels, Gloria E. Hoffman,
Brinda N. Kalro, Lyndon M. Hill, Kenneth S. McCarty, Jr.,
Jules Sumkin, and Michael P. Federle

Secondary amenorrhea has multiple causes (see Fig. 2-1). Therefore, a rational and systematic approach to delineating the diagnosis, *ie*, a complete differential diagnosis, is the cornerstone to management. This chapter is organized in a "head to toe" approach to emphasize that reproductive function cannot be considered in isolation, because amenorrhea often heralds other conditions that involve an interdisciplinary perspective to treat. Central causes of amenorrhea are considered first, because the central input from the gonadotropin-releasing hormone pulse generator is so crucial to ovulation and the maintenance of menstrual cyclicity. Pituitary causes of amenorrhea and anovulation are discussed next, followed by ovarian and uterine causes. Other causes external to the hypothalamic-pituitary-gonadal axis are reviewed last.

The history and physical examination are essential in making the correct diagnosis. Pertinent historical information to obtain includes the chronology of sexual development, including the age of adrenarche, thelarche, and menarche. The occurrence of irregular menses since menarche suggests polycystic ovary syndrome, whereas the abrupt cessation of menses following weight loss suggests hypothalamic disruption of pulsatile GnRH secretion. The physical examination should include palpation of the thyroid; careful inspection of the skin for acanthosis nigricans, striae, and hirsutism;

Tanner staging; and a pelvic examination. The overall habitus should be noted.

Laboratory evaluation of a woman with anovulation and no clear history or physical signs to direct the investigation should begin with clinical chemistries. Luteinizing hormone, follicle-stimulating hormone, thyroid-stimulating hormone, thyroxine, prolactin, and estradiol levels should be measured in a venous blood sample ideally obtained at least 2 hours after exercise, a meal, or a physical examination and between 10:00 AM and 12:00 PM to exclude menopause, thyroid conditions, and hyper-prolactinemia. The possibility of polycystic ovary syndrome can be evaluated by adding an androstenedione level test. Further evaluation depends on the index of suspicion for more occult, but rare, disorders. Once a diagnosis has been made, the patient must be counseled about therapeutic options.

The merits of a given therapy depend on a firm comprehension of the pathophysiology of the disorder in question. The most common cause of secondary amenorrhea is functional hypothalamic amenorrhea (see Fig. 2-3). The pathogenesis of this common and commonly misunderstood disorder is explored in detail in the "Hypothalamus" section. The goal is to heighten the clinician's awareness of the multiple functional glandular disturbances that accompany this mysterious condition. The limits of hormonal interventions are best understood when one realizes that steroid hormonal management alone will not restore hypothalamic function or reverse accompanying endocrine aberrations. The long-term consequences of stress and stress-related anovulation are just beginning to be understood, so it would not be prudent to assume that this condition is benign. Rather than mask the amenorrhea, which is typically the presenting symptom, with hormonal interventions, the patient must be encouraged to alter problematic attitudes and behaviors. Hormonal intervention is best reserved for those who do not respond to psychosocial and lifestyle management.

Other causes of amenorrhea are usually less attributable to lifestyle per se. Treatments for these disorders are generally more straightforward, except in the case of PCOS. The full spectrum of hyperandrogenic anovulation is discussed in chapter 6 and is illustrated here for purposes of contrast. It is important to remember that functional hypothalamic amenorrhea or stress-related anovulation is largely a diagnosis of exclusion; therefore all other causes of amenorrhea and anovulation must be considered and excluded before embarking on psychosocial or psychotropic interventions.

The diagnostic evaluation and treatment of secondary amenorrhea are the same as for primary amenorrhea with normal breast development and uterus present. Refer to Figure 1-43 for further information on treatment of secondary amenorrhea. This chapter mainly discusses etiology.

ℋYPOTHALAMUS

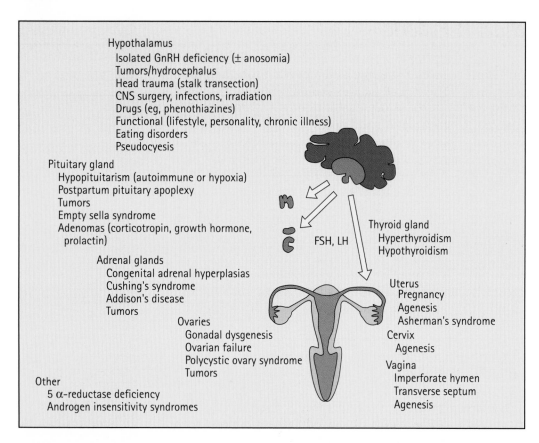

FIGURE 2-1.
Etiologies of amenorrhea. A helpful approach to delineating the cause of secondary amenorrhea is to list potential diagnoses by anatomic level, starting with pelvic causes. In outlining the differential diagnosis, it is helpful to distinguish between amenorrhea (the absence of menses) and anovulation, (the absence of ovulation). Anovulation commonly presents as amenorrhea, but also may be associated with sufficient endometrial stimulation to manifest as oligomenorrhea or even polymenorrhea. CNS—central nervous system; FSH—follicle-stimulating hormone; GnRH—gonadotropin-releasing hormone; LH—luteinizing hormone.

DIAGNOSTIC MODALITIES USED TO DISCERN THE DIAGNOSIS OF AMENORRHEA

History	Hormonal assay
Physical examination	Endometrial biopsy
Clinical chemistries	Magnetic resonance imaging
Karyotype	Provocative testing
DNA analysis	

FIGURE 2-2.
Diagnostic modalities. Modalities shown here may be useful to discern the diagnosis of amenorrhea.

DISTRIBUTION OF CAUSES OF AMENORRHEA IN ONE SERIES

Premature ovarian failure	12
Functional hypothalamic amenorrhea	34
Hyperandrogenism and PCOS	29
Hyperprolactinemia	13
Asherman's syndrome	5
Other	7

FIGURE 2-3.
Distribution of causes of amenorrhea in one series [1]. Numbers are percentages. PCOS—polycystic ovary syndrome.

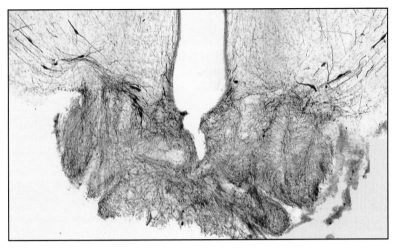

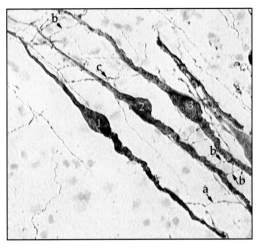

FIGURE 2-4.

Hypothalamus of monkey brain. Median eminence and adjacent basal hypothalamus of a rhesus monkey brain stained for gonadotropin-releasing hormone (GnRH) in brown and counterstained with a methyl-green Nissl stain. GnRH neurons are visible at the borders of the median eminence, within the median eminence, and within the hypothalamus. The dense accumulation of GnRH axons shows the convergence of GnRH axons to the external zone of the median eminence where the portal capillary loops that carry the GnRH to the pituitary are located. Ovarian activity, including folliculogenesis and ovulation, are initiated and maintained by GnRH pulsatility. During the follicular phase, GnRH boluses are released into the portal vasculature at a frequency of about once every 90 minutes. This frequency stimulates pituitary gonadotrophs to synthesize and secrete luteinizing hormone and follicle-stimulating hormone in the appropriate ratio and with effective bioactivity. Gonadotropins, in turn, impinge on the ovary to producetheca and granulosa cell function, permitting folliculogenesis and ovulation if the ovary contains responsive ova.

FIGURE 2-5.

Three gonadotropin-releasing hormone (GnRH) neurons. Interconnections among GnRH neurons are seen as fine processes that extend from one GnRH neuron to another. The letter *a* indicates a bridge between cells 1 and 2, *b* shows bridges between cells 2 and 3, and *c* illustrates a bridge between cell 1 and 3. GnRH neurons originate in the olfactory placode and migrate into the hypothalamus during fetal life. GnRH neurons are intrinsically pulsatile, but they have relatively few synapses or connections. The majority of connections that GnRH neurons form is with other GnRH neurons. These GnRH to GnRH connections permit GnRH neurons to fire synchronously and function as a GnRH "pulse generator," releasing a sufficient bolus of GnRH into the portal vasculature to elicit a pituitary response.

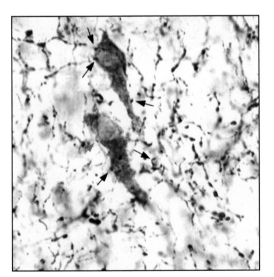

FIGURE 2-6.

Innervation of GnRH neurons. The innervation of GnRH neurons (*brown*) by neuropeptide Y (*blue-black*) revealing apparent contact of neuropeptide Y axons with GnRH neurons. *Black arrows* indicate contacts of neuropeptide Y axons with GnRH neurons. A GnRH axon innervating one of the GnRH neurons is indicated by the *red arrow*. The neuromodulation of GnRH neurons is poorly understood. GnRH neurons pulse synchronously during fetal life, but the GnRH pulse generator is disrupted or inhibited from shortly after birth until puberty. Neuropeptide Y neurons may play a role in the prepubertal hiatus. Neuropeptide Y neurons are activated by metabolic perturbations. Psychogenic and metabolic stressors can disrupt the synchronous firing of the GnRH pulse generator, leading to anovulation. Neuropeptide Y neurons also may play a role in the stress-related inhibition of GnRH drive. Other mechanisms mediating the onset and offset of the synchronous firing of GnRH neurons may involve glial interposition between GnRH appositions such that, although individual GnRH neurons remain pulsatile, they cannot communicate with one another to pulse synchronously.

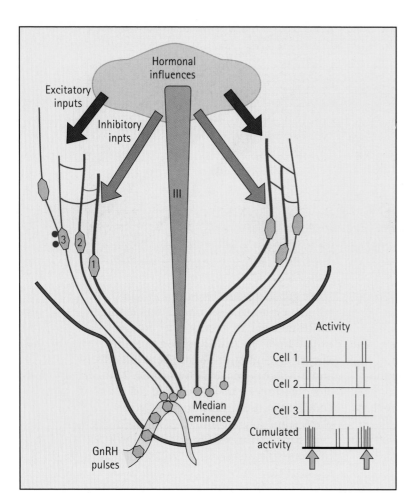

FIGURE 2-7.

GnRH pulse generator and its modulation. The gonadotropin-releasing hormone (GnRH) pulse generator and mechanisms of its control. The hypothetical activity of three of the cells is shown in the *lower right*. When the activity of the cells is summed at the level of the median eminence, bursts of activity that result in pulses of GnRH (*red arrows*) are produced. Some of the factors that influence the firing or release of GnRH also are illustrated. The GnRH neurons shown in this figure receive inputs from other GnRH neurons, both dendritic (in the form of bridges) and axonal (indicated by the terminal from the unlabeled neurons to cell 3). These cells also receive extrinsic excitatory and inhibitory inputs from neurons in various regions of the brain whose activity, in turn, is greatly modified by gonadal steroids. In addition, pulse generator activity can be affected by changes in glial investment of GnRH soma and terminals (not shown). These features temporarily isolate the GnRH cells from extrinsic influences or prevent released GnRH from gaining easy access to the blood.

In general, the function of the GnRH pulse generator in humans is inferred from tracking luteinizing hormone (LH) pulse patterns in the peripheral circulation. For instance, during the luteal phase of the menstrual cycle, there is slowing of LH and GnRH pulse frequency. The slowing of GnRH pulse frequency is mediated by opioidergic neuronal input. Opioidergic neuromodulation of GnRH is induced by exposure to sex steroids, particularly the high doses of estradiol and progesterone that are characteristic of the luteal phase.

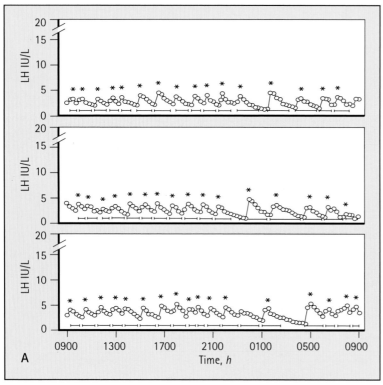

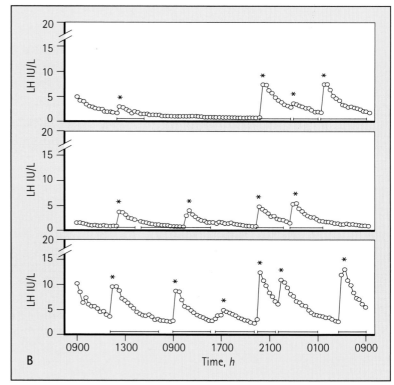

FIGURE 2-8.

Twenty-four-hour luteinizing hormone (LH) pulse profiles. **A**, Twenty-four-hour LH pulse profiles in three eumenorrheic women (EW) with subsequent midluteal progesterone levels higher than 30 nmol/L. Blood samples were drawn at 15-minute intervals for 24 hours and LH was measured in each blood sample by immunofluorometric assay. LH pulses are determined by a computer-assisted algorithm and marked with an *asterisk*. If the theoretical LH pulse frequency is once every 90 minutes, then the number of pulses in a day should be 16, but generally the first and last pulse escape detection.

B, Twenty-four-hour LH pulse profiles in women with stress-related anovulation (SRA). Serial progesterone levels confirmed anovulation. Folliculogenesis requires 11 to 14 days to complete and the LH pulse frequency must be maintained within a normal range during that time. Patients may have frequencies in the normal range, but the frequency is not long enough to permit folliculogenesis to progress to ovulation. If the frequency is intermediate, partial folliculogenesis may occur, resulting in ovulation with a luteal phase that is truncated either in duration or in the amount of progesterone secreted.

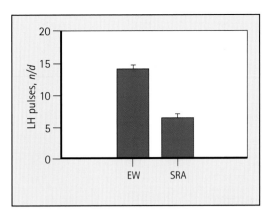

FIGURE 2-9.

Luteinizing hormone (LH) pulse frequency in women with stress-related anovulation (SRA) compared with eumenorrheic women (EW). In women with SRA who are amenorrheic, LH pulse frequency is on average about 50% lower than the LH pulse frequency observed in EW in the early follicular phase (days 3 to 7) [2]. *T bars* indicate ± SEM.

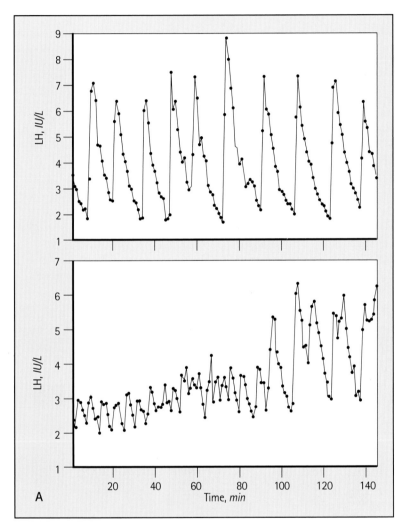

FIGURE 2-10.

Increased luteinizing hormone (LH) pulsatility in women with polycystic ovary syndrome (PCOS). **A**, Twenty-four-hour LH pulse profiles in two eumenorrheic women. Blood samples were obtained at 10-minute intervals for 24 hours, which permits faster pulse frequencies to be more accurately estimated than when blood samples are obtained at 15-minute intervals. **B**, Twenty-four-hour LH pulse profiles in two women with hyperandrogenic anovulation or PCOS. The increased LH pulse frequency is presumed to reflect increased gonadotropin-releasing hormone (GnRH) pulse frequency. Faster GnRH pulse frequencies suppress follicle-stimulating hormone (FSH) release and augment LH release. The anovulation observed in women with PCOS may be in part a consequence of increased GnRH pulse frequency leading to insufficient FSH to sustain folliculogenesis. The hyperandrogenism may be in part a consequence of increased LH stimulation of the ovarian interstitial cell compartment.

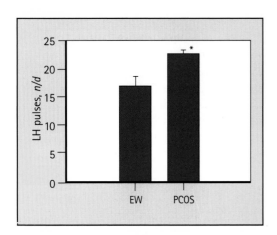

FIGURE 2–11.

Luteinizing hormone (LH) pulse frequencies observed in women with polycystic ovary syndrome (PCOS) versus eumenorrheic women (EW). LH pulse frequencies in women with PCOS are on average about 20% faster than those observed in EW [2]. *T bars* indicate ± SEM.

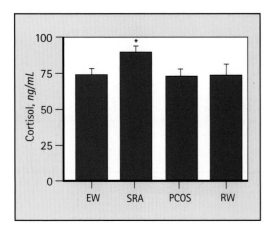

FIGURE 2–12.

Cortisol levels compared. Cortisol levels in eumenorrheic women (EW), women with stress-related anovulation (SRA), women with polycystic ovary syndrome (PCOS), and women who have recovered from SRA (RW). Many investigators have observed that women with SRA have modestly elevated cortisol levels and higher urinary free cortisol levels when compared with eumenorrheic women [3–6]. One interpretation of this observation is that activation of the hypothalamic-pituitary-adrenal (HPA) axis is responsible for the disruption in gonadotropin-releasing hormone (GnRH) drive that is the proximate cause of anovulation. However, women with SRA are aware that they have reproductive impairment, so the increase in cortisol may reflect only heightened worry or concern about health or fertility rather than indicating a causal link between HPA activation and hypothalamic-pituitary-ovarian (HPO) offset. If the increase in cortisol were caused by reproductive anxiety, one would expect that women with other causes of anovulation also would have elevated cortisol levels. As illustrated here, we recently found that women with PCOS have cortisol levels identical to those of EW [7]. Further evidence supporting the concept that activation of the HPA is integral to offset of GnRH drive is the finding that RW have similar cortisol levels to those of EW and PCOS. *T bars* indicate ±SEM.

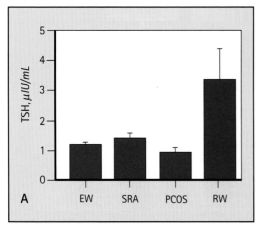 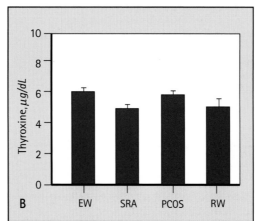 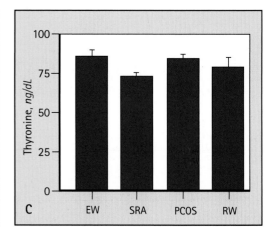

FIGURE 2–13.

TSH levels. Thyroid-stimulating hormone (TSH) (**A**), thyroxine (**B**), and thyronine (**C**) levels in eumenorrheic women (EW), women with stress-related anovulation (SRA), women with polycystic ovary syndrome (PCOS), and those who have recovered from SRA (RW). Women with SRA have lower thyroxine and thyronine levels, but TSH is not elevated, indicating that the hypothalamus is not responding to the lower thyronine and thyroxine levels by raising thyrotropin-releasing hormone (TRH) drive. This pattern is often called "sick euthyroid syndrome" and is seen in hospitalized patients. Women with SRA thus have both hypothalamic hypogonadism and hypothalamic hypothyroidism. Interestingly, the RW group displayed a dramatic increase in TSH levels, although thyroxine and thyronine levels are still somewhat lower than in EW. *T bars* indicate ± SEM.

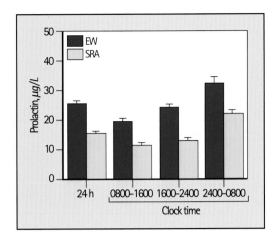

FIGURE 2-14.

Segmental prolactin levels. Twenty-four- and 8-hour segmental prolactin levels in eumenorrheic women (EW) and those with stress-related anovulation (SRA). During each segment, prolactin levels are lower in women with SRA. However, the circadian rhythm and the sleep-induced rise in prolactin are preserved in women with SRA. Prolactin levels in the circulation are increased by estrogen exposure and gonadotropin-releasing hormone (GnRH) stimulation and suppressed by dopamine released into the portal circulation by neurons in the median eminence. Thus, the lower prolactin levels characteristic of women with SRA may be caused by increased dopaminergic tone [8], decreased estrogen levels due to anovulation, and decreased GnRH drive. When obtaining serum chemistry studies to determine the cause of anovulation, a low prolactin level accompanied by a luteinizing hormone to follicle-stimulating hormone ratio less than 1.5 is highly suggestive of SRA. *T bars* indicate ± SEM.

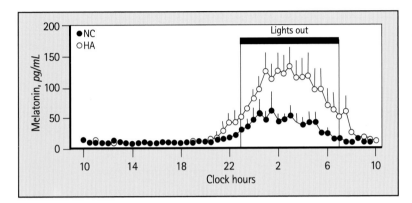

FIGURE 2-15.

Melatonin levels in women with stress-related anovulation (SRA). Melatonin secretion is entrained by the external light–dark cycle. The pineal gland secretes melatonin during the dark phase, presumably to synchronize other neuronal, hormonal, and cellular circadian rhythms. The melatonin secretory profile of women with SRA is amplified but phase intact. Light signals travel from the retina to the hypothalamus before being transmitted to the pineal gland. Thus, one possible explanation for the amplified melatonin rhythm characteristic of women with SRA is altered hypothalamic processing of the light signal [9,10]. *T bars* indicate ± SEM.

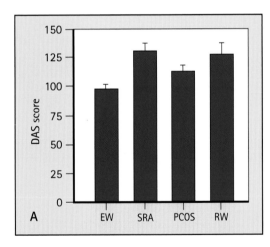

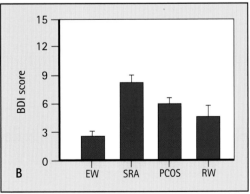

FIGURE 2-16.

Results of surveys using the Dysfunctional Attitudes Scale (DAS) and the Beck Depression Inventory (BDI). **A**, The results of the DAS. This questionnaire surveys coping styles, expectations, outlook, and attitudes. We compared psychiatric and psychologic attributes in eumenorrheic women (EW), women with stress-related anovulation (SRA), women with polycystic ovary syndrome (PCOS), and women who have recovered from SRA (RW). Women with SRA display an amplified, but phase-intact, cortisol rhythm, indicating that the events of daily living elicit a greater response from the hypothalamic-pituitary-adrenal (HPA) axis than that seen in EW, women with PCOS-related anovulation, and RW. Because recovery of ovulation apparently involves restoration of cortisol levels, we have hypothesized that the most effective treatment for SRA would be to reverse the endocrine stress response. To accomplish this reversal, we need to understand the psychologic antecedents that initiate and maintain endocrine arousal [11]. EW had the lowest mean scores, indicating a healthier perspective. Women with PCOS also had low mean scores. In contrast, women with SRA displayed high mean DAS scores, indicating unhelpful attitudes and outlooks. The RW did not receive any formal psychiatric or psychologic intervention. The high DAS mean score in the RW group likely indicates that they remain at risk for HPA axis activation, but while they were participating in the research study, they experienced a decrease in HPA activation sufficient to permit return of gonadotropin-releasing hormone (GnRH) drive.

B, Results from the Beck Depression Inventory (BDI) in the same four groups of women. The DAS inventory is designed to assess psychologic traits, whereas the BDI assesses current mood and attitudes or "state" characteristics. Women with SRA displayed the highest mean scores, but none met criteria for major depression. In contrast to the DAS score, the mean BDI score in the RW group is lower than that of the SRA group, which correlates with the lower cortisol levels seen in the RW group. *T bars* indicate ± SEM.

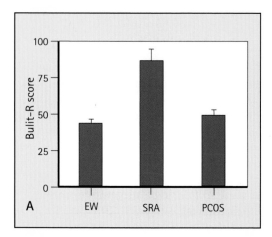

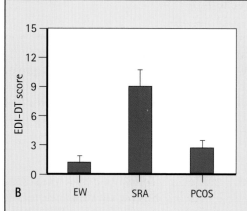

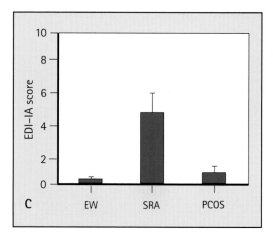

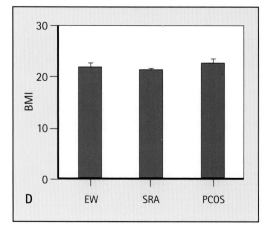

FIGURE 2-17.

Survey results in 3 groups of women. Results of the mean BULIT-R, Eating Disorders Inventory (EDI) subscales, and the role of body mass index (BMI) in eumenorrheic women (EW), women with stress-related anovulation (SRA), and women with polycystic ovary syndrome (PCOS). **A**, Women with SRA do not report bulimic behaviors such as binging, purging, and laxative use, but they do display attitudes toward food that are similar to those of women with bulimia. Although mean scores on the BULIT-R are highest in women with SRA as compared with EW and women with PCOS, the mean scores do not meet clinical criteria for bulimia.

B, Women with SRA also do not meet criteria for anorexia nervosa, but their mean scores on the EDI are higher than those of EW or women with PCOS. Two of the eight subscales are shown. Women with SRA have a higher drive for thinness (DT), which predisposes them to calorie and nutritional restriction and altered thyroidal function such as that shown in Figure 2-13. **C**, Women with SRA also display higher scores on the interoceptor subscale (IA) of the EDI than EW or PCOS. Attitudes toward food are hypothesized to sensitize women to psychologic stressors by increasing endocrine reactivity rather than by causing weight loss.

D, In this study, the BMI of women with SRA was identical to that of EW and women with PCOS. Although distorted attitudes toward food and eating are hypothesized to alter neuroendocrine cascades and increase sensitivity to psychogenic stressors, this sensitization can occur without weight loss. *T bars* indicate ± SEM. BULIT-R–Bulemia Inventory–Revised.

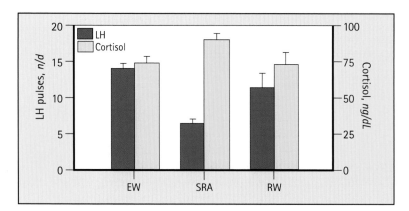

FIGURE 2-18.

Luteinizing hormone (LH) pulse and cortisol concentrations. Mean LH pulse number per 24 hours and mean 24-hour cortisol concentrations in eumenorrheic women (EW), women with stress-related anovulation (SRA), and women who have recovered from SRA (RW). Higher mean cortisol levels correlate with lower LH pulse frequency, suggesting a causal, albeit indirect, link between activation of the hypothalamic-pituitary-adrenal axis (HPA) and suppression of the hypothalamic-pituitary-ovarian (HPO) axis. *T bars* indicate ± SEM.

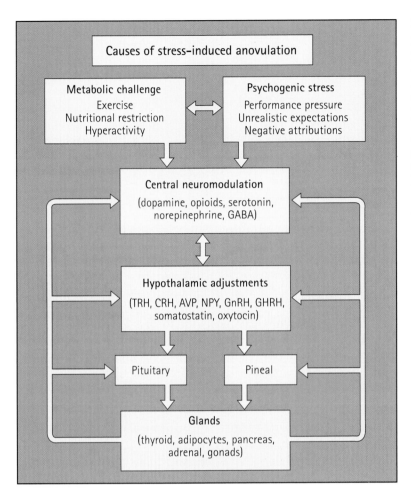

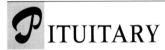

Causes of stress-induced anovulation

Metabolic challenge	Psychogenic stress
Exercise	Performance pressure
Nutritional restriction	Unrealistic expectations
Hyperactivity	Negative attributions

Central neuromodulation
(dopamine, opioids, serotonin, norepinephrine, GABA)

Hypothalamic adjustments
(TRH, CRH, AVP, NPY, GnRH, GHRH, somatostatin, oxytocin)

Pituitary   Pineal

Glands
(thyroid, adipocytes, pancreas, adrenal, gonads)

FIGURE 2-19.

Factors in stress-induced anovulation (SRA). SRA is conceptualized here as syndrome in which psychobiologic characteristics predispose women to sustained alterations in central neural function in response to daily stress. Compensatory hypothalamic adjustments lead to altered pituitary, pineal, and endocrine glandular secretion. The proximate cause of the anovulation is reduced gonadotropin-releasing hormone (GnRH) drive. Synergism exists between stressors that induce metabolic deficits and those that present a psychogenic challenge. AVP—arginine vasopressin; CRH—corticotropin-releasing hormone; GABA— gamma-aminobutyric acid; GHRH—growth hormone– releasing hormone; NPY—neuropeptide Y; TRH—thyroid-releasing hormone.

𝒫ITUITARY

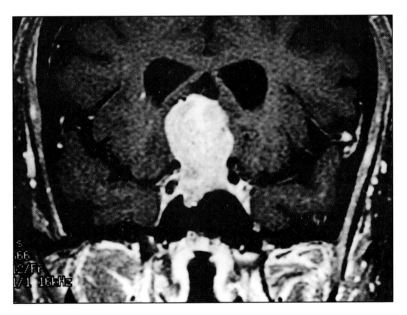

FIGURE 2-20.

Contrast-enhanced, T_1-weighted magnetic resonance image (MRI) in the coronal plane of a large pituitary prolactin-secreting macroade-

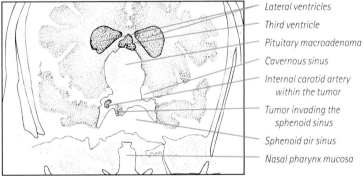

Lateral ventricles
Third ventricle
Pituitary macroadenoma
Cavernous sinus
Internal carotid artery within the tumor
Tumor invading the sphenoid sinus
Sphenoid air sinus
Nasal pharynx mucosa

noma with suprasellar extension into the left cavernous sinus and sphenoid sinus. The internal carotid artery is firmly embedded within the tumor mass. Very large tumors are usually associated with visual field defects (bitemporal hemianopsia is classic) secondary to compression of the optic chiasm that lies above the pituitary gland. A common presenting complaint is an unremitting, dull, generalized headache that is unrelieved by analgesics. These macrodenomas tend to grow slowly, extend locally, and rarely are frankly malignant. Hemorrhage and infarction are more common complications with larger tumors. Coma, circulatory collapse, and irreversible hypopituitarism may result.

010153

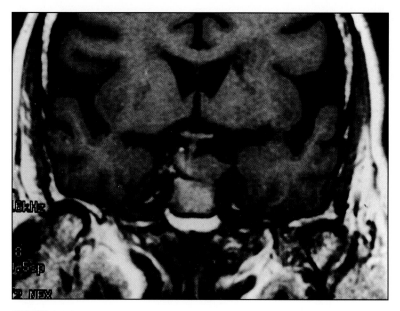

FIGURE 2-21.

T₁-weighted magnetic resonance image (MRI) of pituitary microadenoma enhanced by contrast. The pituitary stalk is deviated only slightly from midline due to mild enlargement

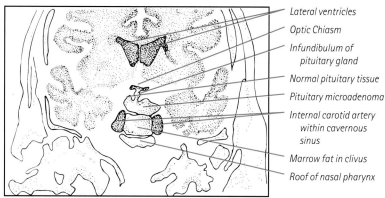

- Lateral ventricles
- Optic Chiasm
- Infundibulum of pituitary gland
- Normal pituitary tissue
- Pituitary microadenoma
- Internal carotid artery within cavernous sinus
- Marrow fat in clivus
- Roof of nasal pharynx

of one side of the gland. Approximately 50% of pituitary adenomas secrete prolactin. Elevated prolactin levels suppress hypothalamic pulsatile gonadotropin-releasing hormone (GnRH) via opioidergic mechanisms and thereby disrupt reproductive function. Luteal insufficiency and anovulation may result. Prolactin levels are higher with macroadenomas (> 10 mm in diameter) than microdenomas. Microadenomas (≤ 10 mm) tend not to enlarge and are polyclonal in origin. Macroadenomas may invade adjacent areas and are monoclonal in origin.

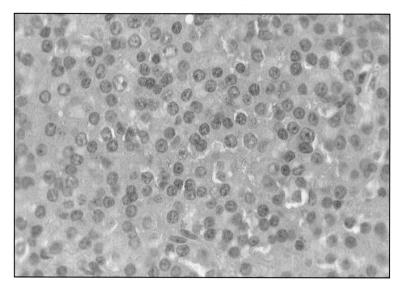

FIGURE 2-22.

Histologic appearance of a pituitary adenoma stained with eosin and hematoxylin. It is virtually impossible to differentiate one type of adenoma from another with routine tissue stains. Specific immunohistochemical staining with antibodies directed against a particular peptide hormone is the only confirmatory method. Adenomas that produce prolactin or growth hormone usually have sheets or cords of uniform cells with dense or sparse granules that stain with eosinophilic stains. The hormone is synthesized by the rough endoplasmic reticulum and is packaged into granules by the Golgi apparatus. Lactotropic cells secreting prolactin have the largest secretory granules. These cells replace normal glandular tissue, the extent of which depends on the tumor size. The stroma may be delicately vascularized. The abundance of granules within the cell correlates directly with the degree of differentiation of tumor cells but not with the secretory capacity of the cells. Prominent nuclei and nucleoli within these cells indicate active protein synthesis.

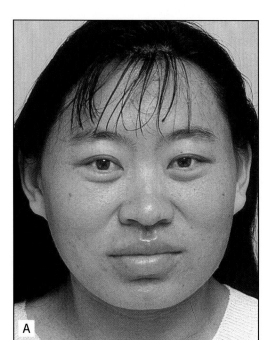

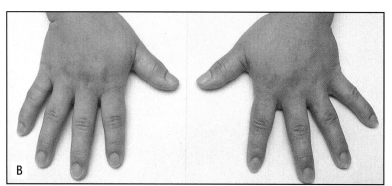

FIGURE 2-23.

Acromegaly. **A,** Facies of a young woman with acromegaly and amenorrhea. In this instance, the amenorrhea was caused by pregnancy, although over 50% of women with acromegaly report menstrual irregularities. The patient had a large, 2-cm pituitary tumor causing bitemporal hemianopsia. Note the coarseness of her facial features, which is caused by dermal hyperplasia. Widening of the jaw resulted in increased interdental spaces and she also had macroglossia caused by connective tissue proliferation.

B, Hands of the same patient. She reluctantly acknowledged an increase in shoe size. Swelling of hands and feet are one of the earliest clinical features of acromegaly.

HYPOTHETICAL RESULTS OF PROVOCATIVE PITUITARY TESTING IN SHEEHAN SYNDROME, STRESS-RELATED ANOVULATION, AND PITUITARY STALK TRANSECTION

Provocative test (releasing factor and pituitary hormone)	Sheehan syndrome	Stress-related anovulation	Stalk transection
TRH-TSH	Low	Normal	Low or normal
TRH-prolactin	Low	Low	Elevated
CRH-ACTH	Low	Normal	Low or normal
GHRH-GH	Low	Normal	Low or normal
GnRH-LH	Low	Normal	Low or normal
GnRH-FSH	Low	Normal	Low or normal

FIGURE 2-24.

Pituitary testing in Sheehan syndrome. Results from provocative pituitary testing in Sheehan's syndrome (postpartum pituitary apoplexy), stress-related anovulation, and pituitary stalk transection. Releasing factors can be simultaneously administered to improve diagnostic yield. ACTH—adrenocorticotropic hormone; CRH—corticotropin-releasing hormone; FSH—follicle-stimulating hormone; GH—growth hormone; GHRH—growth hormone–releasing hormone; GnRH—gonadotropin-releasing hormone; LH—luteinizing hormone; TRH—thyroid-releasing hormone; TSH—thyroid-stimulating hormone.

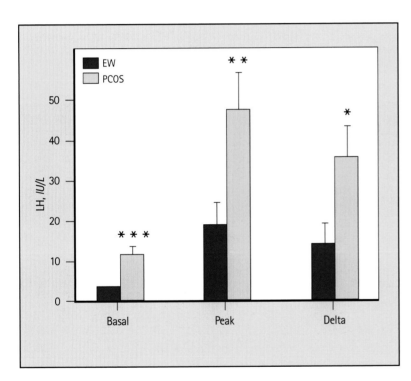

FIGURE 2-25.

Response of LH to GnRH. Mean responses of luteinizing hormone (LH) to an exogenous 100- µg intravenous bolus of gonadotropin-releasing hormone (GnRH) given to eumenorrheic women (EW) and women with PCOS. The increased pituitary release of LH in women with PCOS is probably caused by an increased releasable pool and increased sensitivity induced by persistently increased GnRH drive. *T bars* indicate ± SEM. *Asterisks* indicate statistically significant difference (*Adapted from* Berga *et al.* [2].)

*O*VARY

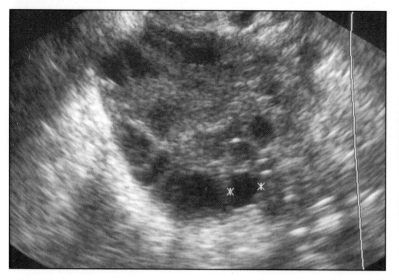

FIGURE 2-26.

Polycystic ovary syndrome. Ultrasound image of ovary with classic features of polycystic ovary syndrome. Note the increased stromal volume with multiple cysts arrayed at the periphery. The failure of follicular progression is a consistent finding in anovulatory women regardless of cause, whereas the increase in stromal volume is classically associated with hyperandrogenic anovulation [12,13].

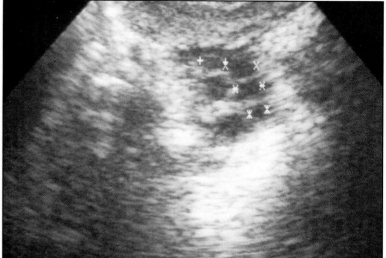

FIGURE 2-27.

Ultrasound of a multifollicular ovary. Multiple cysts are seen but the stromal and overall volume is not increased [14]. This ultrasound pattern is seen in women who are anovulatory owing to decreased gonadotropin stimulation. Women who might display this ultrasound appearance are those with hypothalamic amenorrhea caused by dietary restriction, excessive exercise, or psychologic pressures, and those ingesting oral contraceptives.

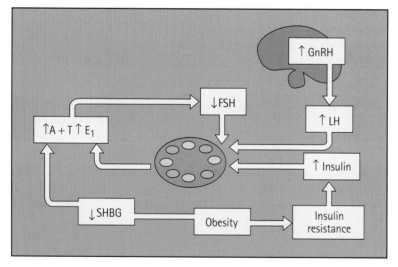

FIGURE 2-28

The pathogenesis of polycystic ovary syndrome (PCOS). The two main causes of anovulation are PCOS and functional hypothalamic anovulation Women with PCOS have increased gonadotropin-releasing hormone (GnRH) input, which increases the luteinizing hormone (LH) to follicle-stimulating hormone (FSH) ratio and inhibits the FSH level to below the threshold needed to sustain folliculogenesis. Thus, small follicular cysts accumulate in the periphery of the ovary. The ovarian stroma, however, hypertrophies because of unremitting LH stimulation that is augmented by hyperinsulinemia. In contrast, women with stress-related anovulation have decreased GnRH stimulation. Follicles in the ovary grow to the gonadotropin-dependent stage and then arrest. The stroma also remains understimulated owing to low levels of both LH and insulin, and thus the overall ovarian volume is much less than that seen in women with PCOS. A—androstenedione; E_1—estrone; SHBG—serum hormone-binding globulin; T—testosterone.

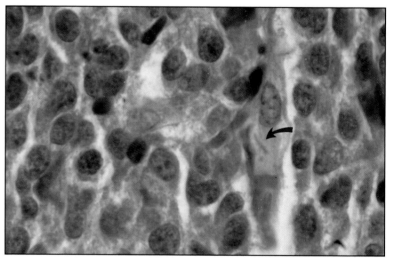

FIGURE 2-29.

Sertoli-Leydig tumor. Image showing Reinke's crystalloids within the cellular cytoplasm (*arrow*). Reinke's crystalloids are aggregates of testosterone in an elongated crystalloid structure. Their presence in the ovary is pathognomonic of a testosterone-secreting tumor.

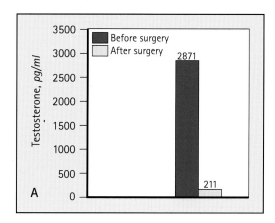
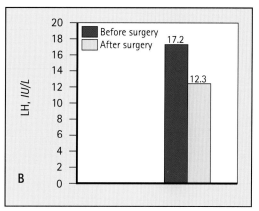
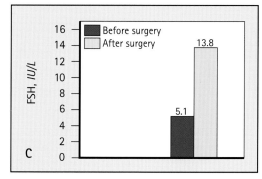
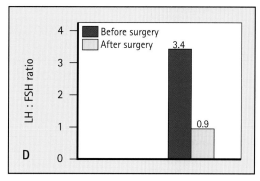
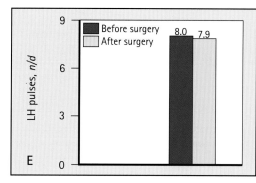

FIGURE 2-30.

Results of surgery for Sertoli-Leydig cell tumor. **A**, Testosterone levels before and after surgery in a woman with a Sertoli-Leydig cell tumor. Selected venous sampling was performed to determine that the site of the excess testosterone secretion was the right ovary. This 20-year-old white woman presented with cessation of lactation (which had been established since delivery 9 months previously), decreasing breast size, new onset of facial acne, deepening of the voice, new hair growth on the inner thighs and below the umbilicus, temporal balding, an increase in clitoral size, and ongoing amenorrhea despite cessation of lactation. Prior to surgery and on day 3 of following her second menses, blood samples were obtained at 10-minute intervals from 8 *am* to 8 *pm* and at 20-minute intervals from 8 *pm* to 8 *am*. Luteinizing hormone (LH), follicle-stimulating hormone (FSH), and testosterone levels were measured in all samples. Note the dramatic fall in testosterone levels following removal of the right ovary. Pathology revealed a Sertoli-Leydig cell tumor, or hilar cell tumor. **B**, LH levels before and after surgery. Note that LH levels fall slightly after removal of the Sertoli-Leydig cell tumor. **C**, FSH levels before and after surgery. Note the significant increase following return of testosterone levels to a normal range. The patient resumed menses promptly. **D**, The LH to FSH ratio changes dramatically after surgery, suggesting that the elevated testosterone levels led to an increase in tonic LH secretion and a suppression of FSH secretion. **E**, LH pulsatility was unaffected by the change in testosterone levels. LH pulse number was in the normal range, about 16 pulses per day, both before and after surgery. These data suggest that excess androgen exposure of extended duration does not modulate gonadotropin-releasing hormone pulsatility in a postpubertal woman.

FIGURE 2-31.

Fetal ovarian cortex with numerous primordial follicles and sparse stroma. Each oocyte is surrounded by a single granulosa cell (*arrow*).

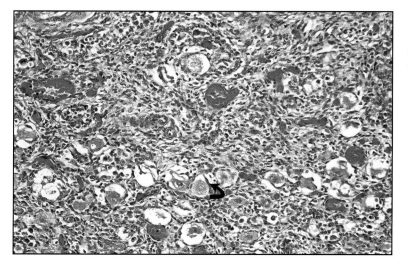

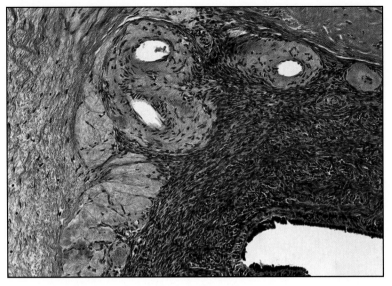

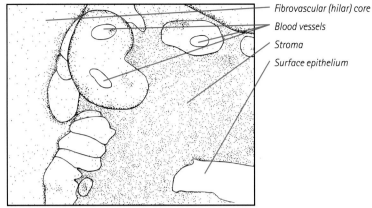

Fibrovascular (hilar) core
Blood vessels
Stroma
Surface epithelium

FIGURE 2-32.
Ovarian cortex with dense stroma devoid of follicles due to menopause. The stroma is interposed between the hilus with fibrovascular core and the cuboidal surface epithelium.

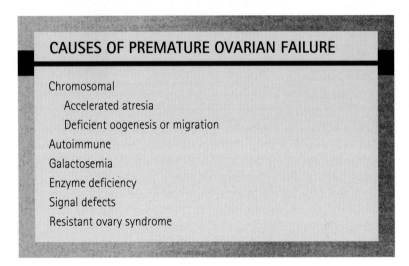

CAUSES OF PREMATURE OVARIAN FAILURE

Chromosomal
    Accelerated atresia
    Deficient oogenesis or migration
Autoimmune
Galactosemia
Enzyme deficiency
Signal defects
Resistant ovary syndrome

FIGURE 2-33.
Causes of premature ovarian failure. The two most common causes are accelerated atresia and autoimmune. Accelerated oocyte atresia is seen in women missing a portion of the long arm of the X chromosome, so it is presumed that the missing DNA encodes for an important regulation of oocyte longevity.

𝒰TERUS

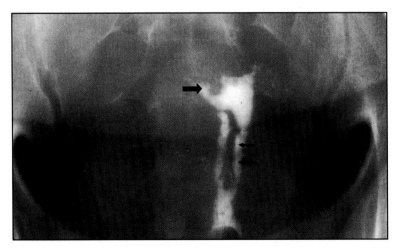

FIGURE 2-34.
Hysterosalpingogram of uterus with Asherman's syndrome. The radiologic contrast is seen as white, and areas of endometrial scarring and adhesion (*arrows*) appear as black areas within the endometrial cavity. Women with Asherman's syndrome may present with amenorrhea if the extent of endometrial denuding is widespread or if menstrual flow is obstructed.

*O*THER CAUSES

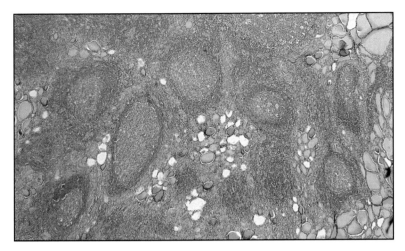

FIGURE 2–35.
Hashimoto's thyroiditis. This disease is characterized by an intense infiltrate of lymphocytes and plasma cells that virtually replace the normal glandular parenchyma. The thyroid gland is diffusely

enlarged but this process is usually painless. This chronic disease eventually renders the patient hypothyroid, although during the process patients may experience a short thyrotoxic phase. This autoimmune attack appears to be a genetically predetermined deficiency in the antigen-specific suppressor T cells that, along with antibody-dependent complement-mediated cytotoxicity, destroys the glandular epithelium and eventually the architecture and function.

Hypothyroidism is often secondary to autoimmune destruction of the thyroid gland. If a goiter is present, it is called Hashimoto's thyroiditis. The incidence of this condition increases with age and is more common in women (female to male ratio, 10:1). Hypothyroidism often is accompanied by menstrual irregularities, menorrhagia being an early common manifestation. Ovarian function can be suppressed by increased prolactin levels due to increased thyroid-releasing hormone drive. Menstrual disturbances also are caused by abnormal endometrial maturation; this mechanism may account for an increase in spontaneous miscarriage. Women with Turner's syndrome are at increased risk for Hashimoto's thyroiditis, as are those with HLA-DR4 antigen.

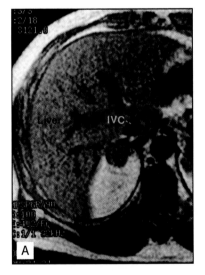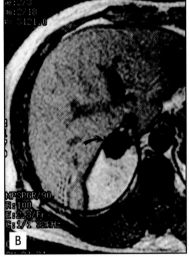

FIGURE 2–36.
Magnetic resonance image (MRI) of adrenal nodule that caused Cushing's syndrome. Ninety percent of Cushing's syndrome are caused by pituitary tumors that secrete adrenocorticotropic hormone, and about 10% to 15% are caused by adrenal tumors (either adenomas or carcinomas). Other causes include ectopic corticotropin secretion by nonpituitary neoplasms, bilateral adrenal hyperplasia, chronic exogenous glucocorticoid adminis-

tration, ovarian tumors, and pituitary corticotropin-releasing hormone–secreting tumors. In women, Cushing's syndrome often presents as amenorrhea accompanied by truncal obesity, muscle wasting, thin skin with easy bruisability and purple striae, hirsutism, acne, hypertension, osteoporosis, glucose intolerance or frank diabetes, lymphocytopenia, hypokalemia, and sometimes frank psychosis. Symptoms of Cushing's syndrome may be mistaken for polycystic ovary syndrome or hyperandrogenic anovulation. Amenorrhea is a common initial symptom because excess cortisol secretion suppresses gonadotropin-releasing hormone (GnRH) drive. The differential diagnosis also includes excess alcohol intake. Diagnostic tests include dexamethasone suppression tests, a 24-hour urinary free cortisol, and corticotropin levels. Abdominal and pituitary imaging is required to localize the tumor site.

A, A right adrenal mass (*arrow*) that has the same magnetic resonance signal intensity as the liver. **B**, Magnetic resonance imaging (MRI) section through the same level using a technique that selectively suppresses the magnetic resonance signal from tissues having both lipid and water components (chemical shift opposed-phase sequence). Note the marked loss of magnetic resonance signal from the adrenal mass (*arrow*) compared with the liver. Adrenal adenomas, unlike metastases, contain large amounts of intracellular lipid, allowing a confident diagnosis to be made by MRI without biopsy. IVC—inferior vena cava.

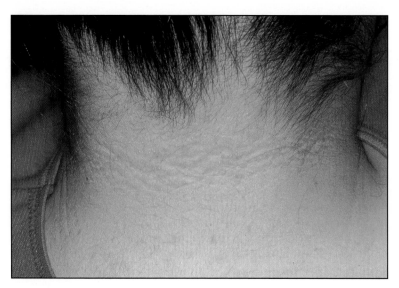

FIGURE 2-37.

Acanthosis nigricans. This skin manifestation of insulin resistance presents as a gray-brown, mossy, or velvety discoloration and thickening of the skin and is often associated with hyperinsulinemia and hyperandrogenism. Histologic features include hyperkeratosis and papillomatosis. Its presence correlates better with insulin resistance than with insulin levels. It is commonly localized to the dorsum of the neck, the groin, axillae, and sometimes under the breasts. High circulating levels of insulin-like growth factor 1 have been implicated as the cause of the skin changes. Typically it is seen in women with polycystic ovary syndrome, but it also may be found in women who are obese, those with diabetes mellitus due to blocking antibodies to insulin receptors, and those with insulin resistance owing to post-receptor defects. Women with insulin-dependent diabetes mellitus who are amenorrheic have been shown to have reduced gonadotropin-releasing hormone (GnRH) secretion [15], which is probably caused by poor glucose control and metabolic stress. In contrast, women with PCOS may have insulin resistance, but GnRH input is increased [16.]

CKNOWLEDGMENTS

Research studies summarized in this chapter were funded by NIH RO1-MH50748 and RR-00056.

REFERENCES

1. Reindollar RH, Novak M, Tho SPT, McDonough PG: Adult-onset amenorrhea: a study of 262 patients. *Am J Obstet Gynecol* 1986, 155:531–543.

2. Berga SL, Guzick DS, Winters SJ: Increased luteinizing hormone and alpha-subunit secretion in women with hyperandrogenic anovulation. *J Clin Endocrinol Metab* 1993, 77:895–901.

3. Berga SL, Mortola JF, Girton L, *et al.*: Neuroendocrine aberrations in women with functional hypothalamic amenorrhea. *J Clin Endocrinol Metab* 1989, 68:301–308.

4. Biller BMK, Federoff JH, Koenig JI, Klibanski A: Abnormal cortisol secretions and responses to corticotropin-releasing hormone in women with hypothalamic amenorrhea. *J Clin Endocrinol Metab* 1990, 70:311–307.

5. Ding JH, Sheckter CB, Drinkwater BL, *et al.*: High serum cortisol levels in exercise-associated amenorrhea. *Annals Intern Med* 1988, 108:530–534.

6. Loucks AB, Mortola JF, Girton L, Yen SSC: Alterations in the hypothalamic-pituitary-ovarian and hypothalamic-pituitary-adrenal axes in athletic women. *J Clin Endocrinol Metab* 1989, 68:402–411.

7. Berga SL, Daniels TL, Giles DE: Women with functional hypo-thalamic amenorrhea but not other forms of anovulation display amplified cortisol concentrations. *Fertil Steril* 1997, 67:1024–1030.

8. Berga SL, Loucks AB, Rossmanith WG, *et al.*: Acceleration of luteinizing hormone pulse frequency in functional hypothalamic amenorrhea by dopaminergic blockade. *J Clin Endocrinol Metab* 1991, 72:151–156.

9. Berga SL, Mortola JF, Yen SSC: Amplification of nocturnal melatonin secretion in women with functional hypothalamic amenorrhea. *J Clin Endocrinol Metab* 1988, 66:242–244.

10. Laughlin GA, Loucks AB, Yen SSC: Marked augmentation of nocturnal melatonin secretion in amenorrheic athletes, but not in cycling athletes: unaltered by opioidergic or dopaminergic blockade. *J Clin Endocrinol Metab* 1991, 73:1321–1326.

11. Giles DE, Berga SL: Cognitive and psychiatric correlates of functional hypothalamic amenorrhea: a controlled comparison. *Fertil Steril* 1993, 60:486–492.

12. Polson DW, Wadworth J, Adams J, Franks S: Polycystic ovaries: a common finding in normal women. *Lancet* 1988, 1:870–872.

13. Pache TD, de Jong FH, Hop WC, Fauser BCJM: Association between ovarian changes assessed by transvaginal sonography and clinical and endocrine signs of the polycystic ovary syndrome. *Fertil Steril* 1993, 59:544–549.

14. Adams J, Polson DW, Abdulwahid N, *et al.*: Multifollicular ovaries: clinical and endocrine features and response to pulsatile gonadotropin releasing hormone. *Lancet* 1985, 2:1375–1378.

15. South SA, Asplin CM, Carlsen EC, *et al.*: Alterations in luteinizing hormone secretory activity in women with insulin-dependent diabetes mellitus and secondary amenorrhea. *J Clin Endocrinol Metab* 1993, 76:1048–1053.

16. Daniels TL, Berga SL: Resistance of gonadotropin releasing hormone drive to sex steroid-induced suppression in hyperandrogenic anovulation. *J Clin Endocrinol Metab* 1997, 82:4179–4183.

CHAPTER 3

Hyperprolactinemia

Michael D. Scheiber and Robert W. Rebar

Prolactin (PRL) was first identified by Riddle *et al.* [1] in the 1930s. However, in humans it proved extremely difficult to separate the lactogenic effects of PRL from those of growth hormone, and research involving human PRL progressed slowly. The identification of human pituitary PRL by Friesen *et al.* [2] and the subsequent development of reliable radioimmunoassays (RIAs) for human PRL in the early 1970s [2] led to a more complete elucidation of the endocrinology and pathophysiology of this hormone.

More recently, the molecular biology of PRL has been quite well defined. The gene has been identified, and several different forms of PRL resulting from posttranslational modification have been recognized. An understanding of the regulatory mechanisms of PRL secretion provides an important foundation for an exploration of both physiologic and pathologic hyperprolactinemia. PRL is unique among the known anterior pituitary hormones in that its regulation is primarily inhibitory. However, the neuroendocrine regulation of PRL secretion is complex.

The clinical consequences of hyperprolactinemia are varied. The classic presentation in reproductive-aged women is galactorrhea in association with amenorrhea, and women with hyperprolactinemia are common in gynecologic and infertility practices. An adequate understanding of the fundamentals of PRL pathophysiology allows the clinician to formulate a rational approach to the diagnosis and treatment of hyperprolactinemia.

Hyperprolactinemia has multiple causes, and the clinical and laboratory evaluation of hyperprolactinemia should be approached in an orderly fashion. Treatment modalities can then be selected appropriately. This chapter provides a brief discussion of all of these areas.

$\mathcal{J}$DENTIFICATION AND STRUCTURE OF PROLACTIN

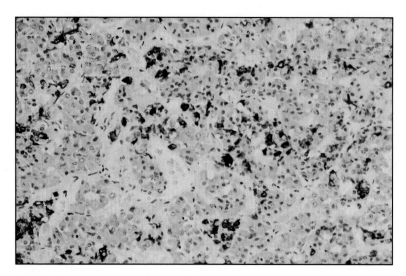

FIGURE 3-1.

Prolactin secretion. Photomicrograph of pituitary cells stained by
avidin-biotin complex immunohistocytochemistry to demonstrate
prolactin (PRL) secretion (diaminobenzidine chromagen, magnification 40×). PRL is made primarily by pituitary lactotrophs (also
known as mammotrophs) in the anterior pituitary. Lactotrophs
normally compose 15% to 25% of the total number of pituitary
cells. During pregnancy and lactation there is considerable hyperplasia and hypertrophy of the lactotrophs, which is largely due to
the stimulatory effects of estrogen. Involution of the lactotrophs
occurs within several months after delivery but is delayed by
breast-feeding. Lactotrophs are acidophils that are indistinguish-
able from somatotrophs (*ie*, those pituitary cells that secrete
human growth hormone) using conventional stains. However,
the lactotrophs can be further classified on the basis of their
electron microscopic appearance; granulated cells correspond to
cells in a resting and storage phase, whereas nongranulated cells
are thought to be in an active secretory state [3]. The corticotrophs,
thyrotrophs, and gonadotrophs comprise the basophilic cell types
in the adenohypophysis. (*Courtesy of* Paul Biddinger.)

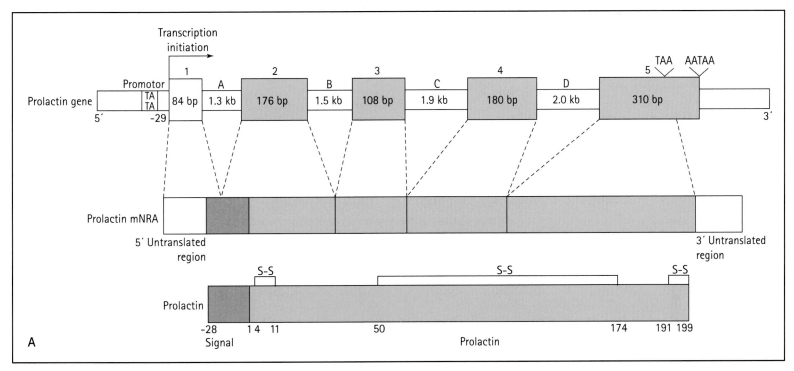

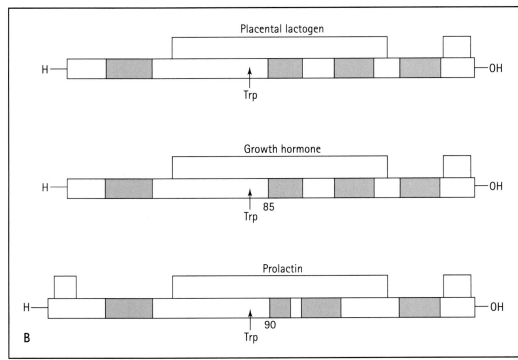

FIGURE 3-2.

Structure of the human prolactin (PRL) gene. **A**, Processing of the human PRL gene. The human PRL gene has been well characterized and is approximately 10-kb long, consisting of five exons separated by four larger introns [4]. There is considerable homology among species in the 5' flanking region, which suggests sites specific for PRL gene regulation. The gene for human PRL has been localized to chromosome 6 [5]. **B**, Homology of the genes for human PRL, growth hormone (GH), and placental lactogen (hPL). The genes for GH and hPL are located on chromosome 17. However, the homology of these three genes suggests a common ancestral gene. Of interest is the observation that, in most mammals, the genes for PRL and GH are located on different chromosomes. The gene for hPL is located on either the chromosome containing the PRL or the GH gene and differs among species [6]. TRP—tryptophan (A *Adapted from* Molitch [3]; with permission.)

REGULATION OF PRL RELEASE

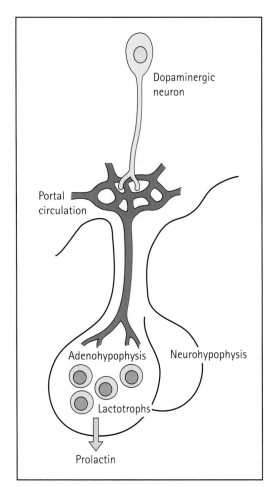

FIGURE 3-3.

Neuroendocrine regulation. The neuroendocrine regulation of pituitary prolactin (PRL) secretion is complex. Unlike most anterior pituitary hormones, the secretion of PRL is under chronic inhibition from the hypothalamus, demonstrated by the fact that interruption of the pituitary stalk results in increased circulating levels of PRL but decreased levels of other pituitary hormones. There are multiple PRL-inhibiting factors (PIFs), but dopamine secreted from neurons in the dorsomedial portion of the arcuate nucleus plays the most important role. Prolactin may inhibit its own secretion directly via negative feedback at the pituitary level or indirectly by increasing dopamine turnover in the hypothalamus [7].

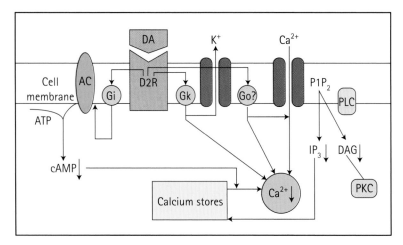

FIGURE 3-4.

Mechanism of action of dopamine on the pituitary lactotrope. Inhibition of pituitary prolactin (PRL) release by dopamine (DA) is mediated through the D2 receptor (D2R) subtype. Activation of this receptor, located on lactotroph cell membranes, results in decreased adenylate cyclase (AC) activity that, in turn, results in decreased intracellular levels of cAMP. This response is coupled through activation of the inhibitory G protein. Mutations or alterations in the genes for the D2 receptor or the G proteins (Gi, Gk, Go) may be involved in the development of pituitary prolactinomas [8]. ATP—adenosine 5' triphosphate; DAG—diacyl glycerol; IP_3—inositol triphosphate; PIP_2—phosphoinositol biphosphonate; PKC—protein kinase C; PLC— phospholipase C. (*Adapted from* Sarapura and Schlaff [9]; with permission.)

SUBSTANCES AFFECTING PROLACTIN RELEASE

Stimulatory	Inhibitory
TRH	Dopamine
VIP	PRL
GnRH	GABA
Serotonin	GAP
Opioid peptides	Endothelin-3
Estrogen	

FIGURE 3-5.

Substances affecting prolactin (PRL) release. Despite the importance of dopamine, multiple other substances may act as either PRL-inhibiting factors (PIFs) or PRL-releasing factors (PRFs). Gonadotropin-releasing hormone(GnRH)–associated peptide (GAP), the 56-amino-acid peptide encoded in the precursor to GnRH, is a potent PRL inhibitor. γ-Aminobutyric acid (GABA) and endothelin-3 have also demonstrated PIF activity. Thyrotropin-releasing hormone (TRH) and estrogen are both potent PRFs and result in the elevated prolactin levels seen in primary hypothyroidism and pregnancy. Vasoactive intestinal peptide (VIP), GnRH, TRH, and serotonin all directly stimulate PRL release. Estrogen acts through stimulation of PRL gene transcription and by inhibiting hypothalamic dopamine release.

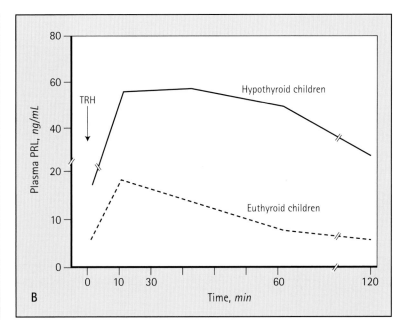

FIGURE 3-6.

PRL response to TRH. The peripheral response of prolactin to intravenous administration of thyrotropin-releasing hormone (TRH). **A**, The mean values of serum prolactin over time in 36 normal men and women after administration of 400 µg of synthetic TRH. *Vertical bars* indicate one SE of mean. **B**, Children with primary hypothyroidism show an exaggerated plasma PRL response to administration of TRH when compared with euthyroid children. TRH is an extremely potent prolactin-releasing factor. (*A adapted from* Jacobs [10]; *B adapted from* Collu as adapted in Mastroianni [11]; with permission.)

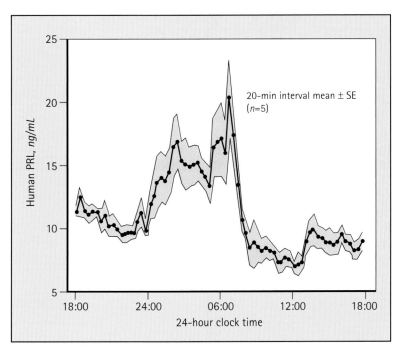

FIGURE 3-7.

Pulsatile secretion. Prolactin (PRL) is secreted in a pulsatile fashion with varying pulse frequencies and amplitudes. There is a diurnal (*ie*, circadian) variation that is not inherent but depends on sleep [12]. PRL levels are highest during nonrapid eye movement sleep. The biologic significance of this sleep-associated rise in PRL is uncertain.

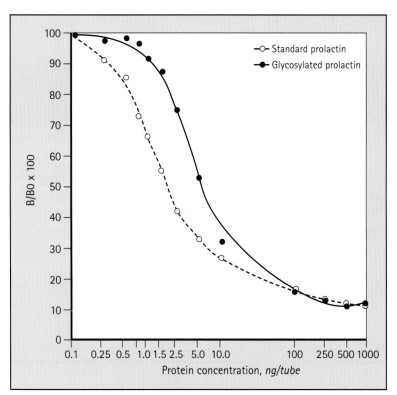

FIGURE 3-8.

Measuring PRL. A standard curve generated by a double-antibody radioimmunassay (RIA) for measurement of standard human prolactin (PRL) (*closed circles*) and glycosylated PRL (*open circles*) in human serum. Historically, PRL was measured using the reverse hemolytic plaque assay or other bioassays, such as the pigeon crop sac or mouse mammary gland assays. These tests relied on the stimulatory effect of PRL on mammary gland tissue to produce changes in organ weight. Today, RIA is the preferred laboratory method for measuring PRL. This figure demonstrates that glycosylated PRL generates a standard curve parallel to that for the major form of circulating human PRL. Thus, most RIAs measure the less biologically active forms of PRL described previously (*eg*, "big PRL" or "big-big PRL") to some extent, thus possibly explaining eumenorrhea and fertility in some hyperprolactinemic patients. B/B_o—bound-to-free ratio. (*Adapted from* Lewis and coworkers [13]; with permission)

CHANGES IN PRL LEVELS

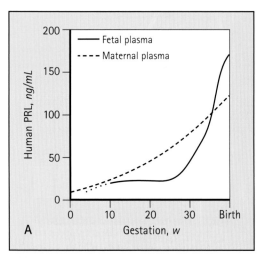 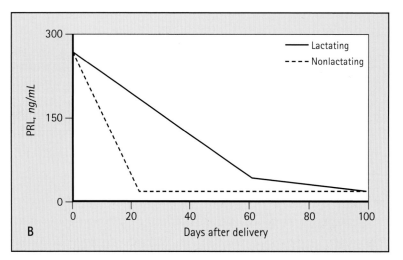

FIGURE 3-9.

Changes in prolactin (PRL) levels. **A**, Serum PRL levels in normal pregnancy. Pregnancy represents a physiologic state of hyperprolactinemia, and PRL rises steadily throughout pregnancy. Levels may peak near 200 ng/mL in the serum at term. These elevated levels prepare the breast for lactation. Lactation, however, does not occur until levels of estrogen fall after delivery. Levels increase in fetal plasma throughout pregnancy as well. Levels are higher in "stressed" pregnancies (as may occur in preeclampsia and diabetes mellitus, for example) than in normal pregnancies. **B**, Postpartum PRL levels in lactating and nonlactating women. PRL levels remain elevated in lactating women for the first 4 to 6 weeks postpartum and then gradually fall to normal basal levels. PRL continues to increase with each episode of suckling in women who exclusively breast-feed. PRL levels will rapidly fall to normal basal levels in the first postpartum week in women who are not breast-feeding. Neonatal PRL levels are elevated at birth, probably due in part to the stimulatory effects of high maternal estrogens, then fall to normal by 3 months of age [15]. PRL levels typically remain elevated for longer periods in highly stressed infants. (*A adapted from* Rebar [14]; with permission).

FACTORS CAUSING TEMPORARY ELEVATIONS IN SERUM PROLACTIN LEVELS

Acute stress (including surgical)	Herpes zoster
Food ingestion	Nipple stimulation
Chest wall stimulation	Suckling
Breast implants	Breast examination
Surgery	Coitus

FIGURE 3-10.

External factors known to influence prolactin (PRL) secretion. Acute stress is well known to induce a brief elevation in PRL levels. Neither prolonged emotional nor physical stress will cause a significant elevation. Food ingestion causes a transient rise in PRL after lunch or dinner, but not breakfast. Nipple or anterior chest wall stimulation from suckling, manipulation, breast implants, surgery, and herpes zoster have all been shown to cause elevated PRL levels. These factors all point to the clinical importance of maximizing laboratory information by drawing serum PRL levels in an awake, nonstressed, fasting state in individuals preferably not on medication, in the follicular phase of a menstrual cycle if cyclic, and prior to breast examination.

DISTRIBUTION OF THE PROLACTIN RECEPTOR

Breast	Seminal vesicles
Liver	Epididymis
Kidney tubules	Lymphocytes
Adrenal cortex	Lung
Prostate	Myocardium
Ovary	Brain
Testes	

FIGURE 3-11.

Distribution of the human prolactin (PRL) receptor. PRL receptors have been isolated in numerous tissues. The human PRL receptor gene has been localized to the short arm of chromosome 5 and is 598 amino acids long. The receptor binds hormone with high affinity and is half-saturated at a hormone concentration of 7 ng/mL [16].

HYPERPROLACTINEMIA AND REPRODUCTIVE DYSFUNCTIONS

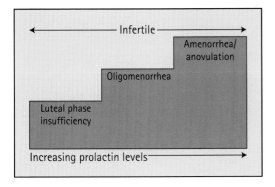

FIGURE 3-12.

Manifestations of hyperprolactinemia. According to Hippocrates, "If a woman has milk and is neither with nor has brought forth her child, her menstruation is suppressed." The manifestations of hyperprolactinemia have long been recognized. The classic clinical presentation of hyperprolactinemia in women is oligo- or amenorrhea associated with galactorrhea. This figure illustrates the spectrum of reproductive dysfunction resulting from hyperprolactinemia. Subtler forms of hyperprolactinemia have been associated with infertility and luteal phase dysfunction. In men, hyperprolactinemia often results in impotence, secondary to hypogonadism. Varying clinical symptoms and findings may result depending on the cause of hyperprolactinemia. (*Courtesy of* Sandoz Pharmaceutical Corp.)

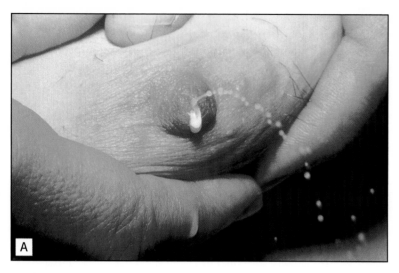

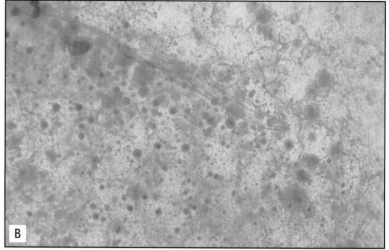

FIGURE 3-13.

Galactorrhea. **A**, Galactorrhea in a nonlactating woman. Galactorrhea is the presence of any amount of milk expressible or spontaneously discharged from one or both breasts. It is often an indicator of hyperprolactinemia. Galactorrhea is inappropriate in the absence of pregnancy or if persistent for more than 1 year after cessation of breast-feeding. **B**, An oil red O stain of galactorrhea showing the characteristic staining of fat globules. A simple smear of breast discharge on a microscope slide identifies the fat globules in breast milk, but they are particularly easy to identify as stained shown here. By definition, milk contains symmetrically round, thick-walled fat globules of varying size. Milk can be clear, white, yellow, or even greenish in color. If cells are present in the smear, a specimen should be sent for cytopathologic evaluation.

CAUSES AND CLINICAL FEATURES

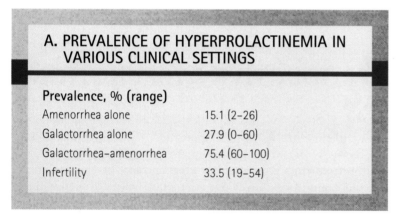

A. PREVALENCE OF HYPERPROLACTINEMIA IN VARIOUS CLINICAL SETTINGS

Prevalence, % (range)	
Amenorrhea alone	15.1 (2–26)
Galactorrhea alone	27.9 (0–60)
Galactorrhea–amenorrhea	75.4 (60–100)
Infertility	33.5 (19–54)

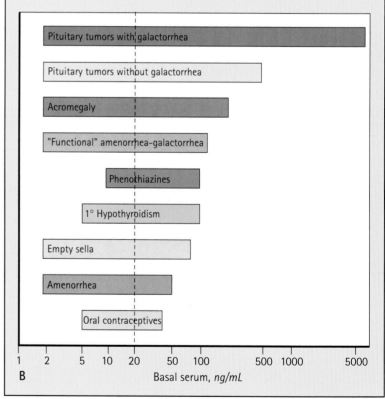

FIGURE 3-14.

Hyperprolactinemia in various clinical settings. **A,** The prevalence of hyperprolactinemia in various clinical settings. Hyperprolactinemia can present with a variety of clinical complaints and findings. This table highlights the high prevalence of hyperprolactinemia in women with amenorrhea and menstrual disorders [17]. **B,** Basal serum prolactin (PRL) levels in various clinical settings. The *dotted line* indicates the upper limit of the normal range. Laboratory variations in measurement of PRL are extremely important, and every clinician must know the range of normal as well as the inter- and intra-assay variation for the laboratory conducting a specific examination. Generally, with double-antibody radioimmunoassay, the range of normal serum PRL is 1 to 15 ng/mL. Values of 16 to 20 ng/mL are considered the extreme upper limit of normal, and levels in this range often warrant a repetition of the assay under the conditions mentioned in Figure 3-11 as well as clinical follow-up. In general, the higher the basal value, the greater the likelihood of a pituitary tumor. This is especially true for values greater than 50 ng/mL. (*Adapted from* Rebar [18]; with permission)

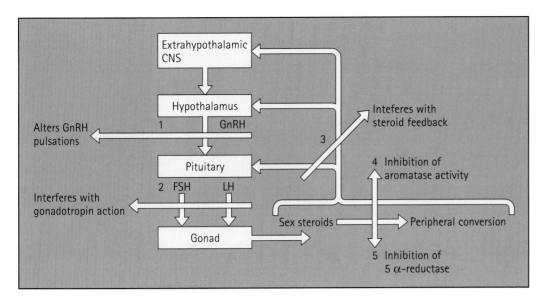

FIGURE 3-15.

Mechanisms by which hyperprolactinemia may interfere with reproductive function. The exact mechanism by which hyperprolactinemia causes menstrual disturbance is largely unknown. One important mechanism is thought to be mediated by dopamine. Increasing levels of prolactin (PRL) stimulate dopamine secretion at the level of the hypothalamus. This, in turn, results in inhibition of gonadotropin-releasing hormone (GnRH) release with a subsequent inhibition of gonadotropin secretion. There is some evidence to suggest that this process is mediated by opioidergic input [19]. A direct inhibitory effect of PRL on luteinizing hormone (LH) secretion has also been proposed. High levels of circulating PRL may interfere with steroid feedback at a central level, or may inhibit enzyme activity in the ovary. CNS—central nervous system; FSH—follicle-stimulating hormone. (*Adapted from* Odell as modified by Molitch [3]; with permission.)

ETIOLOGIES OF HYPERPROLACTINEMIA

Physiologic	Sarcoidosis
Pregnancy	Histiocytosis
Lactation	Pituitary disease
Pharmacologic	Prolactinomas
Neuroleptics	Empty sella syndrome
Phenothiazines	Pituitary stalk lesions
Butyrophenones	Neurogenic
Antidepressants	Chest wall pathology
MAO inhibitors	Spinal cord pathology
Tricyclics	Breast stimulation
Metoclopramide	Other
Reserpine	Idiopathic
Methyldopa	Systemic
Verapamil	Hypothyroidism
Hypothalamic disease	Renal failure
Tumors (craniopharyngioma)	Cirrhosis

FIGURE 3-16.

The different causes of hyperprolactinemia. The differential diagnosis of hyperprolactinemia is long and varied. Initially elevated prolactin (PRL) levels should be repeated under ideal conditions to confirm the diagnosis. Extensive historical information should then be obtained from the patient in an effort to rule out known causes of hyperprolactinemia prior to pursuing further evaluation. MAO—monoamine oxidase.

CHARACTERISTICS OF 28 SCHIZOPHRENIC PATIENTS ON NEUROLEPTIC THERAPY WITH GALACTORRHEA (MEAN ±SD)

Age on reference therapy	30.3±5.9 y
Mean age at first onset	23.2±4.9 y
Previous psychiatric hospitalizations	4.3±4.4
Duration of reference therapy	102.3±90.4 d
Mean value of PRL ($n = 24$)	54.6±52.0 ng/mL
Mean value of PRL ($n = 24$)	37.5±ng/mL
Range of PRL	10–246 ng/mL

FIGURE 3-17.

Characteristics of schizophrenic patients on neuroleptics with galactorrhea. Any medications that affect dopamine regulation can cause changes in prolactin (PRL) homeostasis. Neuroleptic medication blocks the inhibitory effect of dopamine from the hypothalamus, and drugs used to treat Parkinson's disease cause stimulation of PRL release. Both are well-known causes of hyperprolactinemia. The effect of oral contraceptives on the PRL axis is less well documented, but estrogen levels higher than the normal physiologic range may result in hyperprolactinemia. Withdrawal of oral contraceptives and the subsequent rapid decrease in serum estrogen levels may also lead to hyperprolactinemia. In all these groups of patients, the benefits of medication usually outweigh the risks of hyperprolactinemia, especially in asymptomatic women. (*Adapted from* Windgassen and coworkers [20]; with permission.)

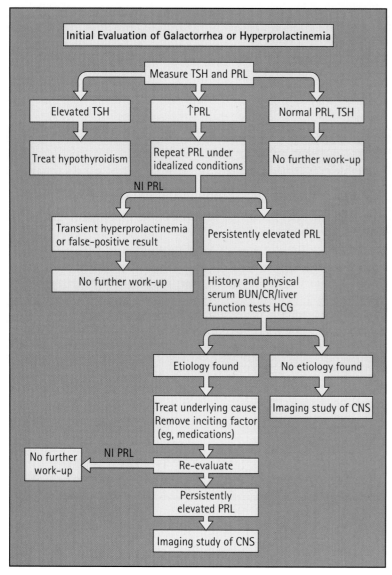

FIGURE 3–18.

Algorithm for the initial evaluation of galactorrhea or hyperprolactinemia. A careful history and physical examination, serum
chemistries (for renal and liver function), sensitive serum
thyrotropin-stimulating hormone (TSH), and a urine pregnancy
test should eliminate most causes of hyperprolactinemia except
hypothalamic–pituitary disease from the differential diagnosis. In
the absence of identifiable factors, radiologic imaging of the hypothalamic–pituitary area is mandatory in patients with hyperprolactinemia. BUN—blood urea nitrogen; CNS—central nervous
system; CR—creatinine; HCG—human chorionic gonadotropin;
NI—normal; PRL—prolactin.

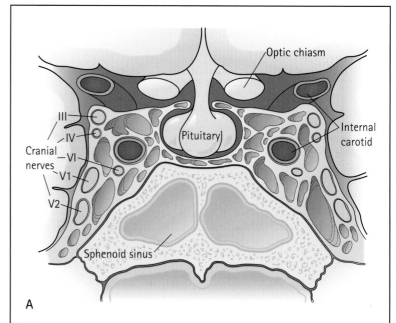

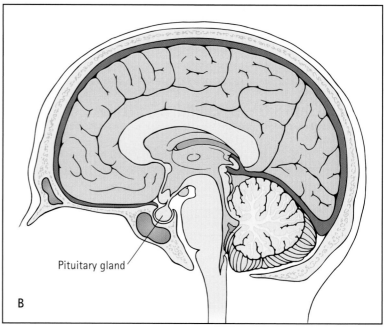

FIGURE 3–19.

MRI of sella turcica. Regional anatomy imaged by magnetic resonance imaging (MRI) or computed tomography (CT) scan as part
of the diagnostic evaluation of hyperprolactinemia. **A,** Cross-
sectional view of the hypothalamic and pituitary region demonstrating the proximity of the pituitary area to the optic chiasm
and sphenoid sinus. **B,** Sagittal view of the same region.
Gadolinium-enhanced high-resolution MRI is the modality of
choice for the evaluation of hyperprolactinemia. The greater resolution of MRI compared with CT scan allows for the identification
of microprolactinomas, many of which are below the resolution
of CT. MRI can detect lesions of 2 to 3 mm diameter. CT may be
slightly superior in the identification of calcified lesions.

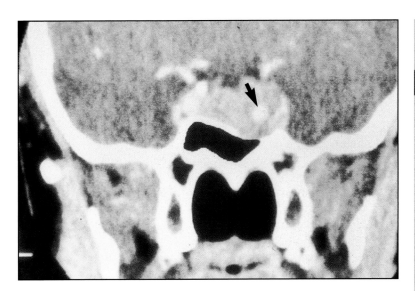

FIGURE 3-20.

Pituitary MRI. Magnetic resonance imaging (MRI) view of a pituitary microprolactinoma (*arrow*) in a 43-year-old woman presenting with amenorrhea, galactorrhea, and climacteric symptoms. Microprolactinomas are those prolactin (PRL)-secreting pituitary tumors measuring less than 1 cm in diameter. They compose about 95% of prolactinomas and rarely spontaneously enlarge or produce effects secondary to compression. Invasion of the dura or sella may occur, and such tumors should be differentiated from true carcinomas. Different autopsy series estimate the prevalence of pituitary prolactinomas to be 15% to 20% [21], thus greatly exceeding that of clinically significant tumors. Treatment is based on symptomatology (*ie*, reversal of galactorrhea, restoration of fertility, and normalization of PRL levels) and on the prevention of long-term sequelae.

BONE MINERAL MEASUREMENTS IN AMENORRHEIC WOMEN

Subject group	Vertebral Mineral, % of Control Subjects	E_2, pg/mL
Control	100	
Hyper-PRL	74.4	37
Hypothalamic Amenorrhea	76.5	46
Primary	83.8	
Secondary	72.8	
Premature ovarian failure	79.1	34

FIGURE 3-21.

Bone mineral measurements in amenorrheic women. This study demonstrates the risk of osteoporosis in women with hypoestrogenism secondary to amenorrhea from hyperprolactinemia. This is one of the most serious long-term sequelae of hyperprolactinemia resulting from pituitary microprolactinomas. Women with hypoestrogenism resulting from hypothalamic amenorrhea or premature ovarian failure also have significant bone loss. (*Adapted from* Cann and coworkers [22]; with permission.)

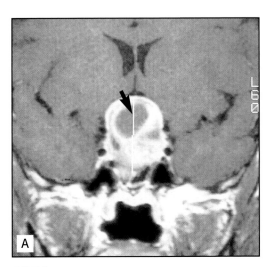 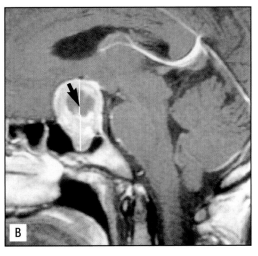

FIGURE 3-22.

Pituitary macroadenoma. **A**, Coronal magnetic resonance imaging (MRI) view. **B**, Sagittal view. This macroadenoma was discovered in a 41-year-old African-American woman who presented with a chief complaint of decreased peripheral vision, primarily in the left eye. Macroprolactinomas are those prolactin (PRL)-secreting pituitary tumors greater than 1 cm in diameter. Patients with macroadenomas are much more likely to present with symptoms related to mass effect such as headache, visual disturbances from optic chiasm compression and nausea. Peripheral visual field testing can be used to evaluate the integrity of the chiasm. Generalized pituitary function testing is warranted in women with macroadenomas. These tumors require treatment regardless of symptoms secondary to their propensity to grow. A distinction must be made between "nonsecreting" pituitary macroadenomas causing hyperprolactinemia secondary to stalk compression and true macroprolactinomas. Generally large macroprolactinomas result in PRL levels greater than 250 ng/mL, whereas stalk compression results in lower PRL elevations (often < 100 ng/mL). Those patients with macroadenomas and PRL levels between 100 and 250 ng/mL present difficult diagnostic challenges. (*Courtesy of* John M. Tew, Jr.)

TREATMENT

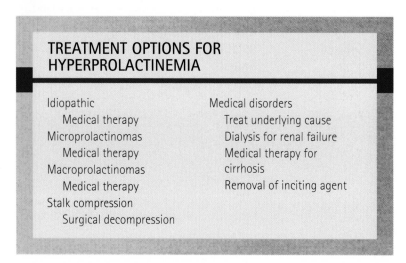

TREATMENT OPTIONS FOR HYPERPROLACTINEMIA

Idiopathic
   Medical therapy
Microprolactinomas
   Medical therapy
Macroprolactinomas
   Medical therapy
Stalk compression
   Surgical decompression

Medical disorders
   Treat underlying cause
   Dialysis for renal failure
   Medical therapy for
   cirrhosis
   Removal of inciting agent

FIGURE 3–23.

Treatment options for hyperprolactinemia. For hyperprolactinemia resulting from idiopathic causes or prolactin (PRL)-secreting pituitary adenomas, treatment modalities include medical therapy, surgical resection, and radiation therapy. Hyperprolactinemia owing to stalk compression is usually treated with surgical decompression if symptoms do not abate with administration of a dopamine agonist. Treatment of hyperprolactinemia resulting from medical conditions (*eg*, primary hypothyroidism or infiltrating diseases) hinges on treatment of the underlying disorder. Drug-induced hyperprolactinemia usually resolves with cessation of the offending agent. Hyperprolactinemia from chronic renal failure often responds to dialysis, whereas that from cirrhosis may be treated medically. The first line of therapy for women with both micro and macro prolactinomas is medical.

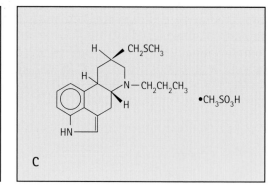

FIGURE 3–24.

Chemical structures of various drugs for treatment of hyperprolactinemia. **A**, Chemical structure of bromocriptine mesylate. It has been the mainstay of medical treatment for hyperprolactinemia for over 20 years. This drug is an ergot-derived dopamine agonist with actions at both the hypothalamic and pituitary levels. Usual doses are 2.5 to 15 mg/d, with larger doses being given in divided doses two or three times per day. **B**, Chemical structure of cabergoline. It recently received approval for usage in the United States from the Food and Drug Administration (FDA), and is an ergoline derivative with a long half-life that allows for twice-weekly dosing. It has a high affinity and selectivity for D2 receptors and appears to be at least as well-tolerated as bromocriptine and slightly more effective in the treatment of hyperprolactinemia [23]. The initial dose is 0.25 mg twice weekly, which is increased up to 1 mg twice weekly according to the patient's prolactin (PRL) level. **C**, Chemical structure of pergolide mesylate. It is as effective and safe as bromocriptine and has the advantages of once-daily dosing and lower cost.

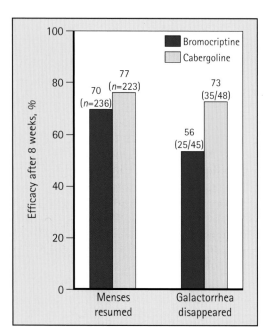

FIGURE 3–25.

Efficacy of medical therapy for hyperprolactinemia. Most patients with hyperprolactinemia will benefit greatly from treatment with dopamine agonist. Therapy leads to suppression of serum prolactin (PRL), restoration of gonadal function, and a reduction in tumor size, if present, in a majority of patients. Success rates of medical therapy vary in the literature, but PRL levels return to normal in approximately 90% of patients with idiopathic hyperprolactinemia or PRL-secreting microprolactinomas. Dopamine agonists will restore ovulation in most female patients; thus barrier contraceptives should be used by those women not desiring pregnancy. Dopamine agonists are probably safe in pregnancy, but their use is usually discontinued when pregnancy is confirmed. Hyperprolactinemia often returns after discontinuation of medical therapy, but spontaneous remissions do occur. The traditional utilization of life-long therapy, especially for idiopathic hyperprolactinemia and microprolactinomas, is being reconsidered. Many clinicians are now discontinuing medical therapy after 1 or 2 years and maintaining close clinical and laboratory follow-up. (*Courtesy of* Pharmacia and Upjohn Company).

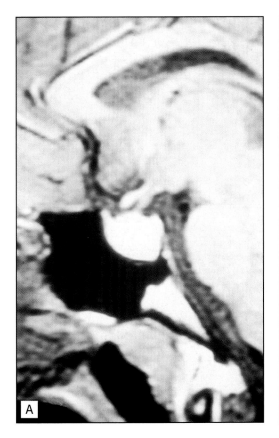 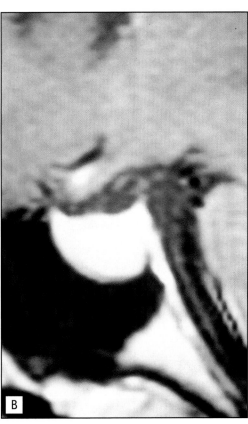

A

B

FIGURE 3-26.

Bromocriptive treatment. Magnetic resonance imaging (MRI) view of macroadenoma before (**A**) and after (**B**) treatment
with bromocriptine. Rapid tumor
shrinkage occurs in 70% to 80% of
patients with macroadenomas who are
treated with dopamine agonist therapy
[24]. Rapid shrinkage of most tumors
occurs in the first 3 months of therapy, but
continued shrinkage may occur up to 12
months or more [24]. Because of the high
percentage of successful responses, medical
therapy has become the treatment of
choice for most macroprolactinomas.
(*Courtesy of* James Leach.)

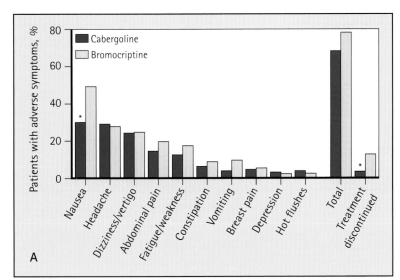 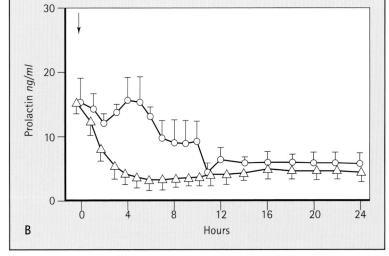

FIGURE 3-27.

Side effects **A**, Relative incidence of side effects in women with
hyperprolactinemia treated with different dopamine agonists. Side
effects of bromocriptine, especially nausea and orthostatic hypotension, can be minimized by starting with very low doses (1.25 mg),
with a snack at bedtime, and slowly increasing the dose every 1
to 2 weeks until therapeutic levels are achieved. **B**, Plasma PRL
levels after oral (triangle) and vaginal (circles) administration of

2.5 mg of bromocriptine. The vaginal administration of bromocriptine has been demonstrated to be effective in reducing serum
PRL levels. Many of the more common side effects of bromocriptine
are reduced with vaginal administration. Since half life is longer
with vaginal administration, once a day dosing is usually sufficient. (*Adapted from* Vermesh [25a]; with permission).

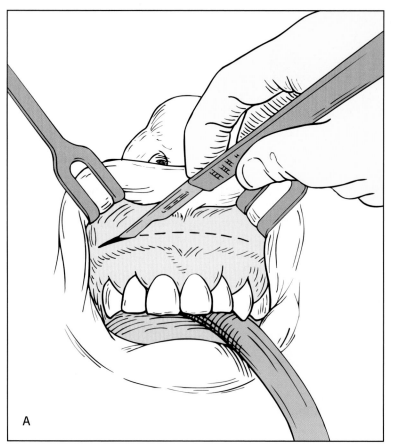

A

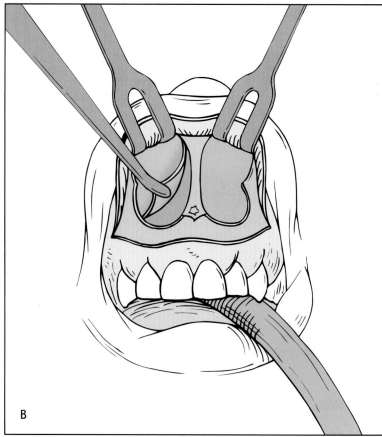

B

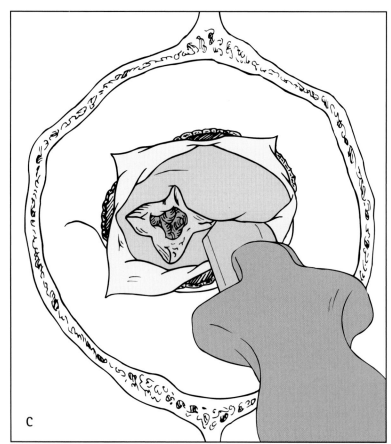

C

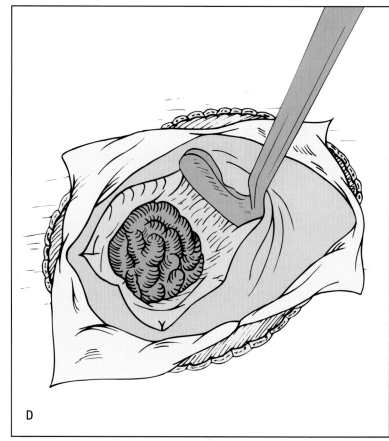

D

FIGURE 3-28.

Surgical approach for transsphenoidal microsurgical resection of pituitary tumors. **A**, A sublabial incision is made above the gingival line. **B**, The muscles of the maxilla are reflected upward and a bilateral submucosal cavity is created. The nasal septum is then partially removed and the sphenoid sinus is eventually entered with a chisel. **C**, The floor of the sella is then entered, and access to the pituitary is gained by incising the dura. **D**, A dissection plane is then developed between the tumor capsule and normal pituitary, thus facilitating removal of the adenoma. Transsphenoidal surgery is successful in up to 80% to 90% of microprolactinomas and may be used in those patients who cannot tolerate medical therapy. Operative success is considerably less with macroprolactinomas. (*Adapted from* Tew and coworkers [26]; with permission.)

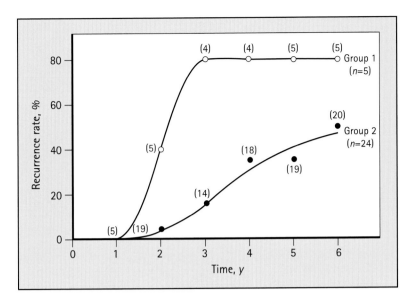

FIGURE 3–29.

Recurrence rates after transsphenoidal removal. Cumulative recurrence rates in patients with microprolactinomas (group 1) or macroprolactinomas (group 2) after initially successful surgery. Numbers in parentheses indicate the numbers of patients seen at each yearly interval. Unfortunately, recurrence rates are as high as 50% with micro- and 80% with macroprolactinomas. Complications of transsphenoidal resection include immediate surgical risks as well as acute and long-term pituitary insufficiency including rhinorrhea, diabetes insipidus, and need to give hMG to induce ovulation as well as ERT for low FSH levels. Given its significant advantages, medical therapy has largely replaced the surgical approach to prolactin-secreting pituitary tumors. (*Adapted from* Serri and coworkers [27]; with permission.)

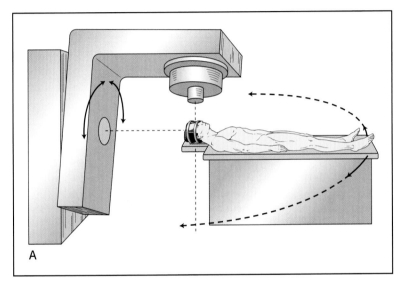

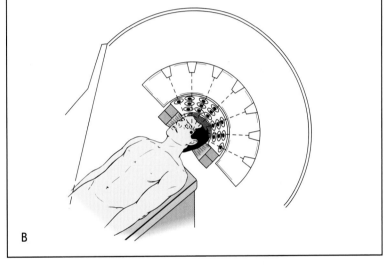

FIGURE 3–30.

Mechanical patient set-up for radiation modalities. **A**, Linear accelerator. **B**, Gamma knife. Radiation modalities have traditionally been reserved for those patients with either persistent or recurrent disease following surgery and medical therapy for those patients unable to undergo surgery or tolerate bromocriptine. Conventional radiation therapy takes 20 or more visits, and has the risks of damage to surrounding tissue, induction of secondary tumors, and resultant hypopituitarism in greater than 50% of patients. Newer forms of radiosurgery, such as the gamma knife, are performed at a single visit and provide more precise localization of photons with subsequent reduced damage to surrounding tissue and a slightly lower incidence of hypopituitarism. As experience is gained with this technique, it may provide an alternative to transsphenoidal surgery in selected patients.

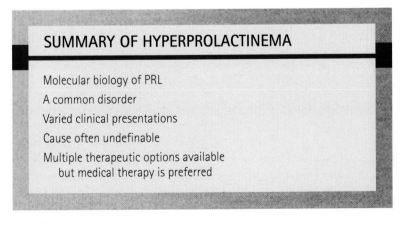

SUMMARY OF HYPERPROLACTINEMA

Molecular biology of PRL

A common disorder

Varied clinical presentations

Cause often undefinable

Multiple therapeutic options available
    but medical therapy is preferred

FIGURE 3–31.

Summary of hyperprolactinemia. Hyperprolactinemia is a common disorder with a wide variety of clinical consequences. The molecular biology of prolactin (PRL) is well understood. However, despite considerable inroads into the understanding of the physiology and endocrinology of PRL, a significant portion of the pathophysiology leading to the clinical consequences of hyperprolactinemia remains to be elucidated. Careful history, physical examination, selected laboratory testing, and radiologic imaging usually provide a clue as to the cause of hyperprolactinemia. Appropriate treatment depends on the cause of the disease and may include treatment of an underlying condition, medical therapy with dopamine agonists or exogeneous estrogen, transsphenoidal or other surgical resections, or radiation modalities. The patient's individual tolerance to therapy and its potential consequences as well as the potential consequences of untreated disease should always be considered when making the best therapeutic decision.

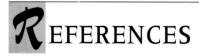

REFERENCES

1. Riddle O, Bates WR, Dykshorn WS: The preparation, identification, and assay of prolactin: a hormone of the anterior pituitary. *Am J Physiol* 1933, 105:191–216.

2. Hwang P, Guyda H, Friesen H: A radioimmunoassay for human prolactin. *Proc Natl Acad Sci U S A* 1971, 68:1902–1906.

3. Moltich ME: Prolactin. In *The Pituitary*. Edited by Melmed S. Cambridge: Blackwell Science, Inc.; 1995:136–186.

4. Truong AT, Duez C, Belayew A, Renard A: Isolation and characterization of the human prolactin gene. *EMBO J* 1984, 3:429–437.

5. Owerbach D, Rutter WJ, Cooke NE, *et al.*: The prolactin gene is located on chromosome 6 in humans. *Science* 1981, 212:815–816.

6. Prager EM, Wilson AC, Lowenstein JM, Sarich VM: Genes for growth hormone, chorionic somatomammotropin, and growth hormone-like gene on chromosome 17 in humans. *Science* 1980, 209:289–292.

7. Zacur HA, Mitch WE, Tyson JE, *et al.*: Autoregulation of rat pituitary prolactin secretion demonstrated by a new perfusion method. *Am J Physiol* 1982, 242:E226–E333.

8. Wood DF, Johnston JM, Johnston DG: Dopamine, the dopamine D2 receptor and pituitary tumors. *Clin Endocrinol* 1991, 35:455–466.

9. Sarapura V, Schlaff WD: Recent advances in the understanding of the pathophysiology and treatment of hyperprolactinemia. *Curr Opin Obstet Gynecol* 1993, 5:360–367.

10. Jacobs LS, Snyder PJ, Utiger RD, Danghaday WH: Prolactin Response to TRH. *J Clin Endocrinol Metab* 1973, 36:1069–1074.

11. Mastroianni L, Coutifaris C: Anatomy and physiology of the hypothalamus and pituitary. In *The FIGO Manual of Human Reproduction*, vol 1 (Reproductive Physiology). Edited by Rosenfield A, Fathalla MF. Park Ridge, NJ: The Parthenon Publishing Group; 1990: 11–21.

12. Rebar RW, Yen SSC: Endocrine rhythms in gonadotropins and ovarian steroids with reference to reproductive processes. In *Endocrine Rhythms*. Edited by Krieger DT. New York: Raven Press; 1979:259–298.

13. Lewis UJ, Singh RNP, Sinha YN, Vanderlaan WP: Glycosylated human prolactin. *Endocrinology* 1985, 116:359–363.

14. Rebar RW: The breast and the physiology of lactation. In *Maternal-Fetal Medicine: Principles and Practice*. Edited by Creasy RK, Resnik R. Philadelphia: WB Saunders; 1989:153–170.

15. Poindexter AN, Buttram VC, Besch P: Circulating prolactin levels: I. Normal females. *Int J Fertil* 1977, 22:1–5.

16. Kelly PA, Djiane J, Edery M: Different forms of the prolactin receptor: insights into the mechanisms of prolactin action. *Trends Endocrinol Metab* 1992, 3:54–59.

17. Molitch ME, Reichlin S: Hyperprolactinemic disorders. *Dis Mon* 1982, 28:1–58.

18. Rebar RW: Practical evaluation of hormonal status. In *Reproductive Endocrinology, Physiology, Pathophysiology, and Clinical Management*, third edition. Edited by Yen SSC, Jaffe RB. Philadelphia: WB Saunders;1991: 830–886.

19. Cook CB, Nippoldt TB, Kletter GB, *et al.*: Naloxone increases the frequency of pulsatile luteinizing hormone secretion in women with hyperprolactinemia. *J Clin Endocrinol Metab* 1991, 73:1099–1105.

20. Windgassen K, Wesselmann U, Schulze Monking H: Galactorrhea and hyperprolactinemia in schizophrenic patients on neuroleptics: frequency and etiology. *Neuropsychobiology* 1996, 33:142–146.

21. Aron DC, Tyrrell JB, Wilson CB: Pituitary tumors: current concepts in diagnosis and management. *Western J Med* 1995, 162:340–352.

22. Cann CE, Martin MC, Genant HK, Jaffe RB: Decreased spinal mineral content in amenorrheic women. *JAMA* 1984, 251:626–629.

23. Webster J, Piscitelli G, Polli A, *et al.*: A comparison of cabergoline and bromocriptine in the treatment of hyperprolactinemic amenorrhea. *N Engl J Med* 1994, 331:904–909.

24. Bevan JS, Webster J, Burke CW, Scanlon MF: Dopamine agonists and pituitary tumor shrinkage. *Endocr Rev* 1992, 13:220–240.

25. Webster J: A comparative review of the tolerability profiles of dopamine agonists in the treatment of hyperprolactinemia and inhibition of lactation. *Drug Safety* 1996, 14:228–238.

25a. Vermesh M, Fossum GT, Kletzky OA: Vaginal bromocriptine: pharmacology and effect on serum prolactin in normal women. *Obstet Gynecol* 1988, 72:693–697.

26. Tew JM, van Loveren HR, Keller JT: *Atlas of Operative Microneurosurgery*, vol 2 (Tumors). Philadelphia: WB Saunders; in press.

27. Serri O, Rasio E, Beauregard H, *et al.*: Recurrence of hyperprolactinemia after selective transsphenoidal adenomectomy in women with prolactinoma. *N Engl J Med* 1983, 309:280–283.

Hyperandrogenism

Laurence C. Udoff, Kenneth H.H. Wong, and Eli Y. Adashi

Androgen excess disorders range from the troublesome but benign problems of excess hair growth and acne to malignant ovarian tumors. The challenge in evaluating a patient with the signs and symptoms of hyperandrogenism is to determine if the androgen excess is an isolated cosmetic problem (*ie*, functional hyperandrogenism), or part of a larger syndrome, such as polycystic ovary syndrome (PCOS) or Cushing's disease. This chapter aims to help the clinician recognize the physical findings that may identify those patients in whom hyperandrogenism is part of a more serious condition. The tables and figures in this chapter were chosen to better explain basic androgen physiology as well as to review current and future treatment strategies for the hyperandrogenic patient.

NDROGEN PRODUCTION AND METABOLISM

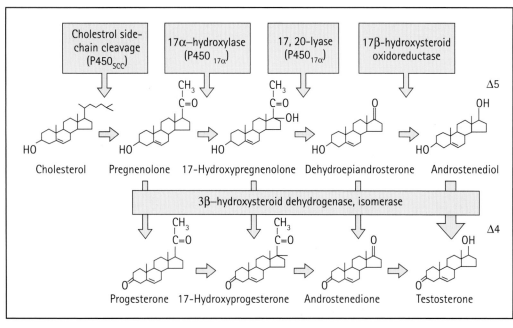

FIGURE 4–1.

Biosynthetic pathways of androgens. Androgens are classically defined as compounds that maintain male sexual behavior in castrated animals (*eg*, testosterone) or more broadly characterized as compounds that are capable of binding to an androgen receptor

and altering the expression of androgen-regulated genes (*eg*, dihydrotestosterone [DHT]). The rate-limiting step in the biosynthesis of androgens is the conversion of cholesterol (formed *de novo* or of low-density lipoprotein cholesterol origin) to pregnenolone by the side-chain cleavage, cytochrome P450. The actual rate-limiting step is the mobilization of cholesterol from intracellular lipid stores to the inner mitochondrial membrane, where the enzymatic reaction occurs. Once formed, pregnenolone crosses the mitochondrial membrane and is exposed to the steroid-metabolizing enzymes on the extramitochondrial side. Androgen biosynthesis proceeds along either one of two pathways: the $\Delta 5$ or $\Delta 4$ pathway. The two primary sites of androgen production are the ovary and the adrenal gland. Androgen synthesis in these tissues is promoted by tropic hormones, luteinizing hormone in the ovary, and adrenocorticotropin in the adrenal gland [1].

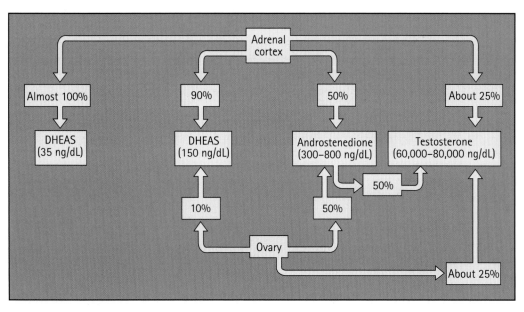

FIGURE 4–2.

Sources and rates of production of circulating androgens in premenopausal adult women. Mean circulating levels of testosterone in normal premenopausal women approximate 35 ng/dL, with a 15% to 20% increase at midcycle due to an increase in ovarian stimulation. Only a small fraction of testosterone circulates as free hormone (1%). The remaining fraction is bound either to sex hormone–binding globulin (SHBG) [69%] or albumin (30%). Testosterone is produced mainly in nonovarian sites at a rate of 0.15 to 0.25 mg/d. Fifty percent of the testosterone produced daily is derived from the conversion of androstenedione to testosterone in such peripheral sites as the liver, spleen, and adipose tissue. The

remaining portion of testosterone is directly secreted in equal amounts by the adrenal gland and the ovary.

Mean circulating levels of androstenedione in normal premenopausal women approximate 150 ng/dL, with a 15% increase at midcycle. The majority of androstenedione circulates loosely bound to albumin (85%); the remaining fractions are either bound to SHBG (8%) or circulate unbound (7%). Androstenedione is equally derived from adrenal and ovarian sources, with a total production rate of 3 mg/d. Given an ovarian production rate of 1.5 mg/d, androstenedione is the major androgen produced by the normal cycling ovary.

Considerably higher circulating levels of dihydroepiandrostenedione (DHEA) and dihydroepiandrostenedione sulfate (DHEAS) are encountered in normally cycling women (3 to 8 ng/mL and 0.5-3 µg/mL, respectively). DHEAS is produced almost exclusively by the adrenal gland at a rate of 11 mg/d. DHEA is produced at a rate of 7 mg/d, mainly derived from the adrenal gland, but also with contributions from the ovary and peripheral sources [2,3].

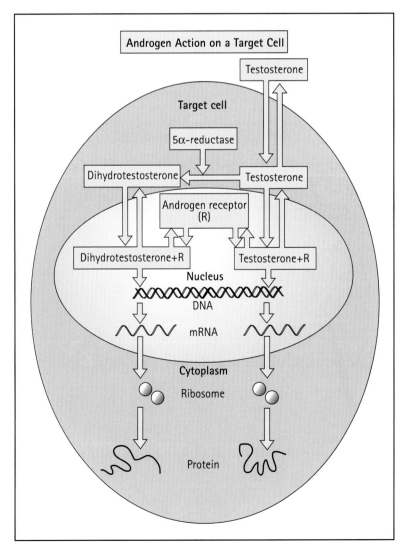

Androstenedione   5α-Androstenedione   Androsterone

Testosterone   Dihydrotestosterone   5α-androstane-3α,17β-diol

FIGURE 4-3.

Metabolism of androgens. The four major circulating androgens— testosterone, androstenedione, dihydrotestosterone (DHEA) and dihydrotestosterone sulfate (DHEAS)— are metabolized in the splanchnic tissues, with the liver being the major site, resulting in a reduction or elimination of biologic activity. These compounds (*eg*, androstenedione) are subsequently conjugated as sulfates and glucuronides and are excreted in the urine [4]. In extrasplanchnic tissues (*eg*, skin), both androstenedione and testosterone can be metabolized to more biologically active compounds, such as dihydrotestosterone and 5αandrostane-3α, 17βdiol [4]. The latter steroid is an excellent marker of peripheral androgen action in hirsute women.

NDROGEN ACTION

Androgen Action on a Target Cell

Testosterone

Target cell

5α-reductase

Dihydrotestosterone ← Testosterone

Androgen receptor (R)

Dihydrotestosterone+R   Testosterone+R

Nucleus

DNA

mRNA

Cytoplasm

Ribosome

Protein

FIGURE 4-4.

Mechanism of androgen action on a target cell. Androgens exert their effect on target cells by binding to specific intracellular receptors. Most tissues, including hair follicles and derivatives of the urogenital sinus and urogenital tubercle, require the conversion of testosterone to dihydrotestosterone for receptor activation. Tissues that favor the direct testosterone pathway are the derivatives of the wolffian duct as well as brain, breast, liver, and muscle. Once formed, the activated receptor ligand complex directly interacts with the promoter regions of the specific target gene, activating a molecular switch that initiates transcription of the downstream androgen-regulated gene. The mRNA encoded by the gene is translated into a protein product that performs some specific intracellular or extracellular function [1].

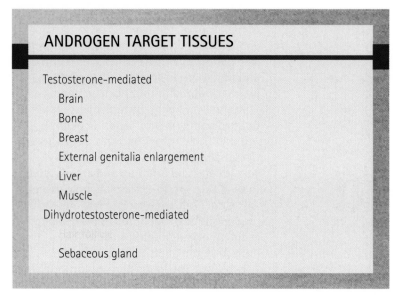

ANDROGEN TARGET TISSUES

Testosterone-mediated
    Brain
    Bone
    Breast
    External genitalia enlargement
    Liver
    Muscle
Dihydrotestosterone-mediated
    Hair follicle
    Sebaceous gland

FIGURE 4-5.

Androgen target tissues. Androgen receptors have been found in various tissues throughout the human body. The precise role that androgens play in these organ systems remains unclear. Preliminary evidence suggests that in the brain, androgens may act to maintain a normal level of sexual desire and responsiveness, and have an impact on affect and cognition. In bone, androgen receptors in osteoblasts may be important for the maintenance of normal bone mineral density. In skeletal muscle, androgens have been shown to stimulate muscle hypertrophy and improve strength. Androgens also have metabolic effects, mainly through the modulation of hepatic activity. Androgen receptors in the skin, when activated by dihydrotestosterone, cause an increase in hair follicle size and growth rate. (*Adapted from* Rittmaster [5].)

LINICAL MANIFESTATIONS OF ANDROGEN EXCESS

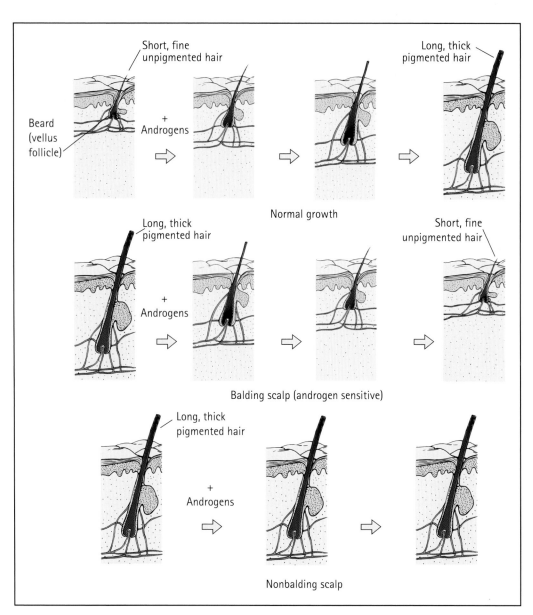

FIGURE 4-6.

Androgens and human hair growth. Current evidence suggests that normal human hair growth is mainly regulated by androgens. Androgens stimulate the gradual replacement of small, fine unpigmented hairs (vellus hairs) by longer, thicker, and more pigmented hairs (terminal hairs) (*top*). This replacement occurs during puberty in the axilla and pubic areas in both sexes, and the beard and suprapubic regions in men. On the balding scalp (*middle*), androgens may have the opposite effect, stimulating the regression of terminal hairs to vellus ones rather than maintaining stable growth (*bottom*) [6].

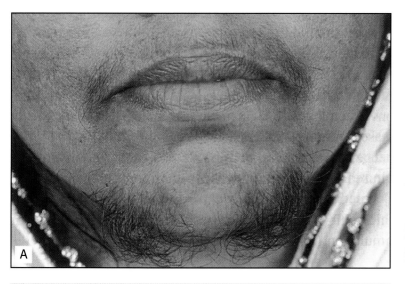

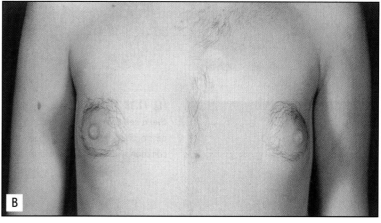

C. CHANGES IN FACIAL AND BODY HIRSUTISM SCORES WITH AGE

Age, y	Site	Score			
		0	1	2	3
15–24	Upper lip	71	19	10	
25–34		61	25	11	3
35–44		47	28	19	5
45–54		40	32	15	10
55–64		36	24	20	16
15–24	Chin	98	2		
25–34		89	5	6	
35–44		84	9	7	
45–54		85	6	6	3
55–64		66	20	10	4
15–24	Lower abdomen	72	18	7	2
25–34		79	12	3	5
35–44		77	20	2	1
45–54		91	4	2	3
55–64		94	4	2	

FIGURE 4–7.

Hirsutism. Hirsutism is defined as androgen-dependent hair growth in locations other than the pubic and axillary regions. Most commonly, this hair growth presents as androgen-dependent hair growth on the upper lip and chin [7] (**A**), around the areolae [8] (**B**), and on the lower abdomen and legs. This subjective characterization is prone to significant variability dependent mainly on patient attitudes and cultural ideals. Ferriman and Gallway attempted to more objectively define hirsutism by devising a standardized scoring system (**C**). According to this scoring system, mild hirsutism is very common and may increase with age [9]. Therefore, the term *functional hyperandrogenism* may be used if the clinical condition refers to socially defined, unwanted manifestations of androgen action that are part of normal variability in women. This condition would be in contrast to women with hirsutism in association with menstrual disturbances, infertility, androgen-secreting tumors, congenital adrenal hyperplasia, or Cushing's syndrome. These designations should in no way diminish the social and psychologic impact that functional hyperandrogenism may have for some women.

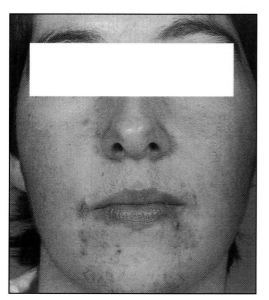

FIGURE 4–8.

Acne. Acne, as an isolated finding, may be considered as part of normal physiology that in some instances is socially unacceptable (as noted previously regarding hirsutism) [8]. Acne occurs when the sebaceous gland becomes plugged owing to an increase in production of sebum. The immune system responds to the chemical (sebum) and bacterial (*Propionibacterium acnes*) stimuli in the gland, resulting in tissue inflammation and follicular rupture [10]. Androgens (dihydrotestosterone [DHT] and testosterone) stimulate sebaceous gland cell division and sebum production; however, several clinical observations suggest that the link between hyperandrogenism and acne is more complex [9]. For example, in men, acne usually disappears after puberty despite persistent elevations in circulating androgens. Additionally, tonically high androgen levels in hyperandrogenic hirsute women often are not associated with acne. To explain these phenomena, it has been proposed that the critical event is a fluctuation in androgen levels, similar to those observed in the midluteal phase of the menstrual cycle when many women will note the development of mild acne. It is important to remember that when acne is found in the presence of hirsutism or other masculinizing features, it may be a sign of a significant medical condition, because acne is associated with androgen excess in approximately 80% of such cases [10].

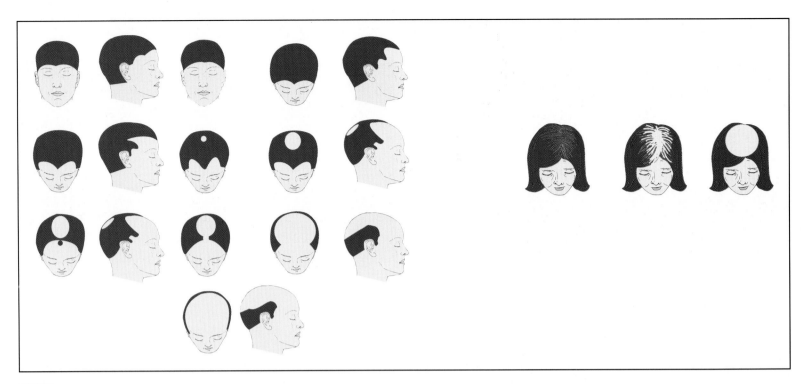

FIGURE 4-9.

Androgenic alopecia. Several patterns of scalp balding have been classically described. The classic pattern in men was described 1951 [7a] (*left*). In 1977, Ludwig noted that women appeared to bald in a different pattern: a diffuse loss over the scalp and preservation of the anterior hair line (*right*) [7b,11]. Further study has revealed that men and women may develop either pattern, with 13% of menopausal women in one series exhibiting signs of frontotemporal recession [12].

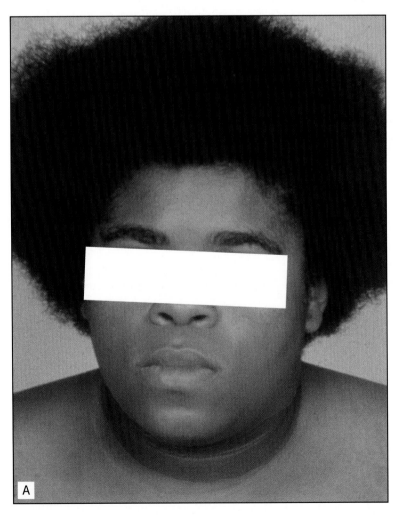

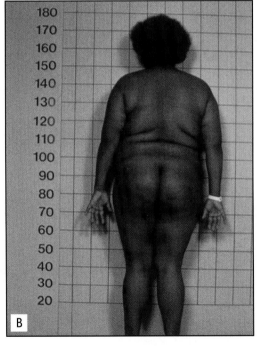

FIGURE 4-10.

Acanthosis nigricans. Hyperandrogenism may be associated with obesity and polycystic ovary syndrome (PCOS—defined as chronic anovulation and hyperandrogenism). Acanthosis nigricans is a common dermatologic condition found in patients with PCOS and obesity. It is characterized by thickened, hyperpigmented skin, usually found in the skin folds of the neck and axillae (**A** and **B**). Histologic features include papillomatosis, hyperkeratosis, and hyperpigmentation. It is considered a cutaneous marker for insulin resistance, also a common finding in PCOS. Acanthosis nigricans may also be associated with one of the severe insulin-resistant hyperandrogenic syndromes [13].

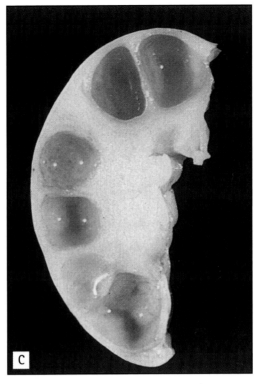

A. CLASSIFICATION OF INSULIN-RESISTANT SYNDROMES ASSOCIATED WITH OVARIAN HYPERANDROGENISM AND DYSFUNCTION

Syndromes of severe insulin resistance
    Congenital-hereditary
        Type A syndrome–HAIRAN syndrome
        Leprechaunism
    Rabson-Mendenhall syndrome
    Congenital lipodystrophies
Acquired
    Possibly HAIRAN syndrome
    Type B syndrome
    Acquired lipodystrophies
States of mild to moderate insulin resistance
    "Typical" PCOS
    Obesity

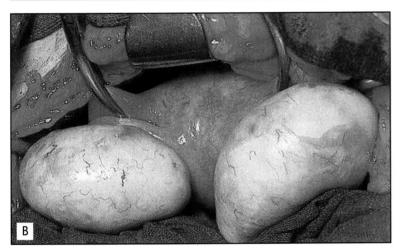

FIGURE 4-11.

Classification of insulin-resistant syndromes associated with ovarian hyperandrogenism and dysfunction. Hyperandrogenism may be part of the constellation of symptoms found in patients with polycystic ovary syndrome (PCOS) (**A**). PCOS is characterized by hyperandrogenism of mostly ovarian origin, with the role of the adrenal gland only recently gaining attention. Classically, patients are anovulatory with enlarged ovaries (**B**) that contain multiple small cortical cysts [8] (**C**).

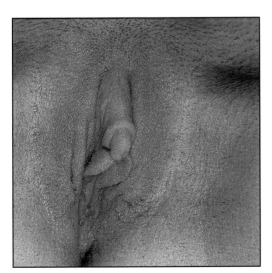

FIGURE 4-12.

Virilization. Clitoromegaly (defined as increased diameter of clitoris to ≥ 8 mm), along with deepening of the voice, breast atrophy, increased muscle mass, central obesity, severe hirsutism, balding, enhanced libido, and amenorrhea may indicate the presence of a masculinizing syndrome (*ie*, virilization). If the symptoms rapidly progress, immediate evaluation is advised because a virilizing tumor of the ovary or adrenal gland may be present. Other causes include ovarian hyperthecosis or drug-induced virilization.

EVALUATION OF HYPERANDROGENIC DISORDERS

DIFFERENTIAL DIAGNOSIS OF ANDROGEN DISORDERS

Adrenal

Adrenal androgen-producing tumors (adenomas, carcinomas)

Congenital adrenal hyperplasia (21-hydroxylase, 11β-hydroxylase, 3β-hydroxysteroid dehydrogenase)

Adrenal hyperplasia assoicated with ovarian disorders

Cushing's syndrome (corticotropin dependent)

  Pituitary corticotropin excess: Nontumor and tumor

  Ecotopic corticotropin-secreting tumors

  Ecotopic corticotropin-releasing factor–producing tumors

Cushing's syndrome (corticotropin-independent)

  Adrenal adenoma

  Adrenal carcinoma

  Adrenal nodular hyperplasia

  Adrenal rest tumor of the ovary

  Exogenous corticoid administration

  Exogenous androgen exposure

Hyperprolactinemia

Hyperthyroidism

Hypothyroidism

Ovary

  Tumors: Sertoli-Leydig, hilus cell, thecoma, luteoma

  Androgen overproduction by follicles (mainly theca)

  Androgen overproduction by activated stroma (stromal thecosis)

Peripheral tissues

  Excess 5α-reductase or 17-ketosteroid reductase

FIGURE 4–13.

Differential diagnosis of androgen disorders. The evaluation of hyperandrogenic disorders begins with a thorough history and physical examination. The goal is to narrow the differential diagnosis [11]. The onset, severity, and rate of progression of symptoms need to be carefully documented. Specific questions should be asked regarding menstrual cyclicity and fertility, the presence of cutaneous manifestations of androgen excess (*eg*, hirsutism, acne, balding), and symptoms associated with severe hyperandrogenism, such as deepening of the voice and changes in libido. The family history needs to be explored for the presence of other family members with similar conditions or diabetes. The physical examination should note the amount and distribution of excess hair growth as well as documenting the other clinical manifestations that could be present, as previously described.

HORMONAL EVALUATION OF HYPERANDROGENISM

Feature evaluated	Findings
Ovulatory menses	Routine hormonal evaluation normal
Oligomenorrhea, mild to severe hirsutism	
Testosterone, ng/kL	<50: PCOS unlikely
	50–200: PCOS likely
	>200 or 2.5× normal: rule out androgen-secreting ovarian tumor by US, CT, or MRI
17-hydroxyprogesterone, ng/dL	>200: rule out CAH (ACTH stimulation test)
DHEAS, μg/dL	>700: adrenal hyperfunction, rule out adrenal tumor, CAH
24-hour urinary free cortisol, μg	>90: possible cushing's syndrome
Dexamethasone (1 mg) suppression test, μg/dL	<5: Cushing's very unlikely
	5–10: Cushing's unlikely
	>10: consistent with Cushing's
Prolactin, μg/mL	<30: consistent with PCOS
	>50: suspicious for prolactinoma
LH and FSH	↑LH, normal FSH: consistent with PCOS
	Normal LH, FSH: nondiagnostic
	↑LH, ↑FSH: consistent with ovarian failure
	↓LH, ↓FSH: consistent with hypothalamic amenorrhea
TSH	↑consistent with hypothyroidism

FIGURE 4–14.

Hormonal evaluation of hyperandrogenism. Laboratory tests should be ordered to evaluate the patient for serious underlying disorders suggested by the history and physical examination. If the patient has only mild to moderate hirsutism, without any other physical manifestations and has normal menstrual cycles and fertility, then no hormonal evaluation is generally necessary. These patients are thought to have functional hyperandrogenism (defined as unwanted manifestations of androgen action that are part of normal variability in women), regardless of whether mild elevations in serum androgens are present. When hirsutism and other clinical manifestations are noted (*eg*, menstrual cycle abnormalities), an initial laboratory assessment should include serum determinations for testosterone, 17-hydroxyprogesterone, and dihydrotestosterone (DHEAS). Patients with menstrual cycle disturbances should also be evaluated for abnormalities in prolactin, thyroid, and gonadotropin hormone secretion. These tests will screen for serious underlying conditions such as polycystic ovary syndrome (PCOS), hypothyroidism, adrenal or ovarian tumors, congenital adrenal hyperplasia, and prolactinomas. Additional tests may be appropriate depending on the clinical suspicion aroused by the history and physical examination. For instance, in a patient with physical findings suggestive of Cushing's syndrome, a 24-hour free urinary cortisol or a dexamethasone suppression test should be obtained. Likewise, in a patient with a pelvic or abdominal mass, or if the symptoms are severe and of rapid onset and progression, a more intensified search for an androgen-secreting tumor is warranted. In general, laboratory assessment of metabolic function (*eg*, fasting glucose, insulin levels, glucose tolerance testing, lipids, growth hormone or insulin-like growth factor levels) are not routinely useful in the evaluation of hyperandrogenism unless it is part of a larger suspected syndrome such as PCOS, acromegaly, or one of the severe insulin-resistance syndromes. CAH—congenital adrenal hyperplasia; CT—computed tomography; FSH—follicle-stimulating hormone; LH—luteinizing hormone; MRI—magnetic resonance imaging; US—ultrasound.

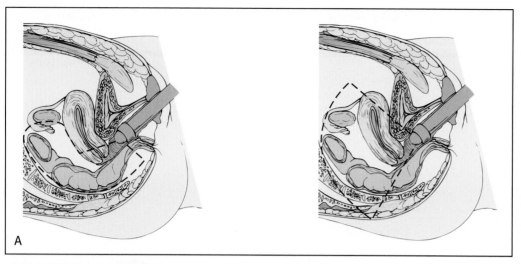
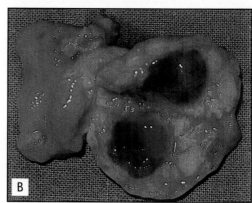
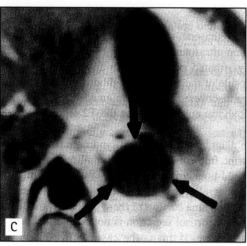
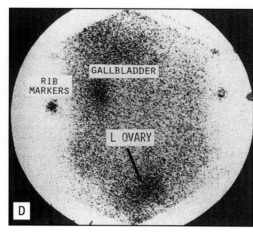

FIGURE 4–15.

Diagnostic imaging in patients with hyperandrogenism. When the history, physical examination, or laboratory testing suggests the possibility of an androgen-producing tumor, various diagnostic imaging modalities may be used. Transvaginal ultrasound (**A**) [14] should identify 90% of all virilizing ovarian tumors (**B**)[8]. Lesions as small as 0.5 cm can be detected. Color Doppler imaging of blood flow patterns may also aid in tumor detection. **C** and **D**, Other imaging techniques include computed tomography (CT) and magnetic resonance imaging (MRI), which also allow for evaluation of the adrenal glands for the presence of an androgen-producing tumor (*eg*, adrenocortical adenoma) [15] . Last, [131]iodomethyl-norcholesterol (NP-59) scintigraphy may provide functional information about a tumor based on preferential incorporation of NP-59 into androgen-producing tumor tissue, in the setting of induced adrenal and thyroid suppression [16].

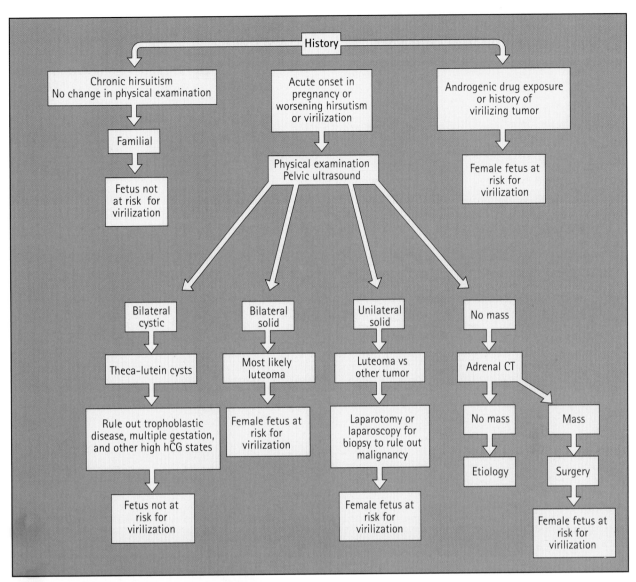

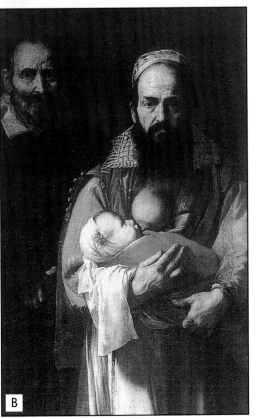

B

FIGURE 4–16.

Gestational hyperandrogenism.(**A**), Importance of history taking in diagnosis of iatrogenic androgen excess in women. Diagnosing drug-induced hyperandrogenism relies mainly on the history of the use of one of the above medications [18]. This history may be difficult to obtain, especially in patients ingesting anabolic-androgenic steroids for sports and fitness, who may want to conceal their drug use. A minimal hormonal evaluation is still suggested because other causes of hyperandrogenism, such as polycystic ovary syndrome, could be present, with symptoms becoming exacerbated by the drug use. CT—computed tomography; hCG—human chorionic gonadotropin.

Gestational hyperandrogenism (acute onset of hyperandrogenism in pregnancy) represents a special case of hyperandrogenism [17] (**B**). It is most often associated with luteomas or theca-lutein cysts. Theca-lutein cysts are almost always bilateral and regress during the postpartum period. They are not associated with fetal masculinization. Luteomas are solid tumors that occur bilaterally in almost 50% of cases. They also regress postpartum, but in instances in which maternal masculinization is present, a female fetus has a 79% risk of virilization. Unilateral ovarian lesions should be presumed malignant until proven otherwise. Almost all of the reported cases of gestational hyperandrogenism have been secondary to an ovarian lesion or drug-related effect.

DRUGS THAT INDUCE IATROGENIC ANDROGEN EXCESS IN WOMEN

Adrogenic anabolic steroids
  Parental preparations
    Testosterone
    Testosterone propionate
    Testosterone enanthate
    Testosterone cypionate
    Nandrolone decanoate
    Nandrolone phenpropionate
    Methanolone enanthate
    Dimeric testosterone
    19-Nortestosterone
  Oral preparations
    Methyltestosterone
    Fluoxymesterone
    Oxymesterone
    Methandostenolone
    Oxymetholone
    Danazol
    Stanozolol
    Oxandrolone
    Ethylestrenol
    Norethandrolone
    Mesterolone
    Methenolone acetate
    Testosterone undecanoate

Synthetic progestin
  Norethisterone
  Norethisterone acetate
  Norgestrel, levonorgestrel
  Ethynodiol diacetate
  Equingestanolol acetate
  Medroxyprogesterone acetate
Antiepileptic drugs
  Phenytoin
  Phenobarbital
  Valproate
Phenothiazines
Corticotropin or ACTH analogue
Metyrapone

FIGURE 4-17

Drugs causing androgen excess. To be complete, evaluation for the presence of an adrenal tumor could be considered, but this is highly unlikely to be the cause. ACTH—adrenocorticotropin. ACTH—adrenocorticotropin.

𝒯 REATMENT

MEDICAL TREATMENT OF HIRSUTISM

Ovarian suppression
  Oral contraceptives with minimal endroenicity
  GnRH analogues
Adrenal suppression
  Glucocorticoids
Antiandrogens
  Spironolactone
  Cyproterone acetate
  Flutamide
  Finasteride

FIGURE 4-18.

Medical options for hirsutism. These options are available for patients with androgen excess characterized mainly by hirsutism [9], with cosmetic results being the main goal of therapy. Hyperandrogenism in association with a serious underlying disorder is treated according to the therapies of choice for that condition. For example, hyperandrogenism cause by an androgen-producing tumor is treated by the surgical removal of the tumor. Likewise, hyperandrogenism caused by congenital adrenal hyperplasia is treated by glucocorticoid replacement. Treatment options for patients with hyperandrogenism and polycystic ovarian disease are discussed elsewhere. When cosmetic improvement is the endpoint of therapy, it must be clearly explained that hirsutism itself is not a disease, and the benefits and risks of any potential treatment must be weighed carefully. Hirsutism is also a chronic disorder that is unlikely to be cured. Treatment regimens may require 6 to 9 months before a response is seen. The rationales for drug treatment include reducing ovarian androgen synthesis, inhibiting adrenal androgen production, and blocking peripheral androgen action. These regimens are also often combined with mechanical methods of hair removal, such as electrolysis. GnRH—gonadotropin-releasing hormone.

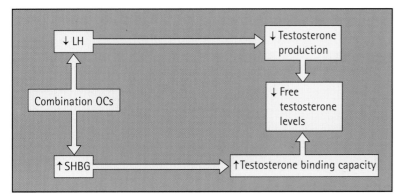

FIGURE 4-19

Rationale for the treatment of hirsutism with oral contraceptives (OCs). OCs have classically been first-line treatment for hyperandrogenism. OCs inhibit gonadotropin secretion and result in a rapid suppression of luteinizing hormone (LH)-dependent hyperandrogenemia [2]. Additionally, the estrogenic component of OCs increase sex-hormone—binding globulin (SHBG) levels, which decreases the amount of bioavailable androgen [2]. Although well-controlled clinical trials have yet to be performed, it is thought that a more estrogenic OC preparation combined with less androgenic progestins may be more effective in controlling hirsutism. The success rate of treating hirsutism with OCs alone is modest. Some reports have shown only 10% of patients with improvement and 50% noting stabilization of symptoms [9].

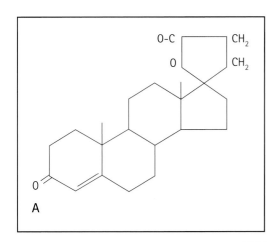

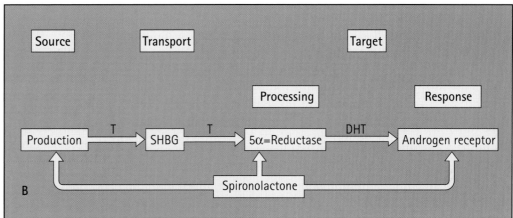

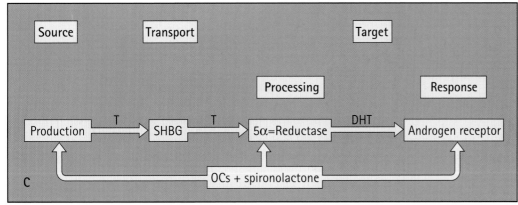

FIGURE 4-20.

Spironolactone as a treatment option for hirsutism. Antiandrogens are another therapeutic option for patients with hyperandrogenism. One drug in this class that is commonly used in North America is spironolactone. Spironolactone (**A**) is an aldosterone antagonist that binds competitively to the androgen receptor with an affinity of 67% compared with dihydrotestosterone (DHT). It is also a weak inhibitor of testosterone synthesis and an inhibitor of 5-α reductase (**B**). The major side effects of treatment include abnormal uterine bleeding, diuresis (although this is limited to the first few days), nausea, fatigue, and possibly headaches at higher doses. Effective contraception during treatment is recommended to avoid possible teratogenic effects. Spironolactone at a dose of 100 mg/d has been shown to decrease the Ferriman-Gallway score by 47% after 1 year [19]. Spironolactone is often combined with oral contraceptives (OCs) to provide peripheral tissue effects to complement the central suppression of androgen production provided for by the OCs and avoid abnormal uterine bleeding (**C**). The progestin compound cyproterone acetate, another potent antiandrogen, is not available in the United States. It has a similar mode of action by blocking the androgen receptor and decreasing ovarian androgen production as well as decreasing to some extent adrenal androgen synthesis. It is also thought to increase testosterone clearance.

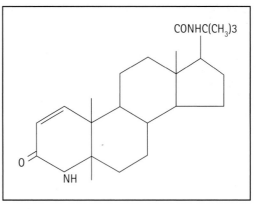

FIGURE 4-21.

Chemical structure of flutamide. Another option for the treatment of hirsutism is flutamide [20]. Flutamide is a nonsteroidal antiandrogen that inhibits the nuclear binding of androgens in target tissues. The absence of changes in circulating androgen levels and the finding of elevations in testosterone levels in patients during flutamide treatment suggest that the mode of action is purely through binding to androgen receptors. The recommended therapeutic dose range is 250 to 500 mg/d. A recent study favored the lower dose because of similar effectiveness, less cost, and the reports of a 0.36% incidence of fatal or nonfatal hepatotoxicity associated with the higher dose [21]. At present, flutamide is mainly used by patients in whom spironolactone is not tolerated, because there has been more clinical experience with spironolactone, and it is less expensive and less toxic.

FIGURE 4-22.

Chemical structure of finasteride. Finasteride is the first of a new class of drugs that selectively inhibit 5-α reductase activity [20]. This inhibition results in the selective blockade of dihydrotestosterone production, peripherally decreasing the amount of hormone available for binding to the peripheral androgen receptor. Few data have been accumulated to document the effectiveness of this treatment. One of the more recent studies recorded a 15% decline in Ferriman-Gallway scores after 9 months of treatment [22]. Therapy has been associated with few if any side effects, but may be less effective than spironolactone [22].

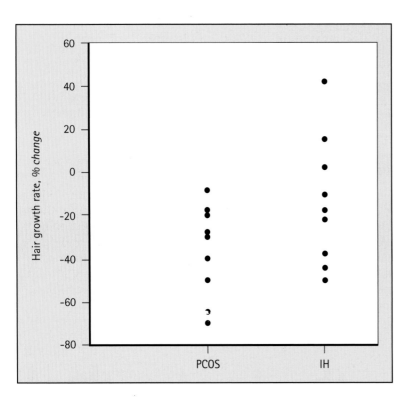

FIGURE 4-23.

Changes in hair growth rates when GrRMa alone was given to women with PCOS and women with idiopathic hirsuitism (IM). Gonadotropin-releasing hormone receptor (GnRH) agonists as a treatment option for hirsutism. GnRH analogues suppress follicle-stimulating hormone and luteinizing hormone secretion via downregulation of the GnRH receptor. As expected by this mechanism of action, women whose hirsutism is mainly caused by ovarian overproduction of androgens will experience the greatest decrease in hair growth (*eg*, polycystic ovary syndrome versus idiopathic hirsutism) [9]. Because estrogen production is also decreased, side effects related to estrogen deficiency will develop including bone loss and hot flashes. These side effects may be controlled by estrogen (and progestin if the patient has a uterus *in situ*) replacement therapy [23,24]. Because of the complexity of this therapeutic option and high cost, this treatment is usually reserved for severe cases not responsive to other measures.

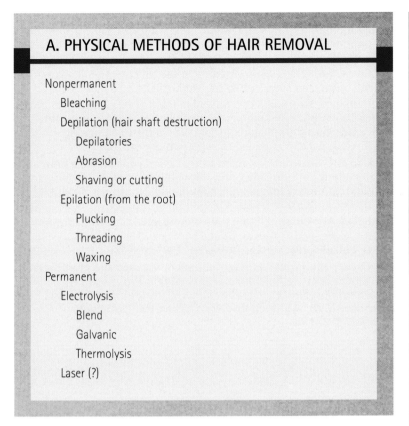

A. PHYSICAL METHODS OF HAIR REMOVAL

Nonpermanent
    Bleaching
    Depilation (hair shaft destruction)
        Depilatories
        Abrasion
        Shaving or cutting
    Epilation (from the root)
        Plucking
        Threading
        Waxing
Permanent
    Electrolysis
        Blend
        Galvanic
        Thermolysis
    Laser (?)

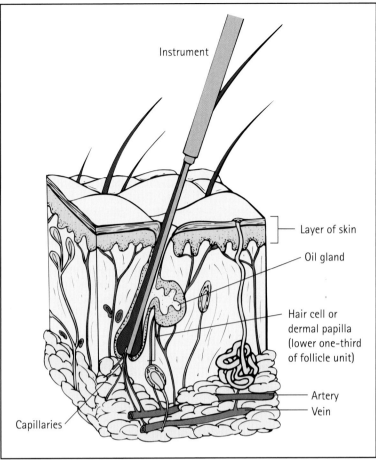

FIGURE 4-24.

Physical methods of hair removal. **A,** Physical methods of hair removal [25] may be the sole treatment for some women or may be combined with various medical therapies as described earlier. Combining physical methods such as electrolysis [25] with hormonal treatment is not recommended until hormonal suppression has been used for at least 6 months, at which point an effect should be noticeable. Although medical treatment may prevent new hair follicles from being stimulated to grow, hair growth that has been previously established will not completely disappear with hormone treatment alone. **B,** Permanent removal of hair can be accomplished only by the electrocoagulation of dermal papillae [26].

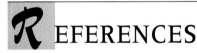 EFERENCES

1. Griffin JE, Wilson JD: The testis. In *Clinical Endocrinology*. Edited by Besser GM, Thorner MO. London: Times Mirror; 1994:11.0–11.26.

2. Speroff L, Glass RH, Kase NG: Hirsutism. In *Clinical Gynecologic Endocrinology and Infertility*. Edited by Mitchell C. Baltimore:Williams & Wilkins;1994: 483–513.

3. Udoff LC, Adashi EY: Androgens, the other class of female hormones. *Postgrad Med* 1996:5–9.

4. Stanczyk FZ: Steroid hormones. In *Infertility, Contraception and Reproductive Endocrinology*. Edited by Mishell DR, Davajan V, Lobo RA. Boston: Blackwell Scientific Publications;1991:53–76.

5. Rittmaster RS. Peripheral actions of androgens. In *Androgen Excess Disorders in Women*. Edited by Azziz R, Nestler JE, Dewailly D. Philadelphia: Lippincott-Raven;1997:63–73.

6. Randall VA. The role of androgens in the regulation of the human hair follicle. In *Androgen Excess Disorders in Women*. Edited by Azziz R, Nestler JE, Dewailly D. Philadelphia: Lippincott-Raven; 1997:115–131.

7. Barth JH. The life-cycle of hair: normal and abnormal growth patterns. In *Reproductive Endocrinology, Surgery and Technology*. Edited by Adashi EY, Rock JA, Rosenwacks Z. Philadelphia: Lippincott-Raven; 1996:1490–1499.

7a.Hamilton JB: Patterned loss of hair in man: types and incidence. *Ann Ny Acad Sci* 1951,53:718-728.

7b.Ludwig E: Classification of the types of androgenetic alopecia (common baldness) occuring in the female sex. *Br J Dermatol* 1977,97:247-254.

8. Adashi EY. The ovary. In *Clinical Endocrinology*. Edited by Besser GM, Thorner MO. London: Times Mirror; 1994:12.0–12.18.

9. Rittmaster RS: Functional hyperandrogenism. In *Reproductive Endocrinology, Surgery and Technology*. Edited by Adashi EY, Rock JA, Rosenwacks Z. Philadelphia: Lippincott-Raven; 1996:1502–1520.

10. Slayden SM, Azziz R: The role of androgen excess in acne. In *Androgen Excess Disorders in Women*. Edited by Azziz R, Nestler JE, Dewailly D. Philadelphia: Lippincott-Raven; 1997:131–140.

11. Wild RA: Hyperandrogenism: implications for cardiovascular, endometrial and breast disease. In *Reproductive Endocrinology, Surgery and Technology*. Edited by Adashi EY, Rock JA, Rosenwacks Z. Philadelphia: Lippincott-Raven; 1996:1618–1634.

12. Greenblatt RB. Hirsutism: ancestral curse or endocrinopathy. In *The Cause and Management of Hirsutism: A Practical Approach to the Control of Unwanted Hair*. Edited by Greenblatt RB, Mahesh VB, Gambrell RD. New Jersey: The Parthenon;1987:17–29.

13. Vidal-Puig A, Moller DE: Classification, prevalance, clinical manifestations, and diagnosis. In *Androgen Excess Disorders in Women*. Edited by Azziz R, Nestler JE, Dewailly D. Philadelphia: Lippincott-Raven; 1997:227–236.

14. Collins JA: Critical technology assessment. In *Reproductive Endocrinology, Surgery and Technology*. Edited by Adashi EY, Rock JA, Rosenwacks Z. Philadelphia: Lippincott-Raven; 1996:1618–1634.

15. Mastorakos G, Chrousos GP: Adrenal hyperandrogenism. In *Reproductive Endocrinology, Surgery and Technology*. Edited by Adashi EY, Rock JA, Rosenwacks Z. Philadelphia: Lippincott-Raven; 1996:1539–1555.

16. Wong IL, Lobo RA: Ovarian androgen-producing tumors. In *Reproductive Endocrinology, Surgery and Technology*. Edited by Adashi EY, Rock JA, Rosenwacks Z. Philadelphia: Lippincott-Raven; 1996:1571–1598.

17. McClamrock HD, Adashi EY: Gestational hyperandrogenism. In *Reproductive Endocrinology, Surgery and Technology*. Edited by Adashi EY, Rock JA, Rosenwacks Z. Philadelphia: Lippincott-Raven; 1996:1599–1616.

18. Cortet-Rudelli, Desailloud R, Dewailly D: Drug-induced androgen excess. In *Androgen Excess Disorders in Women*. Edited by Azziz R, Nestler JE, Dewailly D. Philadelphia: Lippincott-Raven; 1997:613–624.

19. Carmina E, Lobo RA: Peripheral androgen blockade versus glandular androgen suppression in the treatment of hirsutism. *Obstet Gynecol* 1991, 78:845–849.

20. Fruzetti F: Treatment of hirsutism: antiandrogen and 5α-reductase inhibitor therapy. In *Androgen Excess Disorders in Women*. Edited by Azziz R, Nestler JE, Dewailly D. Philadelphia: Lippincott-Raven; 1997:787–798.

21. Muderris IL, Bayram F, Sahin Y, Kelestimar F: A comparison between two doses of flutamide (250 mg/d and 500 mg/d) in the treatment of hirsutism. *Fertil Steril* 1997, 68:644–647.

22. Erenus M, Yucelten D, Durmusoglu F, Gurbuz O: Comparison of finesteride versus spironolactone in the treatment of idiopathic hirsutism. *Fertil Steril* 1997, 68:1000–1003.

23. Heiner JS, Greendale GA, Kawakami AK, *et al.*: Comparison of a gonadotropin-releasing hormone agonist and a low dose oral contraceptive given alone or together in the treatment of hirsutism. *J Clin Endocrinol Metab* 1996, 81:646–651.

24. Carr BR, Breslau NA, Givens C, *et al.*: Oral contraceptive pills, gonadotropin-releasing hormone agonists, or use in combination for treatment of hirsutism: a clinical research center study. *J Clin Endocrinol Metab* 1995, 80:1169–1178.

25. Lucky AW: Physical treatments of unwanted hair. In *Androgen Excess Disorders in Women*. Edited by Azziz R, Nestler JE, Dewailly D. Philadelphia: Lippincott-Raven; 1997:779–786.

26. Fischer KH, Hyatt AL: The anatomy of the skin and physiology of hair growth. In *The Cause and Management of Hirsutism: A Practical Approach to the Control of Unwanted Hair*. Edited by Greenblatt RB, Mahesh VB, Gambrell RD. New Jersey: The Parthenon; 1987:175–198.

Polycystic Ovary Syndrome

Howard S. Jacobs

Polycystic ovary syndrome (PCOS) is the most common cause of a disturbance of the reproductive system in women. Recent advances in ultrasonography have made it possible to detect polycystic ovaries in the ambulent subject. Moreover, by using vaginal probes together with pulsed and color Doppler and computerized reconstruction of the ovary, it is now possible to delineate the morphologic features of the polycystic ovary with some precision. We now recognize the polycystic ovary as one that is usually enlarged by a vascular stroma. The "cysts" are, in fact, usually small- to intermediate-sized follicles that contain oocytes and granulosa cells and can mature in response to ovarian stimulation.

Polycystic ovary syndrome is the association of polycysytic ovaries with specific symptomatology, such as a menstrual disturbance or the consequences of hyperandrogenism. We now know that the syndrome is heterogeneous, with at least two broad sub-groups. One sub-group comprises slim women with regular menstrual cycles, who hypersecrete luteinizing hormone (LH) and who have imparied fertility and a high rate of miscarriage. The other sub-group comprises hyperinsulinemic women with oligomenorrhea and hyperandrogenism. Women in this second group are often obese. Many patients present clinically with symptoms that indicate some overlap between these two forms. It is likely that the heterogeneity of PCOS also embraces other clinical presentations (*eg,* cases associated with congenital adrenal hyperplasia, Cushing's disease, acromegaly). Currently, however, the major factor that we believe leads to clinical expression of PCOS is hypersecretion of insulin. This observation has important implications for our understanding and for management of women with PCOS.

ULTRASOUND FEATURES OF THE POLYCYSTIC OVARY

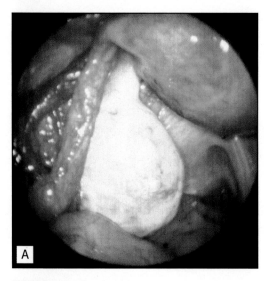

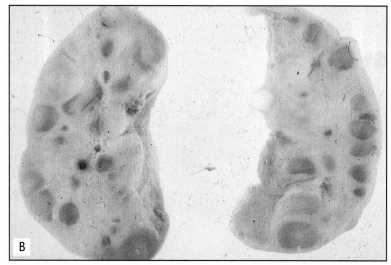

FIGURE 5-1.

Polycystic ovary. **A**, Laparoscopic view. The ovary is larger than normal with a white, thickened capsule. A cyst can be seen on the anterior surface. **B**, Hemisected surgical specimen. The hypercellular medulla can be seen, together with multiple cysts between 2 and 8 mm in diameter. The cysts are arranged in a subcapsular distribution, but are also present throughout the stroma of the ovary.

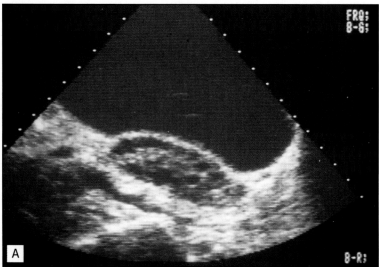

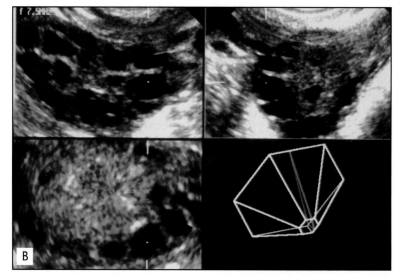

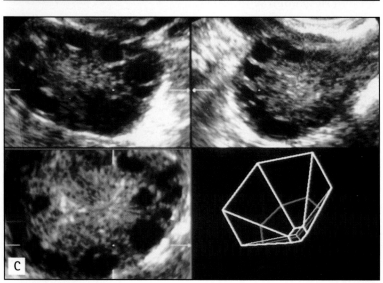

FIGURE 5-2.

Ultrasound images of a polycystic ovary. **A**, Transabdominal ultrasound scan. Note the diagonal electronic calipers. The ovary is larger than normal, the cysts are arranged around the periphery, and the characteristic echodense central stroma readily can be seen. Cysts within the stroma are also discernible. **B**, Transvaginal ultrasound scan. The Combison 530 system (Kretztechnik AG, Zipf, Austria) can create a computerized three-dimensional reconstruction of the ultrasound image. With this technique, the splay of ultrasound from the tip of the probe can be seen in the bottom right-hand panel. The "virtual" plane that has been selected by the operator is colored green. The image reconstructed in that plane is shown within the green box. This technique demonstrates the echodense stroma (*bottom left image*) and the cysts, as seen in the two other images. **C**, Another ultrasound image obtained with the same equipment, but this time the virtual plane selected for analysis is quite different. The polycystic ovary appears to be larger than normal, with an echodense central stroma and the characteristic distribution of cysts and follicles.

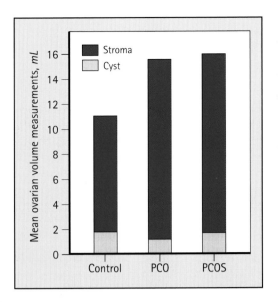

FIGURE 5-3.

Mean ovarian volume measurements. Using the three-dimensional ultrasound technique, it is possible to make accurate measurements of cyst and total ovarian volume and thus derive stromal volume. The increased volume of the polycystic ovary, both in women with asymptomatic polycystic ovaries (PCO) and symptomatic polycystic ovary syndrome (PCOS), is caused by an increase in stromal volume. The volume of the cysts does not vary among the three groups [1].

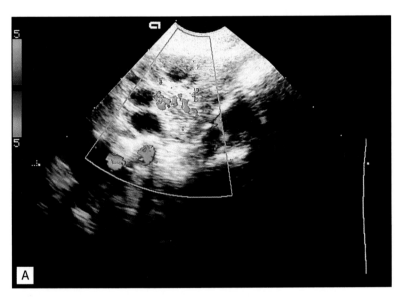

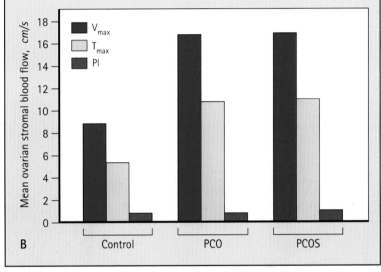

FIGURE 5-4.

Doppler ultrasound studies of vascularity in the polycystic ovary. **A**, Color Doppler ultrasound image of a polycystic ovary. Considerable color, indicating active blood flow, is seen in the stroma, well away from the blood flow that occurs around cysts and follicles. **B**, Ovarian stromal blood flow, whether measured as the maximum velocity (V_{max}) or the timed maximum velocity (T_{max}), is increased in the stroma of polycystic ovaries [2]. There is, however, no detectable difference between control and polycystic ovaries (PCO) in the pulsatility index (PI), *ie*, in resistance to blood flow. These Doppler ultrasound studies indicate that the stroma of the polycystic ovary is highly vascular. This vascularity may be related to the excess vascular endothelial growth factor that has been found in the stroma of PCO (see Figure 5-23). PCOS—polycystic ovary syndrome.

PREVALENCE OF ULTRASOUND FINDINGS OF POLYCYSTIC OVARIES

	Prevalence, *n(%)*
Normal controls	257 (23)
Amenorrhea	73 (26)
Oligomenorrhea	75 (87)
Hirsutism	25 (92)

FIGURE 5-5.

The prevalence of polycystic ovaries, as detected by transabdominal ultrasonography, in normal volunteers and in women with amenorrhea, oligomenorrhea, and hirsutism [3]. Although the high prevalence in women with menstrual disturbances and hirsutism is perhaps expected, note particularly the high prevalence of polycystic ovaries in normal volunteers. Numerous studies have confirmed this important finding—that one fifth of otherwise normal women have the ultrasound findings of polycystic ovaries.

CLINICAL FEATURES

CLINICAL FEATURES OF 1557 PATIENTS WITH POLYCYSTIC OVARY SYNDROME

	Percent
Hirsutism	63.9
Acne	31.6
Acanthosis nigricans	3.6
Infertility	24.8
Menstrual cycle	
Regular	25.0
Oligomenorrhea	51.5
Amenorrhea	21.8
Polymenorrhea	3.0

FIGURE 5-6.

Clinical features of 1557 patients with polycystic ovary syndrome (PCOS) seen at The Middlesex Hospital [4]. The diagnosis was made by ultrasound identification of polycystic ovaries in appropriately symptomatic patients. The particular distribution of symptoms seen in this group of patients no doubt reflects referral bias, because these patients were all seen in a reproductive endocrine rather than a gynecology clinic. Had the information been collected from patients referred to gynecologists, no doubt the prevalence of infertility as a presenting complaint would have been greater. Note that 25% of these women with PCOS had a regular menstrual cycle.

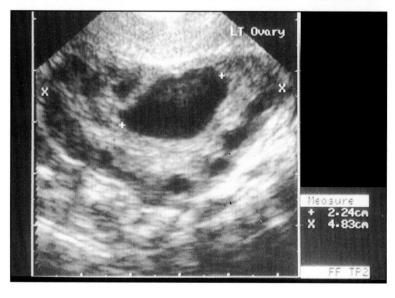

FIGURE 5-7.

Ultrasound image of a dominant follicle in a patient with polycystic ovary syndrome. This woman was complaining of hirsutism but had a regular ovulatory menstual cycle. Note the echodense stroma surrounding the dominant follicle and the failure of the dominant follicle to suppress the cohort of follicles around the periphery. Note the ease with which polycystic ovaries can be identified in the ovulatory woman.

HYPERINSULINISM

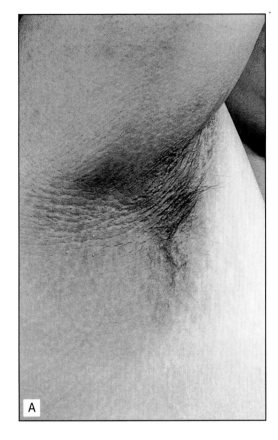

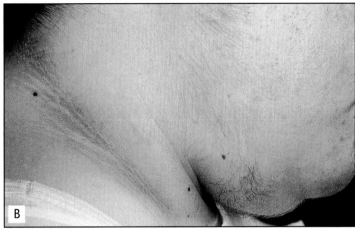

FIGURE 5–8.

Acanthosis nigricans. **A**, One of the first clues to the occurrence of hyperinsulinism and insulin resistance in women with polycystic ovary syndrome (PCOS) was the finding of acanthosis nigricans in young women with PCOS. This image shows the changes of acanthosis nigricans in the axilla. **B**, Acanthosis nigricans around the neck of a young woman whose hirsutism is evident on her face.

In acanthhosis nigricans, the skin is raised, of velvety appearance and feel, and is hyperpigmented. It is thought to represent the response to excessive exposure of the dermis to insulin [5]. We found acanthosis nigricans in 3.5% of our patients (see Fig. 5-6), but microscopic studies indicate that the histological changes associated with this clinical sign are seen much more commonly.

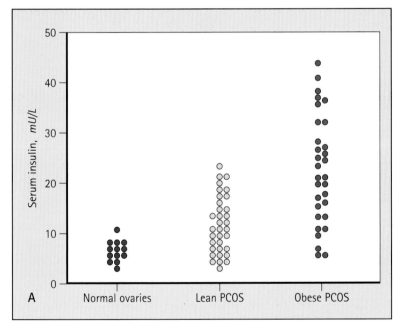

FIGURE 5–9.

Fasting insulin measurements in women with polycystic ovary syndrome (PCOS). **A**, Fasting serum insulin concentrations in normal women with normal ovaries, in women with PCOS who were lean (body mass index between 20 and 22.5 kg/m^2), and in women with PCOS who were obese (body mass index >30 kg/m^2).

Because high fasting insulin levels may be found in the absence of obesity, it is thought that there is a form of insulin resistance specific to PCOS and distinct from that caused by obesity and diabetes mellitus. **B**, Fasting insulin levels and type of menstrual cycle in lean women with PCOS.

(*Continued on next page*)

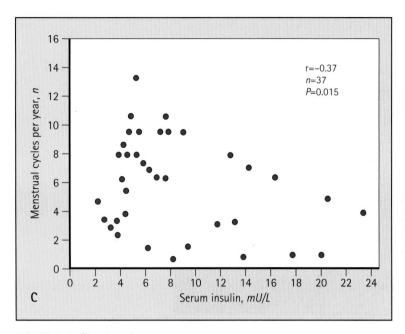

FIGURE 5-9. *(Continued)*
C, Fasting serum insulin and number of menses per year in lean women with PCOS. Both **B** and **C** illustrate the direct relationship of the fasting insulin concentration to irregularity of the menstrual cycle. The higher the fasting serum insulin concentration, the longer the interval between menstrual cycles [6].

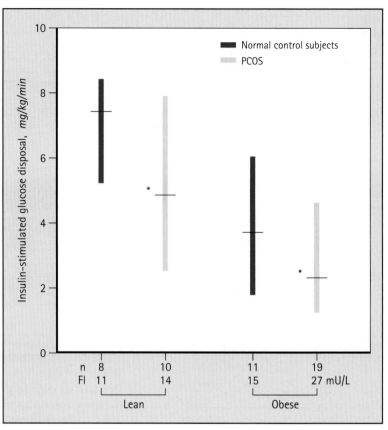

FIGURE 5-10.
Insulin resistance in polycystic ovary syndrome (PCOS) *Asterisk* indicates P<0.01. Dunaif [7], using "clamp" studies to measure the rate of insulin-stimulated glucose disposal, showed that with the rise in the fasting insulin concentration, found a fall in insulin-stimulated glucose disposal. Note the increase in the fasting serum insulin concentration demonstrated in relation to the fall in insulin sensitivity. (*Adapted from* Dunaif *et al.* [8]; with permission.)

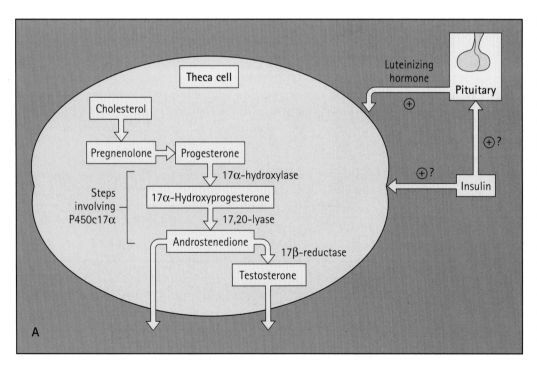

FIGURE 5-11.
The causes and ovarian consequences of hypersecretion of insulin in women with polycystic ovary syndrome (PCOS). **A**, Possible mechanisms of insulin stimulation of ovarian cytochrome P450C17α6 activity and androgen production. The insulin resistance that occurs in women with PCOS is confined to the effect of insulin on glucose disposal. Theca cell sensitivity to insulin remains unimpaired. Thus, the theca cell of the polycystic ovary is chronically exposed to excessive stimulation by insulin [9]. **B**, Conditions causing hypersecretion of insulin in PCOS [10]. Note that serine phosphorylation of the 17,20-lyase component of the cytochrome 9P450c17α enzyme has also been described [11]. The effect is to enhance the androgen-synthesizing component of this enzyme system in the adrenal and the ovary.

(Continued on next page)

B. CONDITIONS CAUSING HYPERSECRETION OF INSULIN IN POLYCYSTIC OVARY SYNDROME

Serine phosphorylation of insulin receptor of 17-20 lyase

Growth hormone and puberty

Obestiy

Diabetes mellitus

FIGURE 5-11. *(Continued)*

Increased serine phosphorylation of the insulin receptor, which inhibits tyrosine autophosphorylation and thereby impairs transduction of the insulin signal, is considered specific to PCOS [7]. The increased insulin requirements at puberty are probably mediated by the increase of growth hormone secretion that underlies the adolescent growth spurt. It probably contributes to the timing of the onset of PCOS, which typically occurs during adolescence. Insulin resistance and hypersecretion of insulin are worsened by obesity and in susceptible family members may be worsened by the development of non–insulin-dependent diabetes mellitus.

*A*NDROGENS

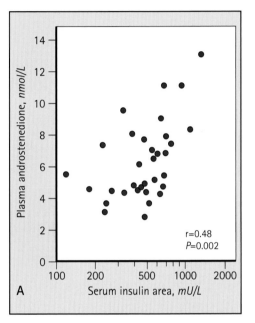

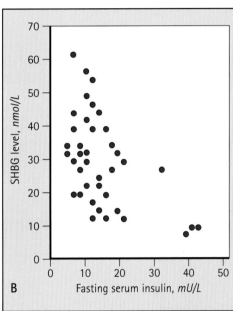

FIGURE 5-12.

Insulin and androstenedione levels in polycystic ovary syndrome (PCOS). **A**, Relationship of serum androstenedione concentrations in lean women with PCOS with the amount of insulin secreted in response to a standard 75-g oral glucose load. The more insulin secreted, the higher the plasma androstenedione level—results consistent with the notion that hypersecretion of insulin activates theca cell androgen production. Androstenedione concentrations are shown in this figure because this steroid is not bound by sex hormone–binding globulin (SHBG), and thus its concentration is not affected by SHBG levels. **B**, Insulin and SHBG in PCOS. The rate of synthesis of SHBG by the liver is reduced by hypersecretion of insulin, so circulating SHBG levels are low in the hyperinsulinemic patient; therefore, for a given amount of testosterone, the free testosterone is increased. This finding means that a normal serum *total* testosterone concentration in a patient with PCOS, particularly if she is obese and insulin resistant, frequently under represents a (raised) testosterone production rate.

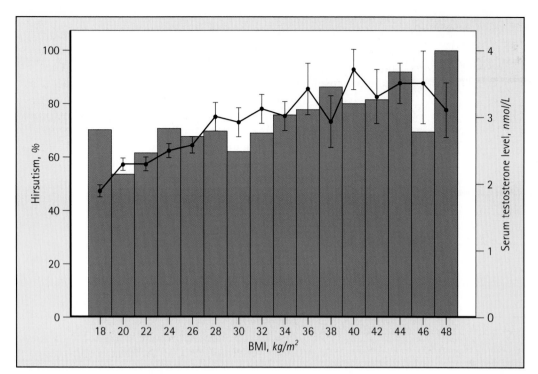

FIGURE 5-13.

Distribution of total serum testosterone concentrations in 1557 women with polycystic ovary syndrome (PCOS) in relation to body weight and the complaint of hirsutism [4]. Despite the effect of obesity on sex hormone–binding globulin synthesis, total testosterone concentrations rise with body weight. The increase in the testosterone production rate in the obese women must have been very great indeed. *T bars* indicate SEM. BMI—body mass index.

$\mathcal{I}$NFERTILITY

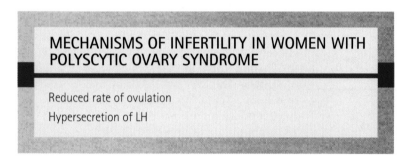

MECHANISMS OF INFERTILITY IN WOMEN WITH POLYSCYTIC OVARY SYNDROME

Reduced rate of ovulation

Hypersecretion of LH

FIGURE 5-14.

Mechanisms of infertility in women with polycystic ovary syndrome. LH– luteinizing hormone.

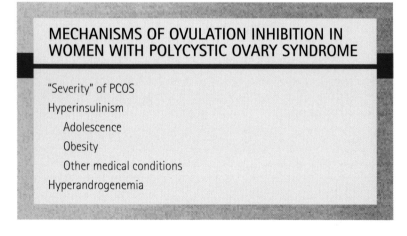

MECHANISMS OF OVULATION INHIBITION IN WOMEN WITH POLYCYSTIC OVARY SYNDROME

"Severity" of PCOS

Hyperinsulinism

    Adolescence

    Obesity

    Other medical conditions

Hyperandrogenemia

FIGURE 5-15.

Mechanisms of ovulation inhibition in women with polycystic ovary syndrome (PCOS). The rate of ovulation in women with PCOS is determined not only by the severity of the condition, but also, by the degree of hyperinsulinism (see Fig. 5-9). Anovulation occurs more frequently in the hyperandrogenized patient. The mechanism is probably mediated by hypersecretion of insulin, which seems to influence both anovulation and excessive androgen secretion.

A. INFERTILITY RELATED TO LUTEINIZING HORMONE CONCENTRATIONS IN 1398 WOMEN WITH POLYCYSTIC OVARY SYNDROME

	Patients, n (% of total)	Mean LH, IU/L
Primary infertility	270 (19.3)	13.7
Secondary infertility	116 (8.3)	11.2*
Proven fertility	108 (7.7)	9.4†
Pregnancy never attempted	904 (64.7)	9.5

*–P= 0.0065; †–P<0.00001

FIGURE 5-16.

Serum luteinizing hormone (LH) concentrations and infertility in women with polycystic ovary syndrome (PCOS). **A**, Infertility related to serum LH concentrations in 1398 women with PCOS [4]. **B**, Graphic representation of LH concentration and percentage of infertility in women with PCOS.

Mean serum LH concentrations were higher in women complaining of infertility compared with those whose fertility had been proven and with those who had never tried to conceive. The mechanism of hypersecretion of LH is uncertain, but there is an increase in both frequency and amplitude of LH pulses [12]. The mechanism, therefore, probably involves both hypothalamic and pituitary control mechanisms. It may also be that in women with PCOS, the hypothalamic LH-releasing hormone pulse generator is genetically programmed to fire more rapidly than in women with normal ovaries. *Asterisk* indicates *P* = 0.0065; *dagger* indicates *P* < 0.00001.

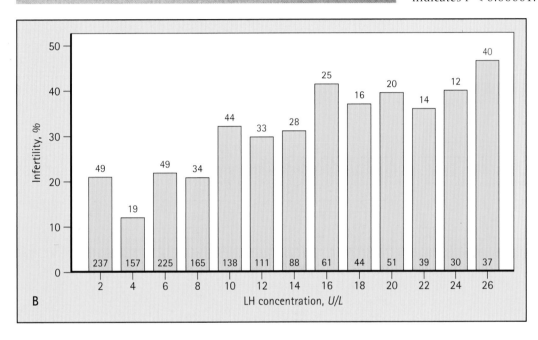

B

A. STUDY DESIGN FOR ASSESSING EFFECTS OF LUTEINIZING HORMONE HYPERSECRETION

Study included 193 women planning to get pregnant

Subjects recruited through television and radio publicity

Subjects underwent interview, examination, and blood test

Serum LH measured on day 8 of regular cycle

polyclonal antiserum for radioimmunossay

LH values up to 10 IU/L were considered normal

B. PREPREGNANCY LUTEINIZING HORMONE CONCENTRATION AND FERTILITY; FISHER'S EXACT PROBABILITY [TWO TAILED]; (P = 0.0158)

	Pregnant, n	Not pregnant, n
Normal LH (n = 147)	130	17
Raised LH (n = 46)	31	15

FIGURE 5-17.

The effects of luteinizing hormone (LH) hypersecretion on fertility and pregnancy outcome. **A**, Description of a field study on the prevalence of LH hypersecretion in women with regular cycles who were planning pregnancy [13]. Approximately 200 women were interviewed, underwent a physical examination, and had a measurement of serum LH on day 8 of a regular menstual cycle. In this study, serum LH concentrations up to 10 IU/L (as measured by a polyclonal radioimmunoassay) were considered normal. The patients were then reviewed 2 years later. **B**, The effect on fertility of having a serum LH concentration above 10 IU/L. Forty-six of the patients had a raised LH and their conception rate was 60% versus 80% in the women whose LH levels were normal. This difference was statistically significant.

(*Continued on next page*)

C. PREPREGNANCY LUTEINIZING HORMONE CONCENTRATION AND PREGNANCY OUTCOME; FISHER'S EXACT PROBABILITY [TWO TAILED]; $P<10^{-8}$		
	Successful, *n*	Miscarriage, *n (%)*
Normal LH (*n* = 130)	115	15 (12)
Raised LH (*n* = 31)	11	20 (65)

D. PREPREGNANCY LUTEINIZING HORMONE CONCENTRATION AND PREGNANCY OUTCOME IN PRIMIGRAVIDAE; FISHER'S EXACT PROBABILITY [TWO TAILED]; P = 0.0078		
	Successful, *n*	Miscarriage, *n (%)*
Normal LH (*n* = 20)	16	1 (6)
Raised LH (n = 5)	2	3 (60)

FIGURE 5-17. *(Continued)*
C, Miscarriage occurred in 12% of the 130 women with a normal serum LH concentration who conceived but in 65% of the 31 women who conceived despite a raised serum LH concentration. This difference was statistically highly significant. **D**, Subgroup analysis of the outcome of pregnancy. In primigravidae, despite the reduction in the number of cases available for study, it was found that hypersecretion of LH was associated with a miscarriage rate of 60%. The results in the two groups were statistically significantly different.

Despite regular ovulatory menstrual cycles, hypersecretion of LH was, therefore, associated with a small but definite impairment of fertility and a major risk of miscarriage. These studies do not, however, indicate whether hypersecretion of LH is a mediator of merely a marker of the risk of miscarriage. Further studies are required for the mechanism to be ascertained.

ONG-TERM CARDIOVASCULAR RISKS

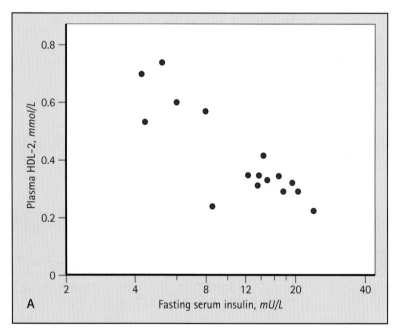

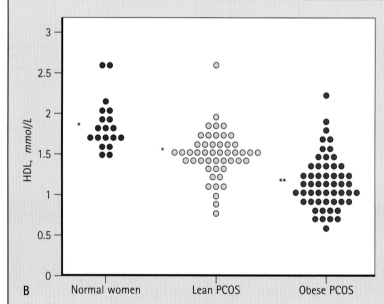

FIGURE 5-18.
Coronary risk factors in women with polycystic ovary syndrome (PCOS). **A**, The impact of hypersecretion of insulin on coronary risk factors in women with PCOS. The concentrations of cardioprotective high-density lipoprotein (HDL)-2 were inversely related to serum insulin concentration in a group of young, slim women presenting with hirsutism and acne, who were found to have PCOS. **B**, Total serum HDL concentrations in women with PCOS, compared with those in women with normal ovaries. There was a greater depression of cardioprotective HDL cholesterol in women with polycystic ovaries, than in normal women, and greater suppression in those women with PCOS who were also obese. *Asterisks* indicate *P<0.01; **P<0.001.

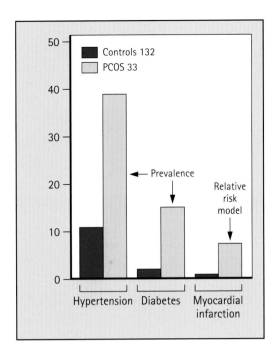

FIGURE 5-19.
Long-term follow-up of women with surgically proven polycystic ovary syndrome (PCOS). The results revealed an increased prevalence of hypertension and diabetes mellitus compared with the normal control subjects [15]. When Dahlgren *et al.* [16] derived a "relative risk" model, their data led them to postulate that PCOS was associated with a six-fold increase in the life-time risk of myocardial infarction. (*Adapted from* Dahlgren *et al.* [16]; with permission.)

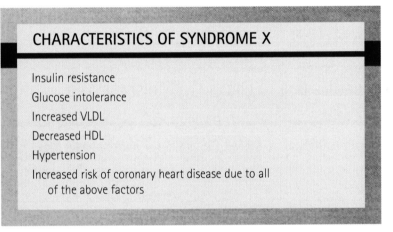

CHARACTERISTICS OF SYNDROME X

Insulin resistance

Glucose intolerance

Increased VLDL

Decreased HDL

Hypertension

Increased risk of coronary heart disease due to all of the above factors

FIGURE 5-20.
Syndrome X and risk of cardiovascular disease [17]. Reaven postulated that the association of insulin resistance with glucose intolerance, and changes in cholesterol metabolism and hypertension, all predisposed individuals to an increased risk of coronary heart disease. Women with polycystic ovary syndrome have many features of syndrome X, *ie*, they have many risk factors for premature development of coronary artery disease. HDL–high-density lipoprotein; VLDL–very low density lipoprotein.

A. LONG-TERM FOLLOW-UP OF WOMEN WITH POLYCYSTIC OVARY SYNDROME

Trace rate	840 of 1028 (82%)
Average age at diagnosis	25.7 y
Average duration of follow-up	28.1 y

B. MORTALITY OF WOMEN WITH POLYCYSTIC OVARY SYNDROME AT LONG-TERM FOLLOW-UP

	Observed, *n*	General population, *n*	SMR (95% CI; 1 = national average)
All causes	48	54.9	0.87 (0.64–1.16)
Circulatory	10	14.3	0.70 (0.34–1.29)
Neoplasms	23	25.4	0.90 (0.57–1.36)
External causes	5	4.2	1.20 (0.39–2.8)
Other	10	11.0	0.91 (0.44–1.67)

C. MORTALITY OF WOMEN WITH POLYCYSTIC OVARY SYNDROME DUE TO CIRCULATORY DISEASE AND DIABETES AT LONG-TERM FOLLOW-UP

	Observed, *n*	General population, *n*	SMR (95% CI; 1 = national average)
All circulatory disease	10	4.3	0.70 (0.34–1.29)
Ischemic heart disease	9	7.2	1.25 (0.57–2.37)
Other circulatory disease	1	7.1	0.14 (0.00–0.79)
Diabetes mellitus	2	0.4	5.1 (0.62–18.5)

FIGURE 5-21.

Long-term follow-up of women with polycystic ovary syndrome (PCOS). **A,** Results of a long-term follow-up study of 1028 women diagnosed surgically as having PCOS before 1970 [18]. The cases were identified by searching records of UK hospitals, and were followed in the UK National Health Service Central Registry until either the end of 1994, death, or age 75 years. **B,** Mortality of women with PCOS at long-term follow-up. We found no increased rate of death from circulatory disease or neoplasms, and the standardized mortality ratios (SMR) for these conditions were not significantly different from those in the general population. **C,** A more detailed analysis of mortality in women with PCOS due to circulatory disease. There was no increased rate of death from ischemic heart disease; however, surprisingly, there was protection from "other circulatory disease" in women with PCOS ("other circulatory disease" refers essen-

tially to women with stroke). These data suggest, therefore, that mortality from stroke is lower in women with polycystic ovaries than in women in the general population. The table also shows the predicted increased rate of death from diabetes mellitus in women with PCOS (see Fig. 5-19).

These results indicate that, despite the association of PCOS with coronary risk factors (see Fis. 5-18 through 5-20), expression of these risk factors in terms of mortality does not occur below age 60. Therefore, some process must exist that protects against fatal coronary heart disease in women under age 60 with PCOS. The most likely factor is estrogen, levels of which are known to be higher in women with polycystic ovaries compared with the normal population. An alternative candidate would be the increased serum vascular endothelial growth factor concentrations that occur in women with PCOS (see Fig. 5-24).

$\mathcal{I}$NTRAOVARIAN EVENTS

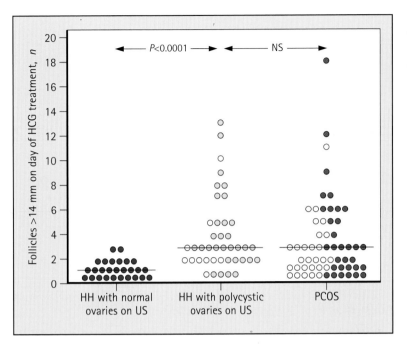

FIGURE 5-22.

The ovarian response to gonadotropin stimulation in a group of anovulatory women with polycystic ovary syndrome (PCOS) who were undergoing induction of ovulation. Human chorionic gonadotropin (hCG) was used to cause ovulation[19]. The results in women with PCOS may be contrasted with those in women with hypogonadotropic hypogonadism (HH) and normal ovaries and also with those in women with HH and polycystic ovaries (identified by ultrasound [US]). The presence of polycystic ovaries in either condition was associated with a significantly greater ovarian response to gonadotropin stimulation. It made no difference whether the patients were treated with human menopausal gonadotropin (*closed circles*) or follicle-stimulating hormone (*open circles*) alone. NS—not significant.

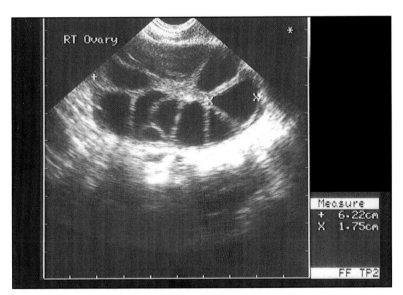

FIGURE 5-23.

The response of a polycystic ovary to gonadotropin stimulation, as seen on ultrasound. In this image there are at least six follicles with a diameter exceeding 16 mm. The thickened stroma between the follicles can readily be seen. In this patient, human chorionic gonadotropin therapy was withheld—otherwise, of course, there would have been a very high risk of multiple pregnancy.

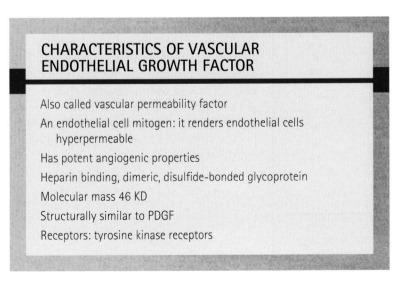

CHARACTERISTICS OF VASCULAR ENDOTHELIAL GROWTH FACTOR

Also called vascular permeability factor

An endothelial cell mitogen: it renders endothelial cells hyperpermeable

Has potent angiogenic properties

Heparin binding, dimeric, disulfide-bonded glycoprotein

Molecular mass 46 KD

Structurally similar to PDGF

Receptors: tyrosine kinase receptors

FIGURE 5-24.

Characteristics of vascular endothelial growth factor (VEGF). This substance is thought to mediate the clinical features of ovarian hyperstimulation syndrome. It may have an important role in the intra-ovarian control of follicle development. PDGF—platelet-derived growth factor.

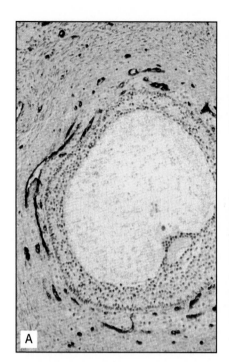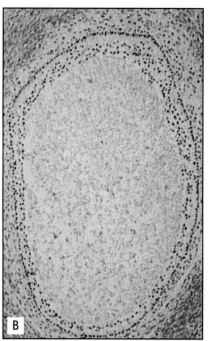

FIGURE 5-25.
Immunostaining of sections of human ovary for vascular endothelial growth factor (VEGF) [20]. **A**, The distribution of the staining indicates some VEGF in theca cells and blood vessels in the normal ovary. **B**, Stain taken from a polycystic ovary, shows a cyst. There is an extraordinary increase in immunostaining for VEGF throughout the theca cells of the hypercellular ovarian stroma.

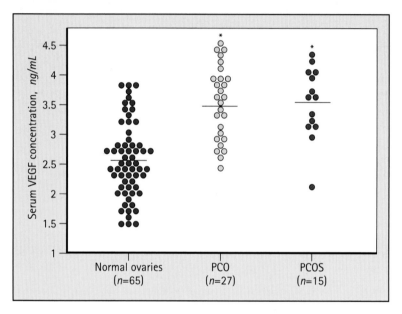

FIGURE 5-26.
Comparison of serum vascular endothelial growth factor (VEGF) concentrations in women with normal ovaries, women with polycystic ovaries (PCO), and women with polycystic ovary syndrome (PCOS) [21]. Serum concentrations of VEGF are raised in women with PCO and, presumably, reflect the extensive immunostaining seen in Figure 5-25 B. *Asterisk* indicates $P < 0.0001$.

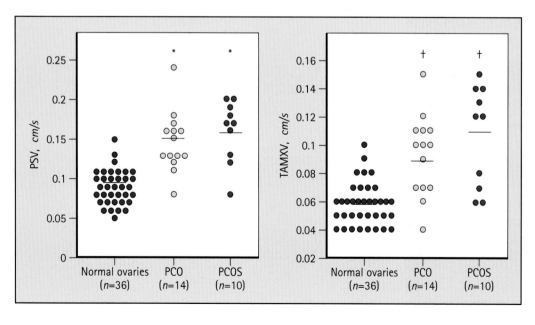

FIGURE 5-27.
Doppler ultrasound study of women with normal ovaries, women with polycystic ovaries, and women with polycystic ovary syndrome (PCOS). The results indicate that women with PCO have increased ovarian blood flow possibly due to increase of ovarian and serum vascular endothelial growth factor (VEGF). *Asterisk* indicates $P = 0.001$; *dagger* indicates $P < 0.001$. PSV—peak systolic blood flow; TAMXV—timed maximal blood flow.

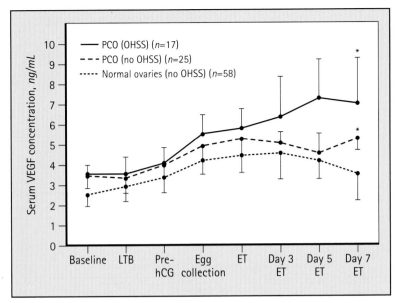

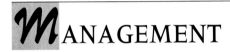

FIGURE 5-28.

Serum vascular endothelial growth factor (VEGF) concentrations during the phase of ovarian stimulation in patients undergoing *in vitro* fertilization (Agrawal *et al.*, Unpublished data). Concentrations are higher at all stages in women with polycystic ovary syndrome (PCOS) comapred with those with normal ovaries, and concentrations are considerably higher in women who go on to develop ovarian hyperstimulation syndrome (OHSS) [22].

These data provide a context for the multiple follicular response to gonadotropin stimulation of the polycystic ovary and remind us of the great danger of multifollicular ovulation, which can result in multiple pregnancy and a high risk of ovarian hyperstimulation. The high levels of VEGF within the polycystic (see Fig. 5-25) suggest that this response is an intrinsic feature of the condition and therefore that ovarian stimulation with gonadotropins is inherently dangerous in women with polycystic ovaries (PCO). *Asterisk* indicates $P < 0.0001$; *dagger* indicates $P = 0.002$. *16T bars* indicate ± SEM. ET—embtyo transfer; hCG—human chorionic gonadotropin; LTB—long term buserelin.

$\mathcal{M}$ANAGEMENT

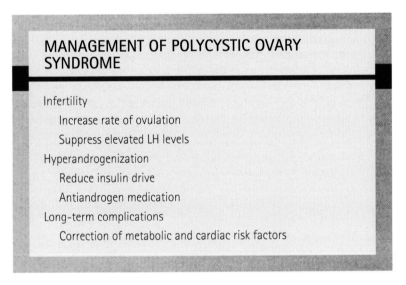

MANAGEMENT OF POLYCYSTIC OVARY SYNDROME

Infertility
    Increase rate of ovulation
    Suppress elevated LH levels
Hyperandrogenization
    Reduce insulin drive
    Antiandrogen medication
Long-term complications
    Correction of metabolic and cardiac risk factors

FIGURE 5-29.

The management of patients with polycystic ovary syndrome depends on the individual patient's complaints. Thus, problems of hyperandrogenism are optimally dealt with by reducing insulin drive to the ovary by the patient undertaking hygienic measures (*eg*, exercise and a reducing diet). Persisting symptoms may be treated by antiandrogens. Infertility is treated by increasing the rate of ovulation (in part by reducing insulin drive) and reducing hypersecretion of luteinizing hormone (LH). Ovarian stimulation is used for those women who do not ovulate, despite losing weight. Finally, long-term reduction in cardiac risk factors requires attention to a hygenic lifestyle.

REFERENCES

1. Kyei-Mensah AA, Tan SL, Zaidi J, Jacobs HS: Relationship of stromal volume to serum androgen concentrations in patients with polycystic ovary syndrome. *Hum Reprod* 1998, in press.

2. Zaidi J, Campbell S, Pittroff R, *et al.*: Ovarian stromal blood flow in women with polycystic ovaries: a possible new marker for diagnosis? *Hum Reprod* 1995, 10:1992–1996.

3. Adams J, Polson D, Franks S: Prevalence of polycystic ovaries in women with anovulation and idiopathic hirsutism. *BMJ* 1986, 293:355–359.

4. Balen AH, Conway GS, Kaltsas G, *et al.*: Polycystic ovary syndrome: the spectrum of the disorder in 1741 patients. *Hum Reprod* 1995, 10:2107–2111.

5. Conway GS, Jacobs HS: Acanthosis nigricans in obese women with polycystic ovary syndrome: disease spectrum not distinct entity. *Postgrad Med J* 1990, 66:536–538.

6. Conway GS: Polycystic ovary syndrome: clinical aspects. *Baillieres Clin Endocrinol Metab* 1996, 10:263–281.

7. Dunaif A: Molecular mechanisms of insulin resistance in PCOS. In *Androgen Disorders of Women*. Edited by Azziz R, Nestler JE, Dewailly D. Philadelphia: Lippincott-Raven Publishers; 1997:485–496.

8. Dunaif A, Segal KR, Futterweit W, Dobrjansky A: Profound peripheral insulin resistance, independent of obesity, in polycystic ovary syndrome. *Diabetes* 1989, 38:1165-1174.

9. Nestler JE: Insulin and ovarian androgen excess. In *Androgen Disorders of Women*. Edited by Azziz R, Nestler JE, Dewailly D. Philadelphia: Lippincott-Raven Publishers; 1997:473–483.

10. Jacobs HS: Environmental factors in PCOS. In *Androgen Disorders of Women*. Edited by Azziz R, Nestler JE, Dewailley D. Philadelphia: Lippincott-Raven Publishers; 1997:339–456.

11. Geller DH, Auchus RJ, Miller WL: The role of P450c17 in androgen biosynthesis. In *Androgen Disorders of Women*. Edited by Azziz R, Nestler JE, Dewailley D. Philadelphia: Lippincott-Raven Publishers; 1997:473–315–327.

12. Soule SG: Neuroendocrinology of the polycystic ovary syndrome. *Baillieres Clin Endocrinol Metab* 1996, 10:205–221.

13. Regan L, Owen EJ, Jacobs HS: Hypersecretion of LH, infertility and spontaneous abortion. *Lancet* 1990, 336:1141–1142.

14. Conway GS, Agrawal R, Betteridge DJ, Jacobs HS: Risk factors for coronary artery disease in lean and obese women with the polycystic ovary syndrome. *Clin Endocrinol* 1992, 37:119–126.

15. Dahlgren E, Janson P-O, Johasson S, *et al.*: Women with polycystic ovary syndrome wedge resected in 1956-1965: a long term follow up focussing on natural history and circulating hormones. *Fertil Steril* 1992, 57:505–513.

16. Dahlgren E, Janson P-O, Johasson S, *et al.*: Polycystic ovary syndrome and risk for myocardial infarction: evaluated from a risk factor model based on a prospective population study of women. *Acta Obstet Gynecol Scand* 1992, 71:599–604.

17. Reaven GM: role of insulin resistance in human disease. *Diabetes* 1988, 37:1595–1607.

18. Pierpoint T, McKeigue PM, Isaacs AJ, Jacobs HS: Mortality of women with polycystic ovary syndrome at long term follow up. *J Clin Epidemiol* 1998, in press.

19. Shoham Z, Conway GS, Patel A, Jacobs HS: Polycystic ovaries in patients with hypogonadotropic hypogonadism: similarity of ovarian response to gonadotropin stimulation in patients with polycystic ovarian syndrome. *Fertil Steril* 1992, 58:37–47.

20. Kamat BR, Brown LF, Manseau EJ, *et al.*: Expression of vascular endothelial growth factor vascular permeability factor by human granulosa and theca lutein cells: role in corpus luteum development. *Am J Pathol* 1995, 146:157–165.

21. Agrawal R, Sladkevicius P, Engmann L, *et al.*: Serum vascular endothelial growth factor concentrations and ovarian stromal blood flow are increased in women with polycystic ovaries. *Hum Reprod* 1998, 13:651-655.

22. Agrawal R, Chimusoro K, Payne N, *et al.*: Severe ovarian hyperstimulation syndrome: serum and ascitic fluid concentrations of vascular endothelial growth factor. *Curr Opin Obstet Gynecol* 1997, 9:141–144.

Dysfunctional Uterine Bleeding: Evaluation and Treatment

Patricia J. Sulak and Paul M. Yandell

Abnormal uterine bleeding (AUB) is a common reason for women to seek medical attention. The most important aspect of the evaluation is the history. One must first determine if the patient actually has abnormal bleeding. Knowledge of the characteristics of bleeding patterns that occur normally during the reproductive years is necessary when assessing patients' complaints. After menarche, menses may be irregular for months to years as the hypothalamic-pituitary-ovarian axis matures. During this time, further evaluation and treatment is not necessary unless the patient is having prolonged episodes of bleeding or excessive amounts of bleeding that is bothersome to the patient or is causing anemia. At the opposite end of the reproductive spectrum, perimenopausal women will also experience menstrual changes that are often normal and require no evaluation or treatment. During the early perimenopausal stage, menstrual cycles may decrease in number of days because of a shortening of the proliferative phase. Patients may become alarmed when menses are 21 to 24 days apart rather than the customary 28- to 30-day cycle. They are often subjected to invasive procedures such as endometrial biopsy, hysteroscopy, curettage, and even hysterectomy for a condition that is normal for this stage of the reproductive spectrum. Endometrial biopsy should be considered if menses are prolonged, heavy, or less than 21 days apart. The perimenopause can span many years before final ovarian failure. In late perimenopause, menses should become lighter and further apart as ovulation becomes erratic. Only 10% of women will experience an abrupt cessation of regular menstrual flow without prior menstrual irregularity. Because the majority of women will undergo alterations in their menstrual cycles, it is important to understand what constitutes a normal change and what mandates further diagnostic evaluation.

Although many diagnostic tests and procedures are available for the evaluation of AUB, it is important that we perform only those tests that are medically indicated, avoiding unnecessary inconvenience, discomfort, morbidity, and health care expenditures. Initial evaluation often involves only a thorough history, physical, and minimal (or no) tests or procedures. Procedures such as a transvaginal ultrasound or hysteroscopy are often indicated when attempts at medical management fail.

The treatment of AUB must be tailored to the patient, with multiple factors considered, including the cause of the bleeding, age of the patient, and concomitant gynecologic problems. Hormonal therapy is the mainstay of treatment, with oral contraceptives (OCs) being the primary initial modality in most patients because of safety, efficacy, and other noncontraceptive benefits. OCs are also the only preventive therapy for AUB. Patients on OCs rarely "develop" AUB and have a much lower incidence of heavy menses, irregular menses, and anemia compared with nonusers. For patients at low risk for endometrial cancer, surgical intervention is indicated only after failure of medical management.

This chapter details the characteristics of normal and abnormal uterine bleeding. A wide array of diagnostic modalities will be discussed, along with the indications, risks, and benefits of hormonal regimens.

ARIABILITY AND DOCUMENTATION OF THE MENSTRUAL CYCLE

NORMAL MENSTRUAL CYCLES

Requirements

Intact, properly functioning hypothalamic-pituitary-ovarian system

Estrogen-induced proliferative endometrium in first half of menstrual cycle

Ovulation at midcycle with progesterone production from the corpus luteum

Progesterone-induced secretory endometrium in second half of cycle

If pregnancy does not occur, hormones decline, and withdrawal bleeding occurs

Characteristics

Can vary greatly among women

Can change dramatically from cycle to cycle

Normal cycle length: 21–35 d

Menstrual length: ≤ 7 d

Average blood loss: 35 mL (range, 20–60 mL)

FIGURE 6-1.

Normal menstrual cycles. Normal menstrual cycles require proper functioning of the hypothalamic-pituitary-ovarian axis, with ovulation occurring at regular intervals. "Normal" bleeding can vary greatly among women and over time in any individual woman. Some women may cycle every 21 days whereas others do so every 35 days. Women may complain that their cycles are "irregular" because they do not occur around the same time of each month, when in fact these women are experiencing a normal menstrual cycle.

A. DOCUMENTING MENSTRUAL CYCLE LENGTH

Must instruct patients on "what is normal"

Determined by counting the number of days from the first day of menstrual flow (not the last day) to the first day of the next menstrual flow

The first day of menstrual flow is defined as cycle day #1

FIGURE 6-2.

Documenting bleeding. Investigators have established that there is poor correlation between the patient's subjective complaint of heavy bleeding and actual measured blood loss through collection of sanitary products and elaborate extraction methods. Because actual measurement of menstrual blood loss is inconvenient, time-consuming, expensive, and lacks correlation with the patient's complaints, other methods of assessing the degree of bleeding are necessary. Measurement of hemoglobin will detect evidence of anemia.

(Continued on next page)

B. MENSTRUAL CYCLE RECORD

Month \ Day	1	2	3	4	5	6	7	8	9	10	11	12	13	14	15	16	17	18	19	20	21	22	23	24	25	26	27	28	29	30	31
Jan																															
Feb																														X	X
Mar			S	B	B	B	S																		B	B	B	S			
Apr															S	S	B	B	S												X
May									B	H	S	S	S																		S
Jun	B	B	S																												X
Jul																															
Aug																															
Sep																															X
Oct																															
Nov																															X
Dec																															

S—Spotting; B—Bleeding; H—Heavy

FIGURE 6-2. *(Continued)*
A simple menstrual calendar allows the investigator to see exactly when bleeding is occurring, length of menses, and, to some extent, the amount of bleeding. This also allows one to determine if the patient is having cyclic versus noncyclic bleeding to assess ovulatory status. Calendars can also be used to monitor response to treatment.

A, How to use the menstrual calendar. **B,** Patient complaining of periods "every 2 weeks," sometimes "two a month." The completed menstrual calendar reveals normal, cyclic menses every 21 to 24 days. "Heavy flow" is defined as passing clots or soaking through a pad or tampon every 2 hours or less.

DEFINING ABNORMAL BLEEDING

DEFINITIONS OF ABNORMAL UTERINE BLEEDING

Menorrhagia or hypermenorrhea: excessive (> 80 mL) or prolonged (> 7 d) bleeding that occurs at regular intervals
Metrorrhagia: bleeding occurring at irregular intervals < 35 d
Menometrorrhagia: prolonged uterine bleeding occurring at irregular intervals
Polymenorrhea: uterine bleeding occurring at regular intervals of < 21 d
Oligomenorrhea: uterine bleeding occurring at intervals from > 35 d to 6 mos
Amenorrhea: no menses for at least 6 mos
Intermenstrual bleeding: bleeding of variable amounts occurring between regular menstrual periods
Dysfunctional uterine bleeding: abnormal uterine bleeding with no demonstrable organic cause (usually secondary to anovulation)
Anovulatory bleeding: abnormal uterine bleeding secondary to anovulation (preferable to the term *dysfunctional uterine bleeding*)

FIGURE 6-3.
Definitions of abnormal uterine bleeding (AUB). To communicate with other health care providers, it is important that accurate terms are used to describe AUB. Hypermenorrhea and menorrhagia are synonymous terms and should be used to describe heavy or prolonged bleeding associated with presumably ovulatory cycles. When bleeding is initially being evaluated and the type and cause of bleeding is uncertain, it is preferable to simply use the term "abnormal uterine bleeding."

CAUSES OF ABNORMAL BLEEDING

CAUSES OF ABNORMAL UTERINE BLEEDING

Anovulation or oligo-ovulation
Menorrhagia/hypermenorrhea
Disorders of blood coagulation
Medications
Reproductive tract pathology

FIGURE 6-4.

Causes of abnormal uterine bleeding. Patients may have more than one cause of their abnormal bleeding. Although the cause may be obvious on initial presentation, often the actual pathology may not become apparent until initial therapy has failed and subsequent procedures are performed.

ANOVULATION OR OLIGO-OVULATION

Pathophysiology
  Lack of progesterone leads to unopposed estrogen stimulation of
    the endometrium, which leads to endometrial growth surpassing
    estrogen support. The result is irregular shedding of the
    endometrium and resultant unscheduled bleeding, and potential
    for development of endometrial hyperplasia or cancer.

Causes
  Perimenarcheal
  Perimenopausal
  Polycystic ovarian syndrome
  Endocrine disorders (thyroid, pituitary, adrenal)
  Anorexia nervosa
  Excessive exercise
  Stress
  Psychotropic drugs
  Brain tumors

Progestin challenge
  Purpose is to assess endogenous estrogen status of the patient
  Types
    MPA, 5-10 mg for 7-10 d
    Progesterone in oil 100-150 mg intramuscularly
  Results
    If no withdrawal bleeding, patient is probably estrogen deficient
      (other possibilities include cervical stenosis or Asherman's syndrome)
    If withdrawal bleeding, patient is producing sufficient estrogen to
      maintain bone density
Management depends on estrogen status
  If estrogen present
    Monthly progestin withdrawal
    Low-dose combination oral contraceptives
    If pregnancy desired, ovulation induction with clomiphene citrate
  If estrogen deficient
    Hormone replacement (estrogen and progestin)
    Low-dose combination oral contraceptives

FIGURE 6-5.

Anovulation and oligo-ovulation. Anovulation and oligo-ovulation are common causes of abnormal uterine bleeding. If the ovaries continue to produce estrogen, but ovulation and the resultant production of progesterone is not occurring at regular intervals, irregular shedding of a dyssynchronous endometrium can occur from the endogenous unopposed estrogen. Patients can be anovulatory but estrogen deficient. For example, in the setting of anorexia nervosa or excessive exercise, amenorrhea or oligo-amenorrhea are caused not only by lack of progesterone production but also lack of estrogen production.

To assess endogenous estrogen status, medroxyprogesterone acetate (MPA) 10 mg a day for 7 days or an injection of 100 mg of progesterone in oil can be used. Bleeding cannot occur after the administration of a progestin unless the endometrium is estrogen primed. Lack of bleeding after completing a course of progestin medication usually signifies estrogen deficiency. A low serum estradiol level of < 30 pg/mL would confirm estrogen deficiency. Other possible reasons for no withdrawal bleeding, such as outflow tract obstruction, Asherman's syndrome, or pregnancy can be assessed by history and physical examination. Estrogen deficiency (serum estradiol < 30 pg/mL) in a young reproductive-age woman is a significant risk factor for serious disease states, including coronary heart disease and osteoporosis. If bleeding occurs after the progestin is administered, sufficient endogenous estrogen production is confirmed (serum estradiol level usually > 40 pg/mL). Patients with

unopposed endogenous estrogen production without endogenous or exogenous progesterone are at increased risk for irregular bleeding and endometrial neoplasia.

Persistent anovulation can lead to significant health consequences. If reproductive-age women are having oligo-amenorrhea or amenorrhea, the cause must be investigated and the endogenous estrogen status of the patient determined. Not having regular menses in the reproductive years can signify estrogen deficiency or unopposed estrogen, both of which must be treated to prevent serious health prolblems. Reproductive-age women should have regular menses unless they are using oral contraceptives, levonorgesterol implants, or depomedroxyprogesterone acetate intramuscular injections. These medications can produce oligo-amenorrhea or amenorrhea secondary to the progestational effects on the endometrium but are not associated with significant estrogen deficiency.

Treatment depends on estrogen status. If a reproductive-age woman is estrogen deficient, she must be counseled on the possible sequelae and offered estrogen in the form of hormone replacement therapy (HRT) or oral contraceptives. If the patient is producing sufficient estrogen, then monthly progestin (MPA 10 mg/d × 10–14 d) can be given or she can be placed on a combination oral contraceptive, all of which are progestin dominant and promote endometrial thinning. If conception is desired, treatment with clomiphene citrate should usually induce ovulation and endogenous progesterone.

MENORRHAGIA OR HYPERMENORRHEA

Heavy or prolonged bleeding that occurs at regular intervals (*ie*, ovulatory)

Abnormal prostaglandin levels in the endometrium

Decrease in prostaglandin $F_{2\alpha}$ (vasoconstrictor) and thromboxane (platelet aggregator)

Increase in prostaglandin E_2 (vasodilator) and prostacyclin (platelet inhibitor)

Diagnosis
- Subjective
  - Patient history
- Objective
  - Examination during heaviest flow
  - Menstrual calendar
  - Anemia

FIGURE 6-6.

Menorrhagia and hypermenorrhea. It is estimated that at least 10% of patients experience subjective heavy menses associated with ovulatory cycles. Several investigators have documented alterations in endometrial prostaglandins in women with menorrhagia compared with those with normal menstrual flow. In the endometrium, prostaglandins that have vasodilatory and platelet inhibition properties are found in greater ratio than those with vasoconstrictive and platelet aggregatory characteristics, resulting in a coagulation environment that promotes greater bleeding.

The clinical diagnosis of menorrhagia is commonly subjective, based on the patient's history. Elaborate methods to document actual blood loss are expensive, time consuming, inconvenient, and often do not substantiate the patient's complaints. Objective evidence of hypermenorrhea can be obtained by direct observation of heavy flow during examination, documentation of anemia, and use of a semiquantitative menstrual calendar to document the number of days and description of flow.

SOME DISORDERS OF BLOOD COAGULATION

Von Willebrand's disease

Idiopathic thrombocytopenic purpura

Leukemia

Prothrombin deficiency

Systemic illnesses (cirrhosis, sepsis)

FIGURE 6-7.

Disorders of blood coagulation. Although many patients present with a previously diagnosed disorder of blood coagulation, a bleeding tendency should be suspected if patient inquiry reveals bleeding at other sites, after procedures, or if there is a failure to respond to medical management. These disorders are frequently found in adolescents who experience excessive menstrual blood loss, especially in the first spontaneous menses.

MEDICATIONS CAUSING ABNORMAL UTERINE BLEEDING

Hormone preparations
    Oral contraceptives
        Noncompliance
        Pill type: 20 µg > 30–35 µg > 50 µg
        Tobacco abuse
        Endometritis
        Polyps
        Leiomyomata uteri
        Concomitant medications (eg, antiepileptics)
    Hormone replacement therapy (continuous regimen)
        Depo-medroxyprogesterone acetate (DMPA)
        Levonorgestrel implants
Psychotropic drugs
Anticoagulants

FIGURE 6–8.

Medications that may cause abnormal uterine bleeding (AUB). Hormone preparations are the most common medications that cause AUB. Oral contraceptives commonly cause irregular "breakthrough" bleeding during the first few months of use. If irregular bleeding persists after 6 months of use, several etiologic factors should be considered. Especially with today's low-dose oral contraceptives (OCs), it is very important that patients not only take their OCs daily, but also take them at the same time each day. A delay of several hours can often lead to breakthrough bleeding in some patients. As estrogen and progestin doses in OCs have decreased, breakthrough bleeding has increased. In general, 20 µg OCs have a greater incidence of breakthrough bleeding than 30- to 35-µg OCs, which have a greater incidence than 50-µg pills. Although there are not many comparative trials, levonorgesterol and new progestin OCs appear to have a lower incidence of breakthrough bleeding. A significantly increased incidence of breakthrough bleeding is also seen in women who use OCs and smoke, most probably secondary to the effects of nicotine on estrogen metabolism. Endometritis, particularly due to *Chlamydia*, is more commonly seen in women with breakthrough bleeding on OCs compared with women with no breakthrough bleeding on OCs. Endometrial lesions such as polyps and fibroids should also be considered to be present in women with persistent breakthrough bleeding on OCs despite excellent compliance and changes in OC preparations. These lesions can often be detected by transvaginal sonography. Endometrial thickness should be relatively thin (≤ 5 mm) in patients on OCs. A thickened appearance may be secondary to a polyp or submucosal fibroid, which can be further delineated with saline infusion sonography. Concomitant medications such as antiepileptic drugs and rifampin can cause breakthrough bleeding because of microsomal enzyme stimulation in the liver.

Although cyclic or sequential hormone replacement therapy (HRT) regimens often produce regular withdrawal bleeding after the administration of a progestin, continuous HRT regimens with daily estrogen and progestin are often associated with irregular bleeding. Approximately 60% to 70% of patients are amenorrheic at 6 months, and 30% to 40% will continue to have irregular bleeding for longer periods or indefinitely. Irregular bleeding on continuous HRT regimens can often be managed by decreasing the estrogen, increasing the progestin, or converting to a cyclic regimen. If irregular bleeding on a continuous HRT regimen persists despite hormonal adjustments, then an organic lesion must be ruled out (polyp, fibroid, neoplasia).

Depomedroxyprogesterone acetate (DMPA) intramuscular injections often cause irregular bleeding. Approximately 60% will be amenorrheic at 1 year with use of 150 mg intramuscularly every 3 months; the remainder will continue to have irregular bleeding for longer intervals. Once DMPA injections are discontinued, most patients do not spontaneously resume ovulation until about 6 months, with approximately 20% not ovulating at 1 year after their last injection. Similarly, levonorgesterol implant users have an 80% incidence of irregular bleeding during the first year of use, which decreases with each year of use.

Psychotropic agents such as tricyclic antidepressants can cause irregular bleeding. Anticoagulants such as warfarin and heparin can also cause heavy menses.

REPRODUCTIVE TRACT DISORDERS

Pregnancy
   Threatened or incomplete abortion
   Ectopic pregnancy
   Gestational trophoblastic disease
Ovarian tumors
   Gonadal stromal neoplasms
   Persistent corpus luteum (Halban's syndrome)
Vaginal abnormalities
   Polyps
   Infection
   Atrophic vaginitis
   Trauma
   Foreign bodies
   Cancer
Cervical abnormalities
   Eversion
   Cervicitis (infection)
   Polyps
   Cancer
   Trauma
Uterine lesions
   Endometrial polyps
   Submucosal leiomyomas
   Endometritis
   Adenomyosis
   Hyperplasia or cancer
   Intrauterine devices

FIGURE 6–9.

Reproductive tract disorders. The most common cause of abnormal bleeding in reproductive-age women is an abnormal pregnancy, which can be evaluated by a sensitive pregnancy test and sonography. Ovarian, vaginal, and cervical abnormalities can usually be detected on physical examination. Uterine lesions are a common cause of abnormal uterine bleeding. Intermenstrual bleeding may be indicative of polyps, leiomyomas, or endometritis. Menorrhagia may be secondary to an intrauterine device or adenomyosis. Patients at risk for endometrial cancer should undergo office endometrial sampling.

ENDOMETRIAL CANCER

Most common gynecologic malignancy (34,600 new cases and 6000 deaths anticipated in 1997)
Most patients between age 50–59
25% prior to menopause; 5% before age 40
75% have stage I disease
Risk factors
   Endogenous
      Early menarche
      Late menopause
      Obesity
      Chronic anovulation
      Nulliparity
      Estrogen-secreting tumors
      Diabetes mellitus
   Exogenous
      Unopposed estrogen replacement therapy
      Tamoxifen
Abnormal uterine bleeding (as warning sign)
   Postmenopausal bleeding
   Perimenopausal bleeding that is heavy, prolonged, cycles < 21 d
   Premenopausal chronic anovulatory bleeding

FIGURE 6–10.

Endometrial cancer. Although most patients with endometrial cancer are menopausal, about one fourth of cases occur prior to menopause. Most of these patients have known risk factors for endometrial cancer, which should prompt the clinician to rule out endometrial neoplasia.

DIAGNOSTIC EVALUATION

EVALUATION OF ABNORMAL BLEEDING

History	Physical examination
Age	Vital signs
Parity	Body habitus
Cyclic versus noncyclic bleeding	Evidence of endocrinopathies
Singular versus chronic episodes	Hirsutism
Duration and amount of bleeding	Hyperprolactinemia
Method of birth control	Hypothyroidism
Marital status/sexual history	Hyperthyroidism
History of bleeding disorders	Cushing's syndrome
Medical illnesses	Abdominal examination
Medications	Pelvic examination
	Breast examination

FIGURE 6–11.

Evaluation of abnormal uterine bleeding (AUB). Evaluating the patient with AUB will largely be dependent on the findings of the history and physical examination. Historical factors to establish abnormality (*eg*, onset, duration) and associated symptoms suggesting pregnancy, endocrine disorder (primary thyroid), hyperprolactinoma, genital tract infection, neoplastic process, or coagulopathy should be obtained. Physical examination in a nonpregnant premenopausal woman with probable anovulatory bleeding should include a thyroid examination as well as breast examination to evaluate for galactorrhea suggestive of pituitary adenoma. Abnormal bleeding occurring in a nonpregnant, premenopausal patient previously controlled on oral contraceptives warrants cervical cultures or an empiric trial of antibiotic treatment as a low-grade endometritis can present as new-onset breakthrough bleeding.

All patients with AUB should have a vaginal speculum examination to rule out vaginal or cervical sources for the bleeding. A Pap smear should be obtained if not performed in the past year. Bimanual pelvic examination should be performed to assess uterine size, position, mobility, and tenderness, as well as evaluating for abnormal adnexal structures.

DIAGNOSTIC TESTS USED IN THE EVALUATION OF ABNORMAL UTERINE BLEEDING

Pregnancy test: in reproductive-age women

Complete blood count and platelet count: if profuse or chronic heavy bleeding

Pap smear: if no documentation of one in past 12 mos

Cervical cultures: if at risk for sexually transmitted diseases or persistent breakthrough bleeding on oral contraceptives

Coagulation studies: if suspicious history, family history, or excessive bleeding not responsive to medical management, especially in teenagers (prothrombin time, partial thromboplastin time, bleeding time, platelet count)

Hormone tests

  Thyroid stimulating hormone (TSH): if menorrhagia, anovulation, or signs or symptoms of thyroid dysfunction are present

  Prolactin: if anovulatory, plus galactorrhea, headaches, and/or visual field defects

  Follicle-stimulating hormone: usually not necessary in perimenopausal patients. Fluctuations in FSH can occur and estrogen deficiency can be diagnosed by patient symptoms and a negative progestin challenge. An FSH test is useful in patients who are estrogen deficient and either desire pregnancy or are less than 35 years of age.

  Serum estradiol: can be considered if the progestin challenge test is negative in a young woman.

  Testosterone and DHEA-S: if hirsutism is severe or acute in onset; if evidence of virilization

FIGURE 6–12.

Diagnostic tests used in the evaluation of abnormal uterine bleeding (AUB). A young reproductive-age woman complaining of heavy cyclic menses may not require any evaluation other than standard pelvic examination and Pap smear prior to initiating therapy. An obese older reproductive-age woman with a long history of chronic anovulatory noncyclic bleeding may require a more extensive evaluation before treatment is initiated. Clinicians should be selective in the ordering of diagnostic tests in the evaluation of AUB. A luteinizing hormone (LH) level or serum progesterone is rarely, if ever, helpful in the management of AUB. Hormonal tests can be expensive and should only be ordered when necessary and when the results will assist in management. A follicle-stimulating hormone (FSH) level or serum estradiol is not indicated in most patients with a positive progestin challenge, because the patient is probably not estrogen deficient. Estrogen deficiency can usually be diagnosed by patient symptomatology and no withdrawal bleeding after a progestin challenge. An elevated FSH or low serum estradiol level (< 30 mg/mL) would confirm the diagnosis of estrogen deficiency. Whether the FSH is increased as with ovarian failure or decreased or normal as with hypothalamic hypogonadotropic conditions, hormone replacement needs to be considered if the patient is estrogen deficient to prevent such sequelae as osteoporosis, heart disease, and estrogen deficiency symptoms. Also, an FSH level can be confusing in young perimenopausal patients because of fluctuating values. Ovulation may resume and the patient is potentially fertile. If patients less than 35 years of age are found to be estrogen deficient, an FSH level may be beneficial to diagnose premature ovarian failure and then rule out a mosaic chromosomal pattern with a Y component, necessitating gonadectomy to prevent possible malignancy. If future fertility is desired, an FSH level may be necessary to assess follicular reserve. DHEA-S—dehydroepiandrosterone sulfate; TSH—thyroid-stimulating hormone.

DIAGNOSTIC PROCEDURES USED IN THE EVALUATION OF ABNORMAL UTERINE BLEEDING

Office procedures
    Endometrial biopsy
    Transvaginal sonography
    Saline infusion sonography
    Diagnostic hysteroscopy
Operative procedures
    Dilation and curettage
    Operative hysteroscopy

FIGURE 6-13.

Diagnostic procedures used in the evaluation of abnormal uterine bleeding (AUB). A number of diagnostic procedures are available for the evaluation of AUB. These include office-based procedures and procedures performed in the operating room. Operative procedures are intended to be both diagnostic and therapeutic. Selection of the most efficacious and cost-effective method requires knowledge of the strengths and weaknesses of each. Availability, expertise, and charges for these procedures vary greatly.

DIAGNOSTIC PROCEDURES FOR ABNORMAL UTERINE BLEEDING IN PREMENOPAUSAL PATIENTS

If at risk for endometrial hyperplasia or cancer
    Endometrial biopsy
If bleeding not responsive to medical management (to rule out
    intrauterine lesion)
    Transvaginal ultrasonography
    Saline infusion sonography
    Hysteroscopy

FIGURE 6-14.

Diagnostic procedures for abnormal uterine bleeding. Patients at increased risk for endometrial neoplasia should be evaluated with office endometrial sampling. Although measurement of the endometrial thickness with transvaginal sonography is useful in postmenopausal patients to assist in determining the need for endometrial sampling, it has not been shown to decrease the need for sampling in premenopausal patients. Patients in whom medical management fails require further procedures to rule out the presence of an endometrial lesion.

BIOPSY

EVALUATION OF PREMENOPAUSAL ABNORMAL UTERINE BLEEDING USING ENDOMETRIAL BIOPSY

Indication
    Detection of endometrial hyperplasia/cancer
    Detection of endometritis
Advantages
    Limited equipment and training
    Low cost
    Low risk
Disadvantages
    Missed focal intraluminal lesions
    Cervical stenosis (uncommon in premenopausal patients)

FIGURE 6-15.

Evaluation of premenopausal abnormal uterine bleeding (AUB) with endometrial biopsy (EMB). EMB is indicated for patients at risk of developing endometrial hyperplasia or cancer. It has replaced dilation and curettage performed for this indication because of similar detection rates (*eg*, sensitivities of 90%–95%) and markedly decreased costs. EMB also avoids conduction or general anesthetic risks associated with dilation and curettage. Rarely, EMB detects evidence of an unsuspected endometritis in a premenopausal patient with AUB. These patients commonly have resolution of AUB following antibiotic treatment.

Endometrial biopsy requires limited equipment and training. It is generally well tolerated and carries minimal risk to the patient. Utilization of soft polyurethane sampling devices minimizes the major risk of uterine perforation and decreases patient discomfort. EMB is designed to detect "global changes" in the endometrium. Because of the small 2- to 4-mm diameter sampling devices and the blinded technique, focal intraluminal lesions such as polyps and submucous myomas are generally missed. These focal lesions are common causes of AUB, especially in patients in whom medical treatment has failed. The presence of severe cervical stenosis is uncommon in premenopausal women, but may occasionally prevent office EMB.

INDICATIONS FOR AN ENDOMETRIAL BIOPSY IN PREMENOPAUSAL PATIENTS

Older than age 40 with AUB

Younger than age 40 with AUB and significant risk factors for endometrial cancer (eg, chronic anovulatory bleeding, obesity)

Abnormal perimenopausal bleeding: heavy, prolonged, or intervals of fewer than 21 days

Patients in whom medical management of AUB fails and who have not previously undergone biopsy

Atypical endometrial cells or atypical glandular cells of undetermined significance (AGCUS) on Pap smear

Normal endometrial cells on Pap smear are an abnormal finding in the second half of the menstrual cycle (consider EMB if risk factors for endometrial cancer)

Patients suspected of having endometritis (empiric antibiotic treatment without EMB may be acceptable)

FIGURE 6–16.
Indications for an endometrial biopsy (EMB) in premenopausal patients with abnormal uterine bleeding (AUB). Premenopausal patients with AUB and risk factors for endometrial cancer are best evaluated with office endometrial sampling. Office EMB is designed to evaluate for the presence of endometrial hyperplasia and cancer. It is not intended to evaluate for focal intraluminal lesions such as polyps or submucous myomas, which are common causes of AUB. Patients older than 40 years of age with AUB should have an EMB prior to attempts at hormonal management. Approximately 25% of endometrial cancers occur in premenopausal women, but only 5% occur in women less than 40 years of age, and these are almost always confined to women with histories of chronic anovulation with unopposed endogenous estrogen production (eg, polycystic ovarian syndrome or infertility, obesity, glucose intolerance). If histologic evaluation of the endometrial sampling is benign (ie, no evidence of neoplasia), but AUB persists despite treatment, further diagnostic evaluation must be pursued to rule out focal intraluminal lesions such as polyps, submucous myomas, or rarely a missed endometrial hyperplasia or cancer.

Endometrial biopsy should also be performed if a Pap smear reveals atypical endometrial cells or atypical glandular cells of undetermined significance, both of which may be evidence of an underlying endometrial neoplasia. Normal-appearing endometrial cells are a common finding if the Pap smear is performed during the first half of the menstrual cycle, especially during or immediately after menstruation. This is an expected normal finding. Endometrial cells on Pap smear during the second half of the cycle may be an abnormal finding and should prompt consideration of an EMB if the patient has risk factors for endometrial neoplasia.

PERFORMING AN ENDOMETRIAL BIOPSY

Devices

    Flexible suction curettes (eg, Pipelle)

    Rigid, sharp instruments (eg, Novak)

    Suction aspiration (eg, Vabra aspirator)

Procedure

    Determine size and position of uterus

    Visualize and cleanse cervix

    Pass the device through the cervix to the top of the uterine cavity

    Thoroughly sample the entire cavity (if a flexible curette is used, the device should be constantly rotated while moving it several times from the fundus to the internal os of the cervix)

FIGURE 6–17.
Performing an endometrial biopsy (EMB). EMB can easily be performed in the office in reproductive-age women. Flexible suction curettes cause minimal discomfort and have a diagnostic accuracy similar to dilation and curettage. Suction aspiration is useful for therapy if bleeding is profuse.

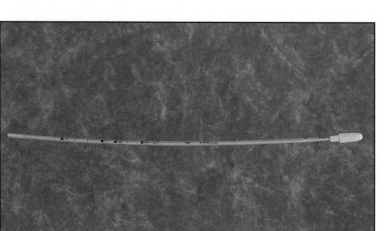

FIGURE 6–18.
Flexible curette. Flexible, polyurethane endometrial sampling devices have provided a reliable means to perform biopsies in an office setting with minimal discomfort and risk. Because these devices are flexible and conform to the direction of the endometrial cavity, they provide a diagnostic accuracy similar to dilation and curettage with much less inconvenience, cost, and discomfort.

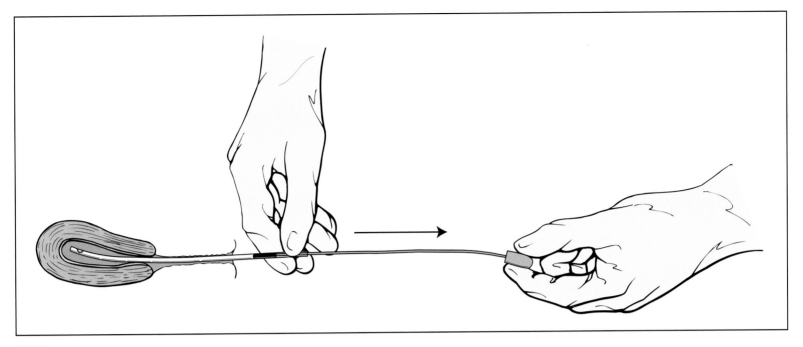

FIGURE 6-19.

Insertion of the catheter. Insert the catheter through the cervix into the uterus until resistance is encountered. While holding sheath, pull piston back completely and without interruption to proximal piston stop, thus creating maximum negative pressure within sheath. Leave piston fully retracted.

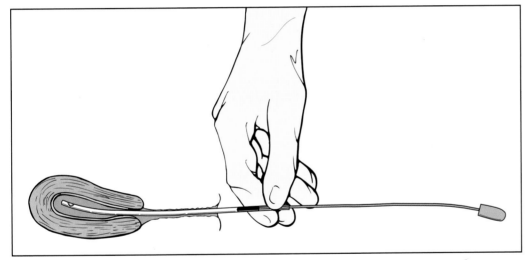

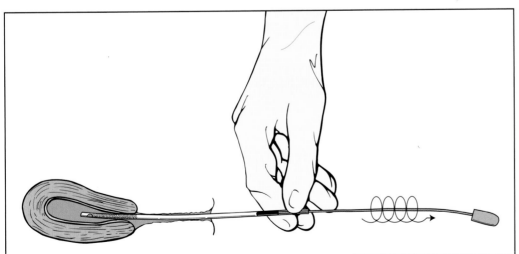

FIGURE 6-20

Sampling of the endometrial cavity. **A**, **B**, and **C**, Simultaneously roll (twist) sheath between fingers while moving sheath back and forth (in and out) between the fundus and internal os three or four times to obtain sample. It has been determined that at least three to four passes should be made to obtain the optimal sample.

(*Continued on next page*)

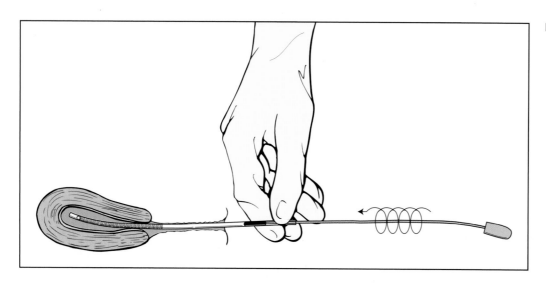

FIGURE 6-20. *(Continued)*

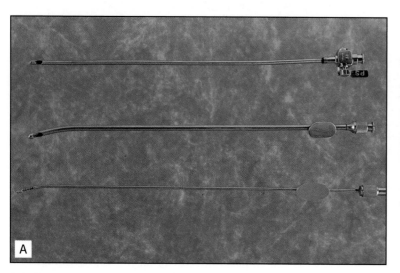

FIGURE 6-21.

Rigid, sharp endometrial sampling devices (**A** and **B**). Rigid, sharp endometrial sampling devices may be necessary to obtain an adequate biopsy, especially if the patient is having profuse bleeding. Use of these devices usually requires anesthetic paracervical block. Because they are not flexible, risk of perforation and damage to internal structures is greater but uncommon if the size and orientation of the uterus is accurately assessed.

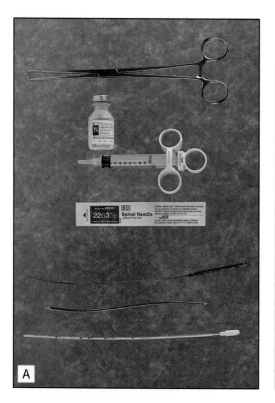

B. PROCEDURE FOR OFFICE ENDOMETRIAL SAMPLING WITH A STENOTIC CERVIX

Place tenaculum on anterior lip of cervix
  Place gently, slowly, and only to the first ratchet
  Lifting cervix upward may open the cervical canal sufficiently to allow passage of the sampling device
Paracervical block (if passage using above not successful)
  10-mL syringe filled with 1% lidocaine or carbocaine without epinephrine
  22-gauge spinal needle
  Inject at 4:00 and 8:00, 3-mm penetration; aspirate to confirm extravascular placement of needle
  Wait 5–10 min to allow full anesthetic effect
Metal dilator (2–3 mm in diameter)
  Can be extremely valuable in relieving any stenosis encountered at the internal os
  A flexible suction curette can usually be passed easily

FIGURE 6-22.

Management of the stenotic cervix. Encountering a stenotic cervix usually does not preclude office endometrial sampling. Patience, anesthesia, and the proper equipment almost always leads to a successful outcome. **A,** Instruments used for office endometrial sampling. *Top,* Tenaculum; *second from top,* lidocaine; *third from top,* spinal needle; *bottom,* dilators. **B,** Outline of procedure used for office sampling.

TRANSVAGINAL SONOGRAPHY FOR THE EVALUATION OF ABNORMAL UTERINE BLEEDING IN PREMENOPAUSAL PATIENTS

Indications

   Premenopausal patients in whom medical management of AUB has failed

   History or examination suggesting possibility of intraluminal lesions

Advantages

   Well tolerated

   Allows evaluation of endometrium, myometrium, and adnexa

   Cost-effective in the office setting

Disadvantages

   Reliability is operator and machine dependent

   High start-up equipment costs

FIGURE 6–23.

Transvaginal sonography. TVS is useful for the evaluation of abnormal uterine bleeding (AUB) in premenopausal patients. TVS uses high-frequency transducers (5–7.5 MHz) to provide high-resolution scans of pelvic structures. The hyperechoic (bright echo) endometrium can be imaged in the longitudinal (or long axis) plane of the uterus and the thickest anterior to posterior dimension measured with electronic calipers to determine the diameter of the endometrial echo complex (ECC). The adjacent hypoechoic myometrium should not be included in this measurement.

In nonpregnant premenopausal patients, pelvic ultrasonography is generally not indicated for the primary evaluation of AUB.

Unlike postmenopausal patients, ECC measurements are rarely helpful because of the endometrial response to endogenous ovarian hormones. An ECC up to 12 to 14 mm may be normal and, except in the very early proliferative phase of the cycle or in women on combination oral contraceptives (OCs), the ECC is rarely less than 5 mm. Further, abnormal pelvic ultrasound findings are poorly predictive of which patients may be effectively treated with medical therapy. Therefore, most nonpregnant premenopausal patients with AUB should undergo medical treatment prior to ultrasonic evaluation. Primary sonographic evaluation of AUB in premenopausal patients should be reserved for those already on OCs or in the early proliferative phase of the cycle on the day of evaluation. Demonstration of an ECC ≥ 5mm in these patients may indicate endometrial pathology and warrants further evaluation with endometrial biopsy (EMB), saline infusion sonography, or office diagnostic hysteroscopy. Patients who are noted on examination to have polyps protruding from the cervix are also at increased risk for polyps in the uterine cavity. Likewise, if the patient is noted on examination to have a fibroid uterus, submucosal fibroids causing AUB may be present.

Office transvaginal sonography (TVS) is well tolerated by patients, producing less discomfort than bimanual pelvic examination. In addition to evaluation of the endometrium, the presence, size, and location of myomata, as well as adnexal pathology, may influence further diagnostic and treatment options.

Reliability of TVS evaluation is both operator and machine dependent. Decisions to substitute ECC measurements for EMB should be made by the physician who performs the ultrasound and is aware of the patient's history and risks of endometrial hyperplasia and cancer. Substitution of ECC measurements for EMB requires imaging of the entire endometrium. Axially positioned uteri or partially obstructing myomas, which prevent complete imaging, invalidate ECC reliability.

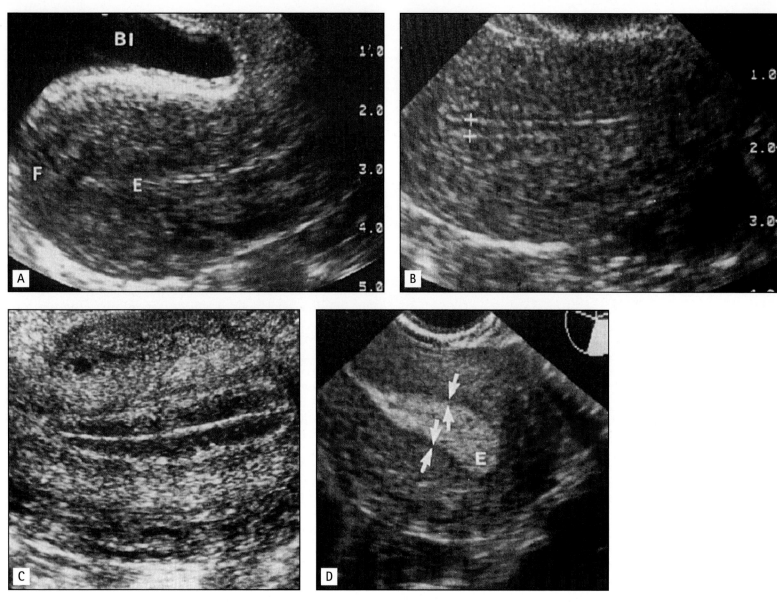

FIGURE 6-24.

Transvaginal sonography (TVS) of the endometrial response to endogenous hormones during the menstrual cycle. Although TVS is useful in the primary evaluation of abnormal uterine bleeding in postmenopausal patients, the endometrium of a premenopausal patient responds to endogenous hormone levels throughout the menstrual cycle and normally has an endometrial thickness of greater than 5 mm except in the early proliferative phase. **A**, Normal uterus cycled 3." **B**, Early proliferative endometrium "8." **C**, Late proliferative endometrium "13." **D**, Secretory endometrium "21."

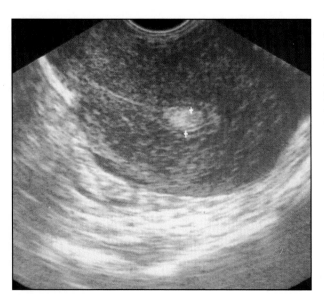

FIGURE 6-25.

Transvaginal sonography (TVS) of an endometrial polyp. In patients in whom medical management fails, TVS may suggest the presence of intraluminal lesions such as polyps or submucosal myomas. During mid to late secretory phase of the menstrual cycle, the endometrial echo appears in a "trilayer pattern," with hyperechoic basalis layers, hypoechoic functionalis layers, and hyperechoic endometrial surfaces. "Disruption" of the endometrial surfaces is consistent (or suspicious) for the presence of endometrial polyps.

SALINE INFUSION SONOGRAPHY FOR THE EVALUATION OF ABNORMAL UTERINE BLEEDING IN PREMENOPAUSAL PATIENTS

Indications

  Premenopausal AUB unexplained by EMB and failed medical
    management

  Alternative for diagnostic hysteroscopy

Advantages

  Well tolerated

  Simple, inexpensive equipment except for TVS

  Evaluation of endometrium, myometrium, and adnexa

Disadvantages

  Uterine enlargement ≥ 10 wk

  Contraindicated with cervical or uterine infection or pregnancy

  Operator and machine dependent

Not a histologic diagnosis

FIGURE 6–26.

Saline infusion sonography (SIS) in the evaluation of abnormal uterine bleeding (AUB) in premenopausal patients. SIS, like office diagnostic hysteroscopy (Dx HSP), is designed to detect focal intracavitary lesions missed by endometrial biopsy or dilation and curettage. When compared with hysteroscopy, SIS performs favorably, with sensitivities greater than 90% to 95%. SIS allows concurrent evaluation of the myometrium and adnexa, which may affect further management decisions.

Saline infusion sonography is well tolerated, with intracervical or paracervical local anasthetic rarely needed. In comparative studies, SIS causes less patient pain and is less expensive than office Dx HSP. Because of the prevalence of office transvaginal sonography (TVS), SIS may be more available than office Dx HSP. If office TVS is available, only relatively inexpensive additional equipment and supplies are needed. These include 1- to 3-mm diameter polyurethane catheters with and without a balloon, 10- to 20-mL syringes, and sterile saline. Balloon catheters are helpful in the 20% to 40% of patients with patulous cervices because they prevent the rapid egress of infused fluid and allow use of low-infusion volumes and pressures. The use of a cine-loop or videotape on the ultrasound machine is helpful in reviewing for small intracavitary lesions and may decrease the need for repetitive saline infusions.

Uterine enlargement greater than 10 weeks may limit SIS if associated with similar endometrial cavity enlargement, because TVS has a focal length of only 6 to 8 cm. Abnormalities occurring outside this distance will not be readily imaged and may be missed. Like Dx HSP or hysterosalpingogram, SIS is contraindicated in the presence of cervical or uterine infection as infusion of intrauterine fluid in these situations may lead to acute pelvic inflammatory disease. Similarly, the presence of a viable intrauterine pregnancy is considered a contraindication for all invasive intrauterine diagnostic procedures such as endometrial biopsy, dilation and curettage, Dx HSP, or SIS. Cervical stenosis may rarely prevent the performance of SIS. Because SIS involves TVS, it is operative and machine dependent. Sonographic findings may suggest the cause of focal intracavitary lesions responsible for AUB, but confirmation requires histologic sampling. Identification of the lesions may allow for "pseudo directed EMB." More commonly, diagnosis is confirmed following operative hysteroscopy scheduled as a result of identification of focal intraluminal lesions by SIS.

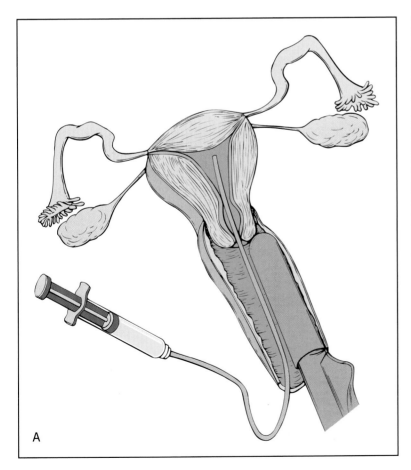

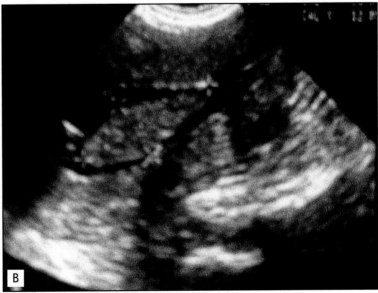

FIGURE 6–27.

Saline infusion sonography. **A,** Instilling sterile saline through a small catheter inserted through the cervix into the uterine cavity while simultaneously performing TVS can help differentiate a thickened endometrium from an intraluminal lesion.

(Continued on next page)

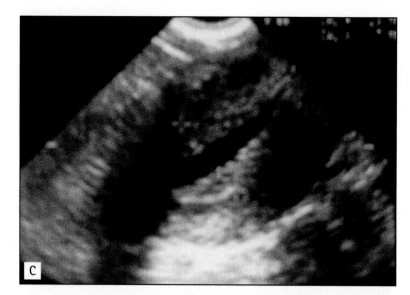

FIGURE 6-27. *(Continued)*
B and **C**, The saline infusion sonography images reveal a focal intraluminal lesion (B) and endometrium on either side of the instilled fluid with no intraluminal lesion (C).

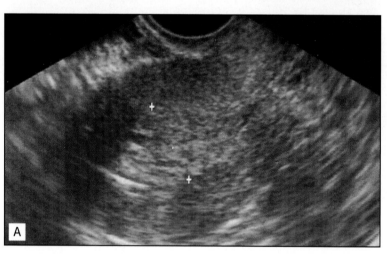

FIGURE 6-28.
Transvaginal sonography (TVS) compared with saline infusion sonography (SIS). **A,** TVS reveals what appears to be a thickened endometrium measuring 18 mm. **B,** SIS clearly delineates an intraluminal lesion (polyp), 15 × 33 mm, with adjacent atrophic endometrium.

HYSTEROSCOPY

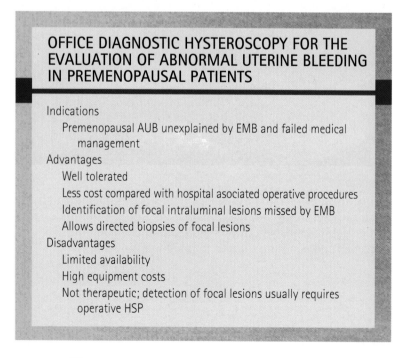

OFFICE DIAGNOSTIC HYSTEROSCOPY FOR THE EVALUATION OF ABNORMAL UTERINE BLEEDING IN PREMENOPAUSAL PATIENTS

Indications
    Premenopausal AUB unexplained by EMB and failed medical
        management
Advantages
    Well tolerated
    Less cost compared with hospital asociated operative procedures
    Identification of focal intraluminal lesions missed by EMB
    Allows directed biopsies of focal lesions
Disadvantages
    Limited availability
    High equipment costs
    Not therapeutic; detection of focal lesions usually requires
        operative HSP

FIGURE 6-29.
Office diagnostic hysteroscopy (Dx HSP) in the evaluation of abnormal uterine bleeding (AUB) in premenopausal patients. Office hysteroscopy (HSP) provides a panoramic view of the endocervical canal and endometrium. This view allows detection and directed biopsy of focal intraluminal lesions missed by endometrial biopsy (EMB). These lesions include polyps, submucous myomata, and rarely focal endometrial hyperplasia or cancer.

Office HSP is well tolerated using the current small 3- to 5-mm diameter flexible hysteroscopes. Local anesthesia with intracervical or paracervical block is recommended. Procedure-associated pain may be further decreased by the use of nonsteroidal anti-inflammatory drugs given 30 to 60 minutes before HSP.

It has been estimated that only 30% of practicing gynecologists perform office HSP. Reasons given for failure to use this modality include 1) high equipment cost, 2) need for operative HSP to remove most focal lesions detected with office Dx HSP, and 3) the availability of SIS, which is a cost-effective substitute for Dx HSP.

WHEN TO CONSIDER OPERATIVE HYSTEROSCOPY FRACTIONAL DILATION AND CURETTAGE

Endometrial sampling is deemed necessary and a stenotic cervix or obstructive mass precludes office EMB

Persistent abnormal uterine bleeding despite medical treatment; cause not resolved with TVS or SIS

Endometrial lesion detected on TVS, SIS, or office Dx HSP

Persistent hyperplasia on EMB despite medical treatment (rule out occult malignancy)

Atypical hyperplasia detected with EMB, especially in perimeno-pausal/postmenopausal patients (rule out occult malignancy)

Therapy for acute profuse bleeding not responsive to medical management

FIGURE 6-30.

When to consider operative hysteroscopy fractional dilation and curettage (D & C) in an operating room. With today's office diagnostic modalities, there is little rationale to perform a D & C for the evaluation of abnormal uterine bleeding (AUB). Operative hysteroscopy with removal of lesions under direct vision has greatly facilitated the treatment of some causes of AUB. Dx HSP—diagnostic hysteroscopy; EMB—endometrial biopsy; SIS—saline infusion sonography; TVS—transvaginal sonography.

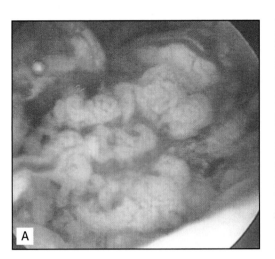 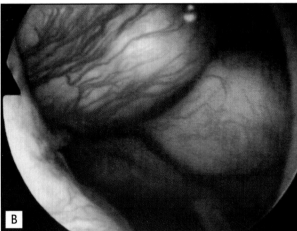

FIGURE 6-31.

Diagnostic hysteroscopy. **A** and **B**, When bleeding is persistent despite medical management and diagnosis is not resolved with endometrial biopsy, transvaginal sonography, or saline infusion sonography, a hysteroscopy should be performed to rule out the presence of intracavitary lesions as noted above.

$\mathcal{T}$REATMENT OF DYSFUNCTIONAL BLEEDING

FACTORS INVOLVED IN DECIDING TREATMENT OF DYSFUNCTIONAL UTERINE BLEEDING

Amount of bleeding

Cause of bleeding

Age of the patient

Medical status

Desire for future fertility

Need for contraception

Coexistent gynecologic problems

Significance to the patient

Results of endometrial biopsy, if performed

FIGURE 6-32.

Factors involved in deciding the treatment of dysfunctional uterine bleeding.

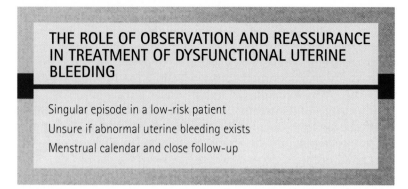

THE ROLE OF OBSERVATION AND REASSURANCE IN TREATMENT OF DYSFUNCTIONAL UTERINE BLEEDING

Singular episode in a low-risk patient

Unsure if abnormal uterine bleeding exists

Menstrual calendar and close follow-up

FIGURE 6–33.

The role of observation and reassurance in treatment of dysfunctional uterine bleeding. If one is unsure from the history if abnormal uterine bleeding actually exists or if this is the first episode in a low-risk patient, endometrial biopsy and treatment may not be necessary. A menstrual calendar and close follow-up may be the most appropriate management.

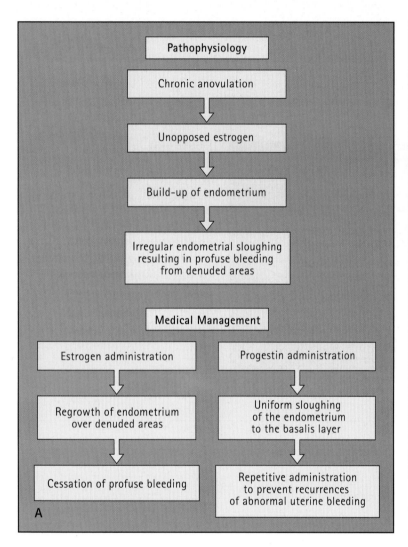

B. TREATMENT REGIMENS FOR PROFUSE BLEEDING IN ANEMIC PATIENTS

COMBINATION OCS

Example: OCs, one tablet 3 × per day for 7 days (one 21-d pill pack); if hemoglobin < 10, continue OCs one a day without a pill-free interval to prevent withdrawal bleeding until anemia is corrected. Thereafter, continue OCs in the standard fashion or administer a monthly progestin.

CONJUGATED ESTROGENS

Example: CEE, 1.25 to 2.5 mg orally 3 to 4 × per day for several days until bleeding has greatly decreased (warn patient to expect light bleeding—the goal is to stop the profuse bleeding). Continue CEE and initiate MPA 10 mg/d and continue until anemia is corrected. Discontinue CEE + MPA and allow a withdrawal bleed. Subsequently place on MPA 10 mg × 10–12 days a month or low-dose OCs.

Example: CEE, 25 mg intravenously if patient is NPO or having nausea or vomiting; given every 3–6 h until bleeding controlled (not to exceed 36–48 h); followed by MPA until anemia corrected. Intravenous route has not been shown to be superior in efficacy to high-dose oral CEE, which is less expensive and easier to administer.

Note: If profuse bleeding persists > 24 h despite medical therapy, operative hysteroscopy, suction aspiration, curettage, or hysterectomy may be indicated.

FIGURE 6–34.

Treatment of profuse bleeding in anemic patients. **A,** Pathophysiology and medical management. **B,** Some examples of treatment regimens.

TREATMENT OF ANOVULATORY BLEEDING

Progestins*

    MPA, 10 mg

    Norethindrone acetate, 5–10 mg

Combination OCs

    Breakthrough bleeding is common the first 3–6 mos

DMPA intramuscular[†]

    150–250 mg intramuscularly every 2–3 mos

Clomiphene citrate or other ovulation-inducing medication if pregnancy is desired

---

*Patient instructed to take the first 10 days of each calendar month if anovulatory or days 14–23 of each menstrual calendar if oligo-ovulatory.
[†]Patient must be instructed that irregular bleeding is common. Approximately 60% will be amenorrheic after 1 year of injections, but the remainder will continue to have irregular bleeding for longer periods.

FIGURE 6-35.

Treatment of anovulatory bleeding. Some form of progestin therapy is necessary for the long-term management of anovulatory bleeding. As discussed, profuse bleeding should initially be controlled with exogenous estrogen followed by estrogen plus progestin. Progestin therapy, such as medroxyprogesterone acetate (MPA), 10 mg for 10 to 12 days each month, is ideal for anovulatory dysfunctional uterine bleeding. This will induce regular withdrawal bleeding if adequate levels of endogenous estrogen are present to stimulate endometrial growth. Combination oral contraceptives are also an excellent treatment for healthy women in addition to providing a multitude of noncontraceptive benefits not present with MPA. Depomedroxyprogesterone acetate is not a first-line therapy because of the high incidence of irregular bleeding with initiation, along with other side effects such as weight gain.

MENSTRUAL CYCLE RECORD

Month	1	2	3	4	5	6	7	8	9	10	11	12	13	14	15	16	17	18	19	20	21	22	23	24	25	26	27	28	29	30	31
Jan										S	S	S	S	S	B	H	H	B	B	S	S	S	S								
Feb																														X	X
Mar																															
Apr			S	S			S	S	B	B	H	B	B	S								S									X
May	P	P	P	P	P	P	P	P	P	P		S	B	B	H	B	S														
Jun	P	P	P	P	P	P	P	P	P	P		S	B	B	B	S	S													X	
Jul	P	P	P	P	P	P	P	P	P	P			B	B	B	S	S														
Aug																															
Sep																															X
Oct																															
Nov																															X
Dec																															

S–Spotting; B–Bleeding; H–Heavy

FIGURE 6-36.

Example of a menstrual calendar of an anovulating woman. This patient complained of very irregular periods (every 2 to 4 months). Progestin was started the first 10 days of each month on May 1 through 10. The result was regular monthly withdrawal bleeding after the progestin was discontinued.

Month	1	2	3	4	5	6	7	8	9	10	11	12	13	14	15	16	17	18	19	20	21	22	23	24	25	26	27	28	29	30	31
Jan																								S	S	S	S	S	S	S	S
Feb	S	S	S	S	S	B	B	B	B	B	B																			X	X
Mar															S	S									B	B	B	B	B	B	B
Apr																															X
May				S	S	B	B	H	B	S	S	S																			
Jun													S	S	S	S	B	B	B	H	H	S				P	P	P	P	P	X
Jul	P	P	P	P	P			S	S	B	B	B	S								P	P	P	P	P	P	P	P	P	P	P
Aug						S	B	B	B	S	S										P	P	P	P	P	P	P	P	P	P	
Sep	S	B	B	S	S									P	P	P	P	P	P	P	P/S	S	B	B	S						X
Oct				P	P	P	P	P	P	P	P				S	B	B	B	S												
Nov																															X
Dec																															

S—Spotting; B—Bleeding; H—Heavy

FIGURE 6-37.

Example of a menstrual calendar of in a woman with oligo-ovulation. This patient complaining of irregular periods was instructed to begin taking the progestin 14 days after the onset of each menses (cycle day 14) and take for 10 days. If menses started while on the progestin, the medication was to be discontinued and reinitiated 14 days later (*see* September 21).

MEDICATION

MEDICATIONS FOR THE TREATMENT OF MENORRHAGIA

Nonsteroidal anti-inflammatory drugs

Combination oral contraceptives

Oral progestins

Depomedroxyprogesterone acetate

Danazol

Gonadotropin-releasing hormone agonists

Medicated intrauterine devices

FIGURE 6-38.

Medications for the treatment of menorrhagia. Although anovulatory dysfunctional uterine bleeding (DUB) is usually easily managed with monthly progestin therapy to oppose endogenous estrogen, ovulatory DUB may be more difficult to treat with progestins alone.

NONSTEROIDAL ANTI-INFLAMMATORY DRUGS USED FOR THE TREATMENT OF MENORRHAGIA*

Ibuprofen, 800 mg 3–4 × daily

Naproxen sodium, 550 mg 3 × daily

Mefenamic acid, 500 mg 3 × daily

Meclofenamate sodium, 100 mg 3 × daily

Beginning day prior to or first day of menses for 3–5 days.

FIGURE 6-39.

Nonsteroidal anti-inflammatory drugs (NSAIDs) used for the treatment of menorrhagia. NSAIDs have been shown to decrease menstrual blood loss associated with ovulation by 20% to 50%. NSAIDs inhibit the synthesis of prostaglandins and also block their action at the receptor site.

COMBINATION ORAL CONTRACEPTIVES USED FOR THE TREATMENT OF MENORRHAGIA

Very effective in decreasing amount of flow

Also effective in lengthening the number of days between cycles in women complaining of menstrual intervals < 28 days

FIGURE 6-40.

Oral contraceptives (OCs) for the treatment of menorrhagia. OCs are first-line therapy for the treatment of ovulatory dysfunctional uterine bleeding in women without contraindications to their use. Although no comparative studies have shown one OC to be superior to another for the treatment of menorrhagia, more androgenic progestins such as levonorgesterol or norgesterol may be the OC of choice in this scenario. Patients should be advised that several months of therapy may be necessary before full benefit is achieved. Nonsteroidal anti-inflammatory drugs (NSAIDs) can also be added during the pill-free interval to assist in decreasing withdrawal bleeding. Women taking OCs who wish to avoid monthly bleeding may also extend the number of active tablets from 3 weeks to 6, 9, or 12 weeks followed by a 1-week pill-free interval, thus reducing the number of bleeding intervals per year.

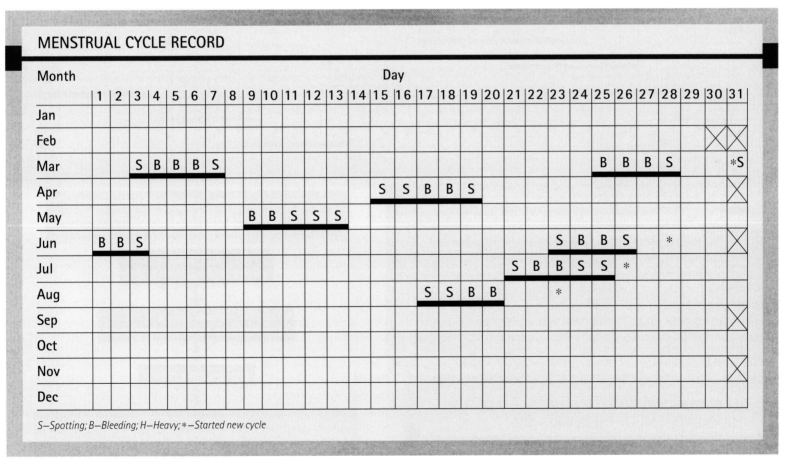

S–Spotting; B–Bleeding; H–Heavy; *–Started new cycle

FIGURE 6-41.

Example of a menstrual calendar of a patient complaining of periods too close together. This patient started on oral contraceptives (OCs) on May 31. (*Asterisk* indicates first day of OC pack). The OCs lengthened the interval between cycles.

ORAL PROGESTINS FOR THE TREATMENT OF MENORRHAGIA

Medroxyprogesterone acetate, 10–30 mg/d

Norethindrone acetate, 5–15 mg/d

Regimen

    Given 12 days of each cycle during luteal phase

    Days 14–25 of cycle if menses ≥ 26 days apart

    Days 12–23 of cycle if menses ≤ 26 days apart

FIGURE 6-42.

Oral progestins for the treatment of menorrhagia. Although oral progestins are a commonly prescribed treatment for ovulatory dysfunctional uterine bleeding (DUB), there is little documented efficacy that they significantly reduce menstrual blood flow. The use of progestins is primarily effective for the treatment of anovulatory DUB. If a trial of progestins is initiated for ovulatory DUB, they should be given in relatively high doses in the luteal phase of the cycle for 12 days. Use of nonsteroidal anti-inflammatory drugs during menses may also be beneficial. The patient should be instructed to keep a menstrual calendar to document when they take their progestin and record days of flow quantitatively. If discussion with the patient and review of the calendar reveals no improvement after 3 months, another form of therapy should be attempted.

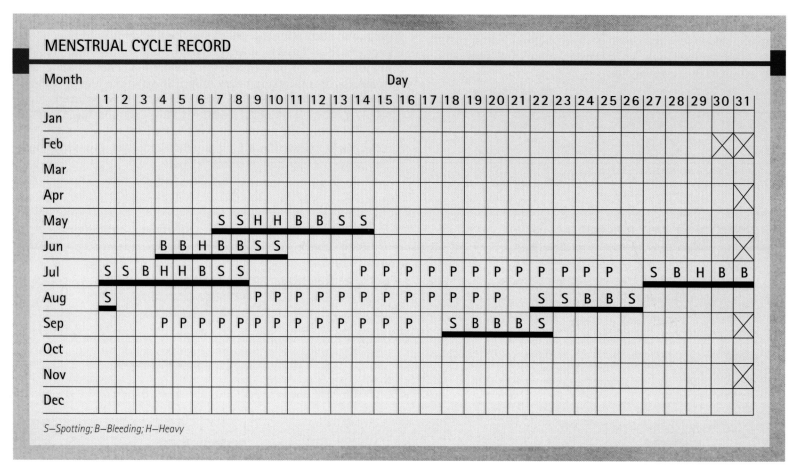

MENSTRUAL CYCLE RECORD

Month	\\ Day 1	2	3	4	5	6	7	8	9	10	11	12	13	14	15	16	17	18	19	20	21	22	23	24	25	26	27	28	29	30	31
Jan																															
Feb																														X	X
Mar																															
Apr																															X
May							S	S	H	H	B	B	S	S																	
Jun				B	B	H	B	B	S	S																				X	
Jul	S	S	B	H	H	B	S	S						P	P	P	P	P	P	P	P	P	P	P	P	P	S	B	H	B	B
Aug	S								P	P	P	P	P	P	P	P	P	P	P	P	P	S	S	B	B	S					
Sep				P	P	P	P	P	P	P	P	P	P	P	P	P	P	S	B	B	B	S									X
Oct																															
Nov																															X
Dec																															

S–Spotting; B–Bleeding; H–Heavy

FIGURE 6-43.

Example of a menstrual calendar of a patient complaining of regular but heavy periods. The patient was given a progestin for 12 days starting 14 days after onset of each period (cycle day 14). The patient also took ibuprofen, 800 mg 3 times daily, starting with onset of flow for 3 to 5 days. The result was decreased amount and number of days of flow.

DEPOMEDROXYPROGESTERONE ACETATE FOR THE TREATMENT OF MENORRHAGIA

Dose: 150–250 mg intramuscularly every 2–3 mos

Disadvantage

    High incidence of irregular bleeding

FIGURE 6-44.

Depomedroxyprogesterone acetate (DMPA) for the treatment of menorrhagia. Intramuscular DMPA can be given as a treatment for ovulatory dysfunctional uterine bleeding. Most patients will eventually become amenorrheic, but this will require up to 1 to 2 years of injections in some patients. DMPA is not a first-line therapy because of its associated high incidence of irregular bleeding and other side effects, including weight gain.

DANAZOL FOR THE TREATMENT OF MENORRHAGIA

Description
    Synthetic steroid derivative with androgenic properties
Dose
    200 mg/d
Disadvantages
    Androgenic side effects
    Expensive

FIGURE 6-45.

Danazol for the treatment of menorrhagia. Danazol is a synthetic steroid derivative of 17 alpha-ethinyltestosterone. It inhibits sex steroid synthesis, competitively binds to androgen receptors and, in high doses, inhibits ovulation. Several studies have documented its effectiveness in reducing menstrual blood loss. Although higher doses (400 mg/d) are more effective in inducing amenorrhea by creating an atrophic endometrium, long-term use is associated with unacceptable androgenic side effects. Reducing the dose to 200 mg/d decreases side effects without altering efficacy. Further reductions to 50–100 mg/d decrease side effects but are not as effective in reducing mean blood loss. Although effective in reducing mean blood loss, long-term use of danazol is not appropriate for most women because of the high incidence of androgenic side effects (acne, weight gain), and the expense of therapy.

GONADOTROPIN-RELEASING HORMONE AGONISTS FOR THE TREATMENT OF MENORRHAGIA

Mechanism of action
    Inhibits ovulation and ovarian steroid production, inducing
        amenorrhea
Dose
    Depoleuprolide, 3.75 mg intramuscularly every month
Disadvantages
    Expense
    Hypoestrogenic state

FIGURE 6-46.

Gonadotropin-releasing hormone (GnRH) agonists for the treatment of menorrhagia. GnRH agonists such as depoleuprolide are very effective in inducing amenorrhea. Long-term therapy as a treatment of ovulatory dysfunctional uterine bleeding (DUB) is not practical because of expense and hypoestrogenic sequelae, including vasomotor symptoms, vaginal dryness, and risk of osteoporosis. If a patient has severe menorrhagia and anemia, GnRH agonists may be used short term to quickly induce amenorrhea and correct the severe anemia.

MEDICATED PROGESTIN INTRAUTERINE DEVICES FOR THE TREATMENT OF MENORRHAGIA

Effective in reducing mean blood loss in ovulatory dysfunctional
    uterine bleeding by 50%–100%
Progesterone: effective for 1 y
Levonorgesterol: effective for 7 y

FIGURE 6-47.

Medicated intrauterine devices (IUDs) for the treatment of menorrhagia. Although copper-containing IUDs may increase mean blood loss, hormonal IUDs have been shown to decrease menstrual blood loss in ovulatory women. The progestin-releasing IUD is effective for only 1 year, with mean blood loss reduction of over 50%. The levonorgesterol-releasing IUD is effective for 7 years, with most patients amenorrheic at 1 year, but is not available in the United States.

SURGICAL TREATMENT FOR ABNORMAL UTERINE BLEEDING

Operative hysteroscopy/fractional D & C
    Direct visualization and removal of intraluminal lesions
Endometrial Ablation
    Menorrhagia not responsive to medical management
    Small intraluminal lesions (submucosal fibroids, endometrial
       polyps) may be removed concurrently
    Future childbearing not desired
    Contraindicated in the presence of endometrial hyperplasia
       or cancer
Hysterectomy
    Failed medical management of AUB
    Severe atypical endometrial hyperplasia
    Other coexistent gynecologic problems (eg, large myomatous
       uterus, prolapse, stress incontinence, endometriosis)

FIGURE 6–48.

Surgical treatment for abnormal uterine bleeding (AUB). Although most cases of AUB can be managed medically, surgical procedures are necessary to remove intraluminal lesions and treat patients in whom medical management is unsatisfactory. Patients in whom medical management fails may be candidates for endometrial ablation, but endometrial neoplasia must first be ruled out.

Endometrial ablation is an alternative surgical therapy for menorrhagia (ovulatory AUB). The presence of AUB due to oligo- or anovulatory cycles is not ideal for endometrial ablation, because residual endometrium will continue to be at increased risk of transformation to adenomatous hyperplasia and cancer unless cyclic progestins are continued postoperatively. Endometrial ablation may be combined with resection of small (< 2 to 3 cm diameter) submucous myomas or polyps in patients with these intraluminal lesions and menorrhagia. Hysterectomy should be considered in patients in whom medical management fails or who have atypical hyperplasia or other coexistent gynecologic problems. D & C—dilation and curettage.

SUGGESTED BIBLIOGRAPHY

Abnormal uterine bleeding: ovulatory and anovulatory dysfunctional uterine bleeding, management of acute and chronic excessive bleeding. In *Comprehensive Gynecology*. Edited by Mishell DR, Stenchever MA, Droegemueller W, Herbst AL. St. Louis: Mosby; 1997:1025–1042.

Cameron IT, Haining R, Lumsden M, *et al.*: The effects of mefenamic acid and norethisterone on measured menstrual blood loss. *Obstet Gynecol* 1990, 76:85–88.

Chamberlain G, Freeman R, Price F, *et al.*: A comparative study of ethamsylate and mefenamic acid in dysfunctional uterine bleeding. *Br J Obstet Gynecol* 1991, 98:707–711.

Cherkis RC, Patten SF, Dickinson JC: Significance of atypical endometrial cells detected by cervical cytology. *Obstet Gynecol* 1987, 69:786–789.

Cherkis RC, Patten SF, Dickinson JC: Significance of normal endometrial cells detected by cervical cytology. *Obstet Gynecol* 1988, 71:242–244.

Chimbira TH, Anderson AB, Turnbull AC: Relation between measured menstrual blood loss and patients: subjective assessment of loss, duration of bleeding, number of sanitary towels used, uterine weight and endometrial surface area. *Br J Obstet Gynaecol* 1980, 87:603–609.

Claessens EA, Cowell CA: Acute adolescent menorrhagia. *Am J Obstet Gynecol* 1981, 139:277–280.

Crosignani PG, Vercellini P, Mosconi P, *et al.*: Levonorgestrel-releasing intrauterine device versus hysteroscopic endometrial resection in the treatment of dysfunctional uterine bleeding. *Obstet Gynecol* 1997, 90:257–263.

Derman SG, Rehnstrom J, Neuwirth RS: The long-term effectiveness of hysteroscopic treatment of menorrhagia and leiomyomas. *Obstet Gynecol* 1991, 77:591–594.

Dysfunctional uterine bleeding. In *Clinical Gynecologic Endocrinology and Infertility*. Edited by Speroff L, Glass RH, Kase NG. Baltimore: Williams & Wilkins; 1994:531–546.

Fraser IS, Pearse C, Shearman RP: Efficacy of mefenamic acid in patients with a complaint of menorrhagia. *Obstet Gynecol* 1981, 58:543–551.

Fraser IS, McCarron G: Randomized trial of 2 hormonal and 2 prostaglandin-inhibiting agents in women with a complaint of menorrhagia. *Aust N Z J Obstet Gynecol* 1991, 31:66–70.

Fraser IS, McCarron G, Markham R: A preliminary study of factors influencing perception of menstrual blood loss volume. *Am J Obstet Gynecol* 1984, 149:788.

Grimes DA: Diagnostic dilation and curettage: a reappraisal. *Am J Obstet Gynecol* 1982, 142:1–6.

Hall P, Maclachlan N, Thorn N, *et al.*: Control of menorrhagia by the cyclo-oxygenase inhibitors naproxen sodium and mefenamic acid. *Br J Obstet Gynaecol* 1987, 94:554–558.

Haynes PJ, Hodgson H, Anderson AB, Turnbull AC: Measurement of menstrual blood loss in patients complaining of menorrhagia. *Br J Obstet Gynecol* 1977, 84:763–768.

Karlsson B, Granberg S, Wikland M, *et al.*: Transvaginal ultrasonography of the endometrium in women with postmenopausal bleeding: a Nordic multicenter study. *Am J Obstet Gynecol* 1995, 172:1488–1494.

Larsson G, Milsom I, Lindstedt G, Rybo G: The influence of a low-dose combined oral contraceptive on menstrual blood loss and iron status. *Contraception* 1992, 46:327–334.

Nygren KG, Rybo G: Prostaglandins and menorrhagia. *Acta Obstet Gynecol Scand* 1983, suppl 113:101–103.

Preston JT, Cameron IT, Adams EJ, Smith SK: Comparative study of tranexamic acid and norethisterone in the treatment of ovulatory menorrhagia. *Br J Obstet Gynaecol* 1995, 102:401–406.

Primary and secondary amenorrhea: etiology, diagnostic evaluation, management. In *Comprehensive Gynecology*. Edited by Mishell DR, Stenchever MA, Droegemueller W, Herbst AL. St. Louis: Mosby; 1997:1043–1067.

Shaw RW: Assessment of medical treatments for menorrhagia [conference proceedings]. *Br J Obstet Gynecol* 1994, 101(suppl 11):15–18.

Stovall TG, Photopulos GJ, Poston WM, *et al.*: Pipelle endometrial sampling in patients with known endometrial carcinoma. *Obstet Gynecol* 1991, 77:954–956.

Tang GWK, Lo SST: Levonorgestrel intrauterine device in the treatment of menorrhagia in Chinese women: efficacy versus acceptability. *Contraception* 1995, 51:231–235.

Vargyas JM, Campeau JD, Mishell DR: Treatment of menorrhagia with meclofenamate sodium. *Am J Obstet Gynecol* 1987, 157:944–950.

Premenstrual Syndrome

Monica McKinnon and
Veronica Ravnikar

Premenstrual syndrome (PMS) is a group of cognitive, somatic, and affective symptoms that present in the luteal phase of the menstrual cycle and remit shortly after the onset of menses. The cause of PMS remains a mystery and is presumably multifactorial. There is increasing evidence that serotonin-mediated brain neurotransmission may be responsible, in part, for PMS symptoms [1]. The serotonin reuptake inhibitors (*eg*, fluoxetine) are the recommended first-line therapy for PMS. Other medical therapy has been shown to be somewhat effective in treating PMS and should be tailored to the individual patient's symptoms and needs. It is obvious that more extensive research is needed to discover the exact mechanism of PMS; however, most women with PMS can be helped with the information and therapies available today.

Regarding surgical treatment of PMS, hysterectomy with removal of the ovaries has been the definitive treatment of severe PMS. If the ovaries are left behind, PMS-like symptoms may still occur. Because surgery is quite radical, medical therapies should be investigated thoroughly before surgical therapy is considered.

SYMPTOMS

A. COGNITIVE AND AFFECTIVE SYMPTOMS OF PREMENSTRUAL SYNDROME

Aggression	Hostility
Altered libido	Insomnia
Anger	Irritability
Anxiety	Lack of concentration
Decreased motivation	Mood swings
Depression	Panic attack
Food cravings	Tearfulness
Forgetfulness	

B. SOMATIC SYMPTOMS OF PREMENSTRUAL SYNDROME

Abdominal bloating	Fatigue
Acne	Headaches
Bloating	Hot flashes
Breast tenderness	Muscle aches
Constipation	Palpitations
Dizziness	Weight gain

FIGURE 7–1.

Symptoms of premenstrual syndrome (PMS). PMS is characterized by a collection of cognitive, somatic, and affective symptoms that repeatedly occur during the luteal phase of the menstrual cycle and remit shortly after the onset of menses. Symptoms can be severe enough to interfere with routine activities and interpersonal relationships. Some of these symptoms include irritability, insomnia, hopelessness, poor concentration, marked anger, abdominal bloating, fatigue, breast tenderness, and fluid retention [2].

A, Cognitive and affective symptoms of PMS. **B**, Somatic symptoms of PMS. **C**, Presenting symptoms for PMS treatment. The patients in this study (*n* = 241) identified their three worst symptoms (percentages equal >100). Note that the affective symptoms—depression, irritability, anxiety—are most predominant. (*Adapted from* Freeman and coworkers [3].)

C. PRESENTING SYMPTOMS FOR PREMENSTRUAL SYNDROME

Symptom (%)	Food cravings (9)
Depression (56)	Anger (8)
Irritability (48)	Backache (6)
Anxiety (36)	Nervousness (5)
Mood swings (26)	Breast tenderness (5)
Headache (23)	Dizziness (3)
Bloating, swelling (22)	Loss of sexual desire (2)
Cramps (21)	Other (11)
Fatigue (19)	

SYMPTOMS OF PREMENSTRUAL DYSPHORIC DISORDER

A. Symptoms must occur during week before menses and remit a few days after onset of menses.

Five of the following symptoms must be present and at least one must be classified 1, 2, 3, or 4

1. Depressed mood
2. Anxiety
3. Lability
4. Irritability
5. Decreased interest in usual activities
6. Difficulty in concentrating
7. Marked lack of energy
8. Marked change in appetite, overeating, or food cravings
9. Hypersominia or insominia
10. Sense of being overwhelmed
11. Other physical symptoms, *eg*, breast tenderness and headaches

B. Symptoms must interfere with work, school, usual activities, or relationships

C. Symptoms must not merely be an exaceration of another disorder

D. Criteria A, B, and C must be confirmed by prospective daily ratings for at least two cycles

FIGURE 7–2.

Symptoms of premenstrual dysphoric disorder (PDD). The American Psychiatric Association has acknowledged this severe form of premenstrual syndrome (PMS) in the *Diagnostic and Statistical Manual of Mental Disorders* edition 4. The term "PMS" now describes a more general variant of the syndrome. However, in most cases "PMS" is generally still used. The criteria for the diagnosis of PDD must include five of 11 specific symptoms. (*Adapted from* the American Psychiatric Association [2].)

EPIDEMIOLOGY AND PATHOPHYSIOLOGY

CAUSES OF PREMENSTRUAL SYNDROME

Serotonin dysregulation

Norepinephrine abnormalities

Hyperprolactinemia

Renin-angiotensin system dysregulation

Vitamin B deficiency

Magnesium deficiency

Theory of sensitization

Hormonal changes

Prostaglandin abnormalities

Abnormal opioid activity

Vitamin E deficiency

Calcium deficiency

Panic threshold hypothesis

FIGURE 7-3.

Proposed causes of premenstrual syndrome (PMS). Approximately 75% of the female population of reproductive age complain of some premenstrual symptoms, most often including dysmenorrhea, irritability, and anxiety (see Fig. 7-1C). Approximately 40% of these women experience true premenstrual dysphoric disorder (PDD) to a certain degree [4]. Regarding the diagnosis of PDD, approximately 4% of menstruating women

meet criteria for diagnosis after prospective symptom charting [5]. Studies have yet to show an unequivocal association between PMS and age, socioecomonic status, parity, diet, exercise, stress, menstrual cycle characteristics, or personality [6].

Although there are many theories of the mechanism of premenstrual syndrome (PMS), the exact cause remains unsolved. The most recent data have shown that serotonin function may be altered in women with PMS or PDD. Because PMS involves an alteration in mood and anxiety, abnormalities in neurotransmitters have been investigated.

Some studies have suggested that abnormalities in the norepinephrine system may play a role [5]; however, more studies are needed to support this theory. Regarding the role of the hypothalamic-pituitary-adrenal axis, the opiate system, prostaglandins, the renin-angiotensin system, vitamins, and minerals, no clear association between these factors and PMS has been documented [5].

Other proposed causes of PMS have focused on the panic threshold hypothesis and the theory of sensitization. The panic threshold hypothesis suggests that as progesterone levels fall in the luteal phase and pCO_2 rises, women with a low threshold for the suffocation alarm system may suffer panic symptoms, and thus PMS symptoms [7]. The theory of sensitization focuses on the fact that the menstrual cycle is a repetitive stimulus, which may explain the gradual worsening of symptoms in some women. To date, however, no empiric evidence has been found in humans to support the theory of sensitization [6]. The cause of PMS is most likely multifactorial and quite complex. It is likely that the cause of PMS will be found to involve the gonadal steroids and their interaction with the neurotransmitter, neuroendocrine, and circadian systems that influence mood, behavior, and cognition [5].

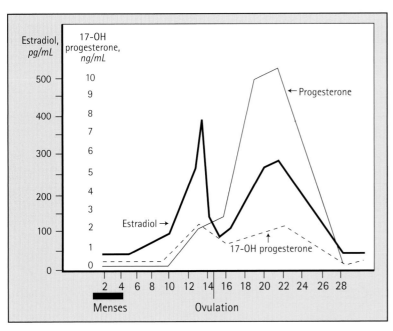

FIGURE 7-4.

Hormonal fluctuation of the menstrual cycle. Estradiol and progesterone levels are shown at various times during the menstrual cycle. Ovarian steroid hormones interact with the central nervous system at multiple levels, although the details of this interaction are not yet clear. Ovarian steroid hormones can directly affect neurotransmitters in the following ways: 1) their synthesis, release, reuptake, and

enzymatic inactivation, and the sensitivity of presynaptic and postsynaptic receptors; 2) they can couple to second messenger systems within the cell and exert influence through genomic action; and 3) they can act directly on the nerve membrane, affecting its excitability [5]. Increasing evidence suggests that serotonin dysregulation may be linked to the cause of PMS. Steiner and colleagues [8] showed that fluoxetine, which selectively inhibits the reuptake of serotonin, was significantly superior to placebo in reducing symptoms of tension, irritability, and dysphoria (see Fig. 7-7A). Sayegh and colleagues [1] recently showed that a carbohydrate-rich beverage designed to increase serum tryptophan (a precursor of serotonin) levels relieves mood and appetite disturbances and also improves certain aspects of memory (Fig. 7-7B).

Many studies in the past have tried to document an association between PMS and changes in hormone levels. Such an association does make sense because the symptoms of PMS coincide with the cyclical changes of progesterone and estrogen. Conversely, however, studies have not found consistent evidence regarding the hypothalamic-pituitary-gonadal axis in women with PMS compared with control subjects [5]. Schmit and colleagues [9], using the antiprogesterone agent RU 486, found that the agent did not eliminate the symptoms of PMS and that PMS could occur in the absence of the luteal phase of the menstrual cycle. The current literature does not support abnormalities in other hormone levels involved in the menstrual cycle as well (follicle-stimulating hormone, luteinizing hormone , prolactin, sex hormone–binding globulin, testosterone) [6]. (*Adapted from* Speroff and coworkers [10].)

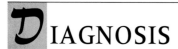

DIAGNOSIS

MENSTRUAL SYMPTOM DIARY

Name: _____

	Date																												
	Day of Cycle	1	2	3	4	5	6	7	8	9	10	11	12	13	14	15	16	17	18	19	20	21	22	23	24	25	26	27	28
	Menstruation																												
	Nervous tension																												
	Mood swings																												
	Irritability																												
	Anxiety																												
	Depression																												
	Crying																												
	Forgetfulness																												
	Confusion																												
	Insomnia																												
	Increased naps																												
	Avoid activities																												
	Feel clumsy																												
	Fatigue																												
	Breast tenderness																												
	Abdominal bloating																												
	Swelling (legs, hands)																												
	Headaches																												
	Migraine headaches																												
	Hot flashes																												
	Abdominal cramps																												
	General aches																												
	Food cravings: salt																												
	sweets																												
	Skin problems																												
	Weight																												
	Basal body temperature																												

Grading of menses
1. Light
2. Moderate
3. Heavy
4. Heavy with clots

Grading of symptoms
0 None
1 Mild (does not interfere with activities)
2 Moderate (interferes with activities)
3 Severe (disabling; unable to function)

FIGURE 7–5.

Menstrual symptom diary. The second important step in the diagnosis is prospective charting by the patient of her symptoms regarding her menstrual cycles. This charting should be performed for at least two to three consecutive menstrual cycles. The patient's daily records should then be reviewed with a focus on the timing and severity of symptoms. To diagnose premenstrual syndrome (PMS), the symptoms should be related to the menstrual cycle: high incidence in the week before menstruation and low incidence in the week that follows menstruation [6]. The severity of the symptoms should be severe enough to disrupt routine activity and there should be an increase from postmenstrual levels [6]. (See Fig. 7-2 for diagnosis of premenstrual dysphoric disorder.)

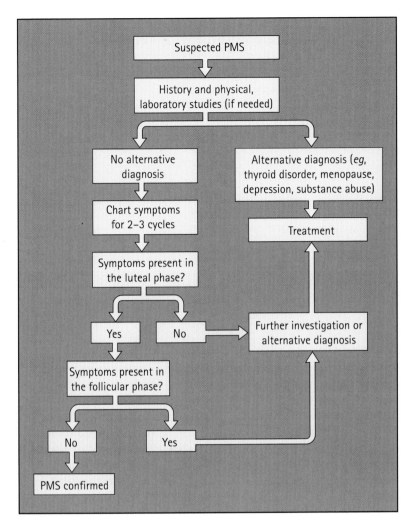

FIGURE 7–6.

Diagnostic procedure for suspected premenstrual syndrome (PMS). A complete history and physical examination must be performed first. A pelvic examination should also be done. The history may show that the patient has another disorder that needs further investigation (*eg*, major depression, personality disorder, panic disorder). No laboratory tests can be performed to make the diagnosis of PMS. Of course, if it seems necessary in a particular patient to rule out other causes for her symptoms, such as menopause or thyroid disease, this should be performed in the initial work-up.

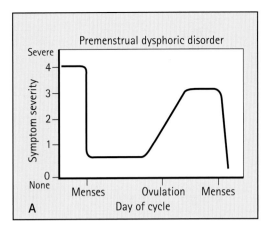

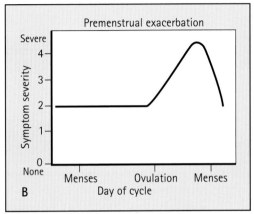

FIGURE 7–7.

Graphic representation of daily symptom charting. **A**, Daily symptom charting results of a woman with premenstrual dysphoric disorder (PDD). Symptoms are absent during the follicular phase, but at ovulation or shortly after, symptoms begin to increase in intensity to moderate-to-severe levels. Symptoms are alleviated within the first few days of menses following the cycle. **B**, Daily symptom charting results of a woman with premenstrual exacerbation. Symptoms (*eg*, depression, irritability) are rated as mild to moderate during the follicular phase. At or shortly after ovulation, symptoms increase in intensity to moderate-to-severe level. After the first few days of menses of following cycle, symptom severity returns to baseline mild-to-moderate level. (*Adapted from* Pearlstein [5].)

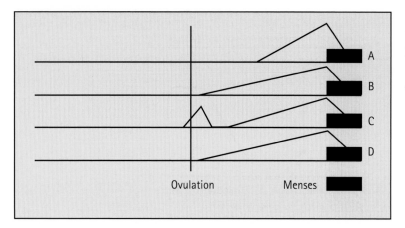

FIGURE 7-8.
Variability in onset and duration of premenstrual symptoms. Most patients experience patterns A or B (symptoms are confined to the luteal phase and terminate rapidly at menstruation). (*Adapted from* Ferin and coworkers [11].)

TREATMENT

PSYCHOSOCIAL INTERVENTIONS FOR PREMENSTRUAL SYNDROME

Education*

    Physiology of the normal menstrual cycle

    Hormones and associated symptoms

Stress management and coping skills †

    Biofeedback

    Self-hypnosis

    Deep-breathing techniques, yoga, other relaxation techniques

Environmental changes

    Alteration of the physical surroundings of the home or office through the use of color, music, plants, artwork, and so on

    Selection of a private, quiet place for "time-out"

    Adequate rest and sleep

    Regular exercise

*Religious and cultural factors may need to be addressed, and the patient's family members and/or significant others should also be educated about the syndrome.
† The patient should avoid planning stressful events during the time when premenstrual symtoms are most prevalent.

FIGURE 7-9.
Psychosocial interventions for premenstrual syndrome (PMS). A number of treatments for PMS have been proposed over the years. The symptoms associated with PMS are usually multiple; therefore single therapy may not be effective. Treatments include diet, vitamins, minerals, exercise, surgery, hormonal manipulation, and pharmacotherapy. Because not all these studies have been subjected to double-blind crossover studies with placebo, the placebo effects are questionable. The current recommendation for first-line therapy at present is serotonergic antidepressants. In addition to existing treatments, several psychosocial interventions—education, stress management, and environmental changes—may also be effective. (*Adapted from* Parker [4].)

PHARMACOTHERAPY FOR PREMENSTRUAL SYNDROME

Agent	Proven benefit	Side effects	PMS symptoms
Diuretics	Negative	Hypotension, electrolyte imbalance	Water retention/bloating
Atenolol	Negative	Hypotension, gastrointestinal upset, depression, insomnia, decreased HDL, increased triglycerides	Anxiety
Prostaglandin inhibitors	Positive	Adnominal pain, diarrhea, gastritis, acute renal failure, interstitial nephritis, nephrotic syndrome	Muscle aches, mastalgia
Bromocriptine	Positive	Gastrointestinal upset, hypotension, arrhythmias	Mastalgia
Serotonergic antidepressants	Positive	Anxiety, insomnia, gastrointestinal symptoms	Psychologic
Tricyclic antidepressants	Positive	Sedation, hypotension, arrhythmias, blurred vision, constipation, seizures, sexual disturbance	Psychologic
Anxiolytics (alprazolam)	Positive	Sedation, addictive potential, additive CNS depression	Psychologic/anxiety
Nonbenzodiazepine anxiolytics (buspirone)	Positive (more trials needed)	Similar to anxiolytics, but reduced side effects	Psychologic/anxiety

FIGURE 7-10.

Pharmacotherapy for premenstrual syndrome (PMS). Studies involving serotonergic antidepressants have thus far proven their efficacy and easy tolerability [6]. In a double-blind crossover study using fluoxetine (20 or 60 mg/d), Steiner and colleagues [8] fluoxetine was found to be effective in decreasing the psychologic symptoms of tension, irritability, and dysphoria in women with premenstrual dysphoric disorder (PDD). This study also showed that 20 mg/d resulted in side-effects that were more similar to placebo, and thus there is no reason to use the higher dose of 60 mg/d [8]. There have also been some studies showing sertraline to be superior to placebo for treatment of PDD [5].

Tricyclic antidepressants have demonstrated a reduction in premenstrual symptoms; however, a higher rate of side-effects has been noted [6]. Anxiolytics have also been investigated for efficacy. The largest study of alprazolam did show modest efficacy for PMS symptoms [12], and it is also convenient that alprazolam is effective if administered only in the luteal phase.

Benzodiazepines cause drowsiness and can be addictive; however, if used in the luteal phase only, dependency has not been shown [12]. Buspirone, a nonbenzodiazepine anxiolytic, has been noted to be effective; however, large trials to confirm these findings are needed [6].

Diuretics can improve bloating and weight gain; however, side-effects with diuretics, such as hypotension and electrolyte imbalances, must be noted. There has not been any proven benefit for the use of diuretics in PMS and therefore they are not recommended [6]. Research does not support the use of atenolol in the treatment of PMS [6]. Prostaglandin inhibitors may relieve some of the somatic complaints of PMS, but they do not treat the affective symptoms and therefore have very limited use. Bromocriptine, a dopamine-receptor agonist, may also be helpful with somatic complaints (mastalgia); however, it does not help mood and anxiety related to PMS [6]. CNS—central nervous system; HDL—high-density lipoprotein.

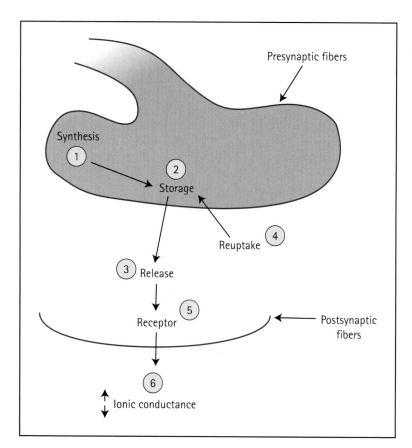

FIGURE 7-11.

Mechanics of serotonin reuptake inhibitors. Serotonin reuptake inhibitors block serotonin uptake at presynaptic nerve endings (site 4). The blocking of serotonin uptake increases serotonin (neurotransmitter) in the synapse and on postsynaptic receptors (site 5). (*Adapted from* Katzung [13].)

FIGURE 7-12.

Chemical structure of fluoxetine. (*Adapted from* Katzung [13].)

HORMONAL THERAPY FOR PREMENSTRUAL SYNDROME

Agent	Proven benefit	Side effects	PMS symptoms
GnRH agonists	Positive (short term only)	Osteoporosis, heart disease, menopausal symptoms	Psychologic/somatic
Danazol	Positive (short term only)	See GnRH agonists	Psychologic/somatic
OCs	Positive/negative	Minimal	Psychologic/somatic
Progesterone	Negative	Minimal	Psychologic/somatic

FIGURE 7-13.

Hormonal therapy for treatment of premenstrual syndrome (PMS). Gonadotropin-releasing hormone (GnRH) agonists disrupt the production of follicle-stimulating hormone and luteinizing hormone and eliminate ovulation and sex steroids. One such medication is Depo-Lupron (TAP Pharmaceuticals Inc: Deerfield, IL). This therapy has been shown to be effective, but has major side-effects if used longer than 6 months. The hypoestrogenic state created by these medications can cause menopausal symptoms, and increases the risk for osteoporosis and heart disease. GnRH therapy with estrogen and progesterone add-back therapy possibly may be used; however, studies have shown that there is some loss of efficacy using this regimen [5].

Regarding oral contraceptives (OCs), there is some evidence that certain patients may benefit; however, the efficacy of OCs in the treatment of PMS has not been proven and is therefore not recommended for first-line therapy [6]. Although progesterone supplementation was once a popular treatment for PMS, there is no evidence from studies that any form of progesterone is more effective than placebo [6]. Therefore, progesterone supplementation for treatment of PMS symptoms is not recommended.

DIETARY MODIFICATION FOR TREATMENT OF PREMENSTRUAL SYNDROME

Agent	Proven benefit	Side effects	PMS symptoms
Carbohydrate-rich beverage	Positive	Nonexistent	Mood, appetite, and cognitive disturbances
Vitamin E	Positive (more studies needed)	Minimal	Mood, appetite
Vitamin B$_6$	Negative	Neurotoxicity	Fatigue, irritability, depression
Calcium	Positive (more studies needed)	Minimal	Depression, irritability, headaches, back pain
Magnesium	Positive (more studies needed)	Minimal	Mood disturbances, water retention
Evening primrose oil	Negative	Minimal	Water retention, weight gain
St. John's Wort (*hypericum perforatum*)	Positive negative (PMS studies needed)	Minimal	Depression

FIGURE 7–14.

Dietary modification for the treatment of premenstrual syndrome (PMS). Although dietary modification has not been evaluated in controlled trials, it does no harm to recommend to patients that they eat well-balanced meals to improve their sense of well-being. Food that is high in sugars and salt should probably be avoided because these foods may promote water retention [4]. The avoidance of caffeine and alcohol is also recommended because they tend to increase anxiety and irritability.

It has been hypothesized that women with PMS may increase their intake of carbohydrate-rich foods in an unconscious attempt to increase their serotonin level. Sayegh *et al.* [1], using a specially formulated carbohydrate beverage known to increase tryptophan and thus serotonin, showed the beverage to be effective in improving mood, appetite, and some cognitive disturbances. One product currently available called "PMS Escape" (Intra Nutria, Framingham, MA) indeed aims at increasing serotonin levels. This over-the-counter carbohydrate beverage is rich in tryptophan and may be beneficial to some patients.

Vitamin E has been of interest in treating PMS. High-dose treatment (400 IU/d) has been associated with a reduction in mood symptoms and food cravings [6]. Vitamin E does not help physical symptoms and there is not enough concrete evidence demonstrating its effectiveness in the treatment of PMS.

There is no good evidence to support the use of Vitamin B$_6$ in the treatment of PMS. Vitamin B$_6$ is also associated with the development of neurotoxicity, even at low doses (50 mg/d) [4]. In light of this information, vitamin B$_6$ is not advocated for the treatment of PMS.

Calcium (1 g/d) may reduce depression, irritability, headaches, and back pain [4], and is recommended for women in the prevention of osteoporosis. Although there have not been many studies on calcium, it is beneficial and may be used for PMS either alone or with other medical treatments. Magnesium (360 mg/d) may improve mood and water retention [4] in PMS; again, more studies are needed. Evening primrose oil has also been studied but is generally considered not to be helpful [5].

A product that has recently become popular in the United States is St. John's Wort. This product is an extract of the plant *Hypericum perforatum* and is available in natural food stores. Hypericum extracts consist of approximately 10 constituents, including naphthodianthrons, flavonoids, xanthones, and bioflavonoids [14]. The mechanism of action of this herb is unclear at this time [14]. St. John's Wort has been used for depression and has been shown in some studies to be superior to placebo for the treatment of depression [14]. Studies have suggested that the side-effects are rare and mild; however, long-term side-effect information is lacking. The comparison of St. John's Wort with other antidepressants is also lacking at this time. In light of the fact that there has been no scientific data in regards to St. John's Wort in the treatment of PMS, this herb cannot be recommended for treatment at this time. This herb may be the treatment of the future because of its effectiveness in the treatment of depression and the low side-effect profile observed thus far.

REFERENCES

1. Sayegh R, Schiff I, Wurtman J, *et al.*: The effect of a carbohydrate-rich beverage on mood, appetite, and cognitive function in women with premenstrual syndrome. *Obstet Gynecol* 1995, 86:520–528.

2. American Psychiatric Association: *Diagnostic and Statistical Manual for Mental Disorders*, edn 4. Washington, DC: American Psychiatric Association; 1994.

3. Freeman E, Sondheimer S, Weinbaum P, *et al.*: Evaluating premenstrual symptoms in medical practice. *Obstet Gynecol* 1985, 65:500–505.

4. Parker P: Premenstrual syndrome. *Am Fam Phys* 1994, 50:1309–1317.

5. Pearlstein T: Hormones and depression: what are the facts about premenstrual syndrome, menopause, and hormone replacement therapy? *Am J Obstet Gynecol* 1995, 173:646–653.

6. Barnhart K, Freeman E, Sondheimer S: A clinician's guide to the premenstrual syndrome. *Med Clin North Am* 1995, 79:1457–1471.

7. Klein D: False suffocation alarms, spontaneous panics, and related conditions: an integrative hypothesis. *Arch Gen Psychiatry* 1993, 50:306–317.

8. Steiner M, Steinberg S, Stewart D, *et al.*: Fluoxetine in the treatment of premenstrual dysphoria. *N Engl J Med* 1995, 332:1529–1534.

9. Schmit P, Nieman L, Grover G, *et al.*: Lack of effect of induced menses on symptoms in women with premenstrual syndrome. *N Engl J Med* 1992, 324:1174–1179.

10. Speroff L, Glass R, Kase N: Regulation of the menstrual cycle *Clinical Gynecologic Endocrinology and Infertility* edn 5. Baltimore: Williams & Wilkins; 1994:183-230.

11. Ferin M, Jewelewicz R, Warren M: The premenstrual syndrome. In *The Menstrual Cycle*. New York: Oxford University Press; 1993:198–204.

12. Freeman E, Rickels K, Sondheimer S, *et al.*: A double blind trial of oral progesterone, alprazolam and placebo in treatment of severe premenstrual syndrome. *JAMA* 1995, 274:51–57.

13. Katzung B: *Basic and Clinical Pharmacology*, edn 5. East Norwalk, CT: Appleton & Lange; 1992: 297–413.

14. Linde K, Ramirez G, Mulrow C, *et al.*: St. John's Wort for depression: an overview and meta-analysis of randomised clinical trials. *BMJ* 1996, 313:253–258.

SELECTED BIBLIOGRAPHY

Barbieri R, Schiff I: *Reproductive Endocrine Therapeutics*. New York: Alan R. Liss; 1988:201.

Prior J, Gill K, Vigna Y: Fluoxetine for premenstrual dysphoria. *N Engl J Med* 1995, 333:1152–1153.

Ragan P: Greater alcohol use in women with PMS. *Am J Psychiatry* 1995, 152:1539–1540.

Rubinow D, Schmidt P: The treatment of premenstrual syndrome: forward into the past. *N Engl J Med* 1995, 332:1574–1575.

Su T, Schmidt P, Danaceau M, *et al.*: Effect of menstrual cycle phase on neuroendocrine and behavioral responses to the serotonin agonist m-chlorophenylpiperazine in women with premenstrual syndrome and controls. *J Clin Endocrinol Metab* 1997, 82:1220–1228.

van Leudsen H: Premenstrual syndrome no progesterone; premenstrual dysphoric disorder no serotonin deficiency. *Lancet* 1995, 346:1443–1444.

Menopause

Donna Shoupe

Natural menopause is defined as permanent cessation of menstruation due to failure of ovarian follicular development in the presence of adequate gonadotropin stimulation. The decline of ovarian function is a gradual process that begins at age 35, when the ovary begins to shrink in size. As ovarian estradiol production gradually declines, early problems associated with estrogen deficiency begin to appear. The transitional period, or perimenopause, lasts from age 40 to 55, during which time there is a progressive decline in estradiol and progesterone production and, to a lesser extent, declines in testosterone and androstenedione secretion.

Over time, the loss of ovarian sex hormone production takes a heavier toll. The perimenopausal and early menopausal complaints of hot flushes, mood swings, depression, and vaginal dryness progress to more bothersome problems of height loss, skin changes, bladder symptoms, and forgetfulness. After a decade of low estrogen levels, the previously silent systemic changes begin to appear as serious medical problems. Surgical menopause, which results in a sudden and total loss of ovarian steroid production, often results in more severe symptoms of estrogen deficiency and accelerated risks of morbidity and death from cardiovascular events, osteoporosis fractures, and dementia.

ℰPIDEMIOLOGY

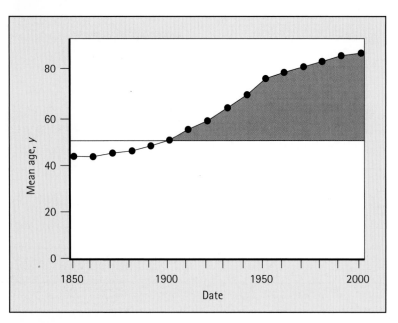

FIGURE 8-1.

Age of menopause and life expectancy. The average life expectancy of US women has risen from approximately 48 years in 1900 to 87.2 years (for women born today). Therefore, one third of a woman's life is spent after the menopause. The number of postmenopausal women has increased from 5 million in 1900 to over 45 million women in 1990. A woman aged 65 years can expect to live to age 84.2 years, and a 75-year-old woman can expect to live another 12 years.

Unfortunately, only 15% to 35% of post menopausal women are currently taking estrogen-replacement therapy (ERT). Compliance rates for short-term use (2 years) range from 20% to 80%, whereas long-term use of ERT is substantially lower and can be as low as under 5% in poorly motivated populations. Except for the highly motivated, financially stable, and educated woman, the assumption should be that women are highly unlikely to take replacement therapy for a lifetime. Improving compliance through better education and easy accessibility to hormone replacement, and ovarian preservation whenever possible, should continue to be a goal.

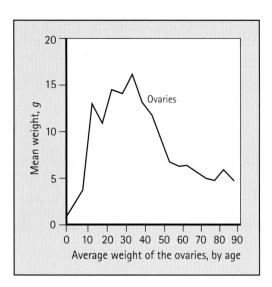

FIGURE 8-2.

Morphologic changes and follicular decline in perimenopause. Ovarian weight increases dramatically during early development and reaches peak amounts from 20 to 35 years of age. At age 35, ovarian weight drops precipitously, closely approximating the age when perimenopausal symptoms begin. Follicular volume decreases as well, although the most dramatic losses occur at much earlier ages.

SYMPTOMS AND SYSTEMIC CHANGES LINKED TO ESTROGEN DEFICIENCY

Symptoms or systemic changes	Phase of menopause
Changes in menstrual pattern	
Shorter or longer cycles	Perimenopause
Lighter or heavier bleeding	Perimenopause
Occasional irregular cycles	Perimenopause
Cessation of bleeding	Post menopause
Somatic symptoms or changes	
Increased frequency or severity of headaches	Perimenopause
Worsening menstrual migraines	Perimenopause
Dizziness	Perimenopause
Skin collagen depletion	Post menopause
Joint pain	Post menopause
Fat redistribution from hips to waist	Post menopause
Increased atherosclerosis	Post menopause
Increased bone loss	Perimenopause and natural menopause
Vasomotor instability	
Night sweats, hot flashes	Perimenopause
Mini–hot flushes	Perimenopause
Hot flushes, night sweats	Post menopause
Psychologic and cognitive disturbances	
Mild-to-moderate depression	Perimenopause and natural menopause
Irritability, mood changes	Perimenopause and natural menopause
Worsening premenstrual syndrome symptoms	Perimenopause
Declines in cognitive function	Post menopause
Urogenital system and sexual dysfunction	
Decreased vaginal lubrication	Perimenopause and natural menopause
Decreased libido, dyspareunia	Perimenopause and natural menopause
Vaginal atrophy, urinary incontinence, urinary tract infections	Post menopause

FIGURE 8-3.

Symptoms and systemic changes linked to estrogen deficiency. Various changes occur in perimenopause and natural menopause. Systems affected include menstrual patterns, somatic changes, vasomotor instability, psychologic and cognitive disturbances, and urogenital and sexual dysfunction.

RANGE OF DAILY OVARIAN SECRETION RATES OF ANDROGENS AND ESTROGENS IN YOUNG POSTMENOPAUSAL WOMEN

	Ovarian Hormone Production	
Hormone	Reproductive age	Post menopause
Estradiol, µg/d	40–80	0–20
Estrone, µg/d	20–50	0–10
Testosterone, µg/d	50–70	40–50
Androstenedione, mg/d	1.0–1.5	0.3–0.6

FIGURE 8-4.

Range of daily ovarian secretion rates of androgens and estrogens in young and postmenopausal women. (*Adapted from* Longcope [1].)

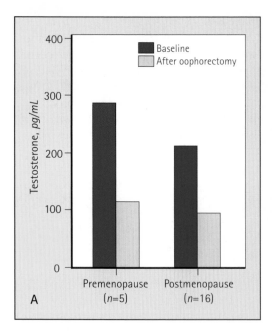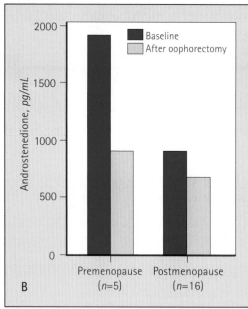

levels in age matched women who have undergone bilateral oophorectomy (12 ng/dL). For up to 4 years after menopause, the ovaries continue to secrete estrogens, and plasma levels of estrogens during the early postmenopausal years are only slightly below the levels in the early follicular phase. This is why the transition or perimenopause generally lasts from age 40 through age 55.

Both ovarian and adrenal production of these hormones falls in the menopause, but substantial quantities still remain. Androgens are important in stimulating bone formation and muscle development and are associated with an increased sense of well-being, lowered bone fracture rates, and improved sexual function. Additionally, androgens are peripherally converted to estrogens and are the primary source of estrogens in the late menopause. In surgically oophorectomized women, the loss of the ovarian contribution to plasma androgens accounts for the more pronounced signs and symptoms of estrogen deficiency that these women undergo.

FIGURE 8-5.

Postmenopausal steroid production. Comparison of testosterone (**A**) and androstenedione (**B**) levels in women of reproductive age with natural and surgical menopause. The typical postmenopausal ovary is not quiescent and clearly not unimportant. In premenopausal years, the dominant hormone of the menstrual cycle is not estradiol, which is measured in picograms, but rather testosterone and androstenedione, which are measured in nanograms and milligrams. Plasma levels of testosterone in naturally postmenopausal women are approximately double (25 ng/dL) compared with plasma

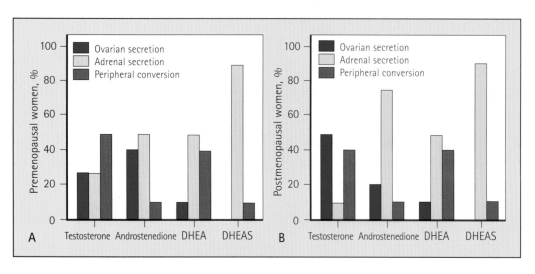

FIGURE 8-6.

Origin of plasma androgens in women. The ovaries and adrenal glands both synthesize the androgens testosterone and androstenedione. Although the adrenals are the primary source of dehydroepiandrosterone (DHEA) and dehydroepiandrosterone sulfate (DHEAS), the ovary also secretes small amounts of DHEA.

In premenopausal women (**A**), approximately 50% of plasma testosterone comes from the conversion of androstenedione in peripheral tissues. However, in postmenopausal women (**B**), ovarian secretion becomes more important and accounts for 50% of total plasma testosterone.

UROGENITAL AND VULVOVAGINAL CHANGES

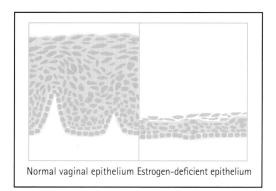

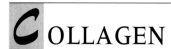

Normal vaginal epithelium Estrogen-deficient epithelium

FIGURE 8-7.

Comparison of normal and estrogen-deficient vaginal epithelium. As estrogen progressively decreases during the perimenopause and post menopause, there is a gradual thinning of the vaginal, urethral, and bladder mucosa. As the severity of urogenital atrophy increases, so do the number of vulvovaginal complaints. Atrophic vaginitis causes itching, burning,

dyspareunia, pain, tightness, discomfort, and vaginal bleeding. The trigone of the bladder and the urethra are embryologically derived from estrogen-dependent tissue, and atrophy can result in urinary urgency, incontinence, dysuria, urinary frequency, or frequent urinary tract infections. Without adequate estrogen, there is attenuation of the elastic supportive tissues around the bladder, urethra, and uterus, resulting in increased risk of developing a cystocele, rectocele, uterine descensus, or urinary stress incontinence.

Systemic estrogen replacement is effective in preventing many of these changes and may be all that is necessary in many postmenopausal women. Local administration of estrogen by vaginal creams or an estrogen-releasing ring may be added for those who, despite taking oral or transdermal estrogen therapy, complain of urinary or vaginal symptoms.

Postmenopausal atrophic vaginitis is often accompanied by a superficial vaginal infection, usually coliform, streptococci, staphylococci, or dipheroids. Other treatments include pelvic floor exercises, pessary, surgery, hygienic lifestyle changes, and vaginal antibacterials and other nonhormonal preparations.

The vagina consists of three layers: the epithelial layer, composed of stratified squamous epithelium with no true glands; a middle muscular layer; and a deep fibrous layer that has evolved from the pelvic fascia. The epithelial cells of the vagina contain the largest number of estrogen receptors of any genital tissue, and respond to ovarian estrogen stimulation. With the progressive fall in estrogen, this layer becomes thinner and the percentage of superficial cells to intermediate and parabasal cells (the maturation index) decreases.

COLLAGEN

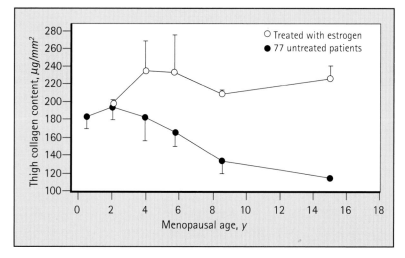

FIGURE 8-8.

Relation between thigh skin collagen content and menopausal age in 52 estrogen-treated women. Collagen makes up about one third of the total body mass. It is a major component of all connective tissues including skin, bone, tendons, ligaments, arteries, uterus, and dentine. There are five structurally and genetically distinct

collagens in the human body, although 90% of the total collagen in the body is type I. Skin and bone are primarily composed of type I, although skin also has type III collagen.

A fraction of the collagen in all tissues is continually degraded and replaced. There are changes in collagen biosynthesis and metabolism with aging. For example, the amounts of glycosylated hydroxylysine and hydroxylysine in type I collagen and the amount of immature and reducible cross-links tend to decrease with age.

Estrogen has a marked beneficial impact on collagen metabolism and the decline of estrogen in the peri- and postmenopausal woman. It is associated with collagen deficiency in the skin, urogenital tract, musculoskeleton system, and vascular system.

After the menopause, skin thickness and collagen content decrease with time, resulting in thin, transparent, flaky skin that easily bruises. These changes can be largely prevented using estrogen-replacement therapy. Approximately 30% of the skin collagen content can be lost during the first 5 years after menopause, although the average decline is 2.1% per year over a period of 10 years. Estrogen can increase skin collagen content in women with low levels initially, but is of prophylactic value only in women treated early in the menopause who have normal levels at the start of treatment [2].

BONE LOSS AND OSTEOPOROSIS

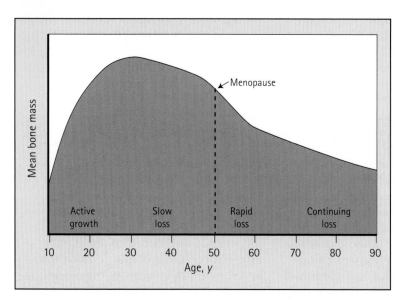

FIGURE 8-9.

Bone loss in women after natural menopause. Osteoporosis is defined as a condition characterized by low bone mass, with microarchitectural deterioration of bone tissue leading to enhanced bone fragility and increased fracture risk. In developed countries, increased life expectancy has placed enormous emphasis on aging-related disorders, and one of the most important of these is osteoporosis. Not only does osteoporosis result in crippling deformities of the spine, it also causes back and hip pain, loss of mobility, necessitates surgical intervention, and is responsible for nearly 45,000 deaths per year in the United States.

Peak bone mass occurs at approximately age 35 to 40 years and is lower in women than in men. After this peak, there is a gradual bone loss in both men and women. This loss is associated with declining estrogen levels, but is particularly associated with women with low calcium intake. Adequate calcium intake (1000 mg/d) during the 4th decade is associated with retention of peak bone mass at the time of the menopause. After menopause there is an accelerated bone loss in women who do not take exogenous estrogen therapy but still maintain adequate calcium intake. (*Adapted from* Wasnich *et al.* [3].)

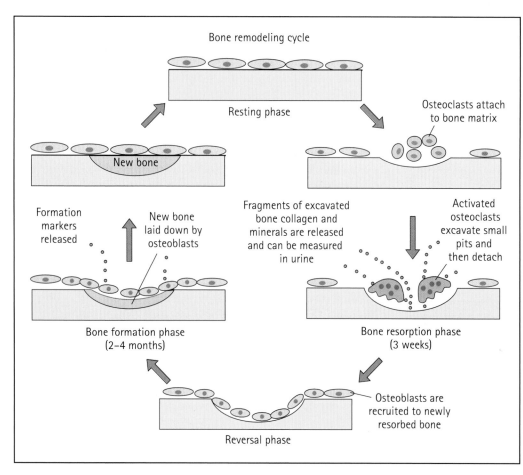

FIGURE 8-10.

Bone balance and normal bone remodeling. Human bone is made up of living tissue that undergoes a continuous process of bone breakdown (resorption) and rebuilding (formation). Trabecular bone, which makes up 25% of the skeleton, is metabolically active and has a high turnover rate. Trabecular or cancellous bone is a spongy network that forms the internal support system within the cortical bone shell. High concentrations of trabecular bone are found in the vertebral bodies, pelvis, and the ends of long bones. These

areas are highly sensitive to excessive rates of bone resorption. Cortical (compact or lamellar) bone forms the outer shell of all bones and makes up 75% of the skeleton. It has a slower turnover rate than trabecular bone. Both trabecular and cortical bone contain organic components (collagen-rich, protein matrix) and an inorganic component (calcium phosphate, hydroxyapatite). During early adulthood, bone resorption and formation are in balance and the total bone mass remains constant. About 3% of cortical bone and 30% of the trabecular bone of the spine is remodeled each year. The biologic processes are not well understood, but each cycle can take several months. Bone resorption and formation appear to be interdependent: a change in one directly affects the other. During post menopausal years, the loss of estrogen results in accelerated bone resorption and formation. Formation, however, is not able to keep up with resorption, resulting in a net loss of bone ranging from 1% to 4% per year.

Bone resorption is carried out by osteoclasts, which are derived from cells within the bone marrow. Bone resorption is carried out on a special surface of the osteoclast known as the "ruffled border." Here, the acid pH solubilizes the mineral component of bone (calcium phosphate or hydroxyapatite crystals) and proteolytic enzymes digest the hydroxyproline-containing protein organic matrix. Small

(*Continued on next page*)

FIGURE 8-10. *(Continued)*

amounts of bone collagen are released into the circulation. Measurement of urinary excretion of deoxypyridinoline, cross-linked N-telopeptides, or hydroxyproline are measures of bone resorption activity. Bone resorption markers can be used to detect present levels of bone resorption and predict bone mineral content and response to therapy.

Osteoblasts synthesize and release protein components of the bone's matrix during bone formation. Bone alkaline phosphatase is released into the circulation, making the bone-specific alkaline phosphatase assay a particularly reliable bone formation marker. A more recently discovered marker for bone formation is osteocalcin (also called bone GLA-protein), a noncollagen protein found in dentin and bone. Serum osteocalcin release is accelerated during postmenopausal increased bone turnover and is decreased following glucocorticoid treatment. Another marker of bone formation is procollagen I extension peptides.

CLINICAL FEATURES OF OSTEOPOROSIS

No early warning signs; fracture often first sign

Gradual height loss due to silent vertebral crush fractures

Dorsal kyphosis

Chronic back pain

Protuberant lower abdomen

Breathing problems; pulmonary dysfunction

Hip fracture; sequella include morbidity, surgery, pain, infections, complications of poor mobility and death

FIGURE 8-11.

Clinical features of osteoporosis. Although there are no early warning signs, the late manifestations of osteoporosis are severe and life threatening.

TREATMENT

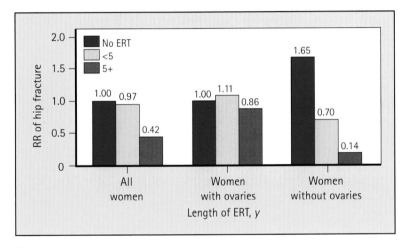

FIGURE 8-12.

Relative risk of hip fracture by years of estrogen use. Use of estrogen-replacement therapy (ERT) is reported to lower the risk of hip fracture by about 50%. The greatest beneficial effect of ERT is seen in oophorectomized women who have elevated rates of bone resorption and hip fracture due to the total loss of ovarian estrogen, androstenedione, and testostereone production compared with women who have undergone natural menopause. (*Adapted from* Paganini–Hill *et al.* [4].)

As estrogen declines during the perimenopause and natural menopause, there is an associated increase in bone resorption due to accelerated osteoclast activity. Osteoblastic bone formation increases, but inevitably rates of bone formation cannot keep up with resorption rates and there is a net loss in bone. Addition of estrogen normalizes osteoclastic resorptive rates and allows formation to catch up. This suppression of osteoclastic activity by estrogen is mediated by cytokines that also increase osteoblastic activity. Progestins also have antiresorptive action, whereas androgens primarily stimulate osteoblastic activity, although they have some antiresorptive effects.

The dose of estrogen should be kept to a minimum to optimize bone protection and minimize bleeding and side effects. The doses

needed to optimize bone preservation vary greatly among individuals. Menopausal women and those who retain their ovaries maintain adequate calcium intake (1000 mg/d) and do adequate weight-bearing activities, and are able to maintain bone balance at much smaller doses than high-risk women, such as those with surgical menopause. Doses as low as 0.3 mg esterified or conjugated estrogens with adequate calcium intake are reported to be protective against bone loss. Dosage regimens need to be individualized based on body weight, ovarian status, age, other menopausal symptoms, and individual preferences. Compliance increases as individual satisfaction increases and as side effects and bleeding decreases. ERT, calcium, and weight-bearing exercises are an effective combination to prevent or treat osteoporosis. In sunny climates, adequate vitamin D (200 to 400 IU/d) is of less concern but should be a consideration, especially in elderly women or those with inadequate sunlight exposure (< 5–10 min/d).

Alendronate is an effective and selective inhibitor of osteoclast activity and is approved for the treatment and prevention of osteoporosis in postmenopausal women. Treatment with alendronate increases bone mineral density by 3% to 5% per year and significantly decreases loss of height and vertebral fracture rate. Although use of alendronate and estrogen together has not been well studied, current data demonstrate that the combination is safe and effective. Recently, raloxifene, a benzothiophene derivative and a selective estrogen receptor modulator was approved by the US Food and Drug Administration for prevention of osteoporosis. Use of daily raloxifene in three osteoporosis prevention studies resulted in a 2% to 3% increase in bone mineral density compared with calcium-supplemented placebo after 24 months. The effects on fracture rates are not yet known. Although the effects of raloxifene on bone and serum cholesterol are similar to estrogen, its main advantage over estrogen is that it has no estrogenic effect on uterine tissue, thus avoiding bleeding problems. Data also indicate that it may lower the risk of breast cancer through antiestrogenic action. Beneficial effects on the cardiovascular and central nervous systems have not been shown.

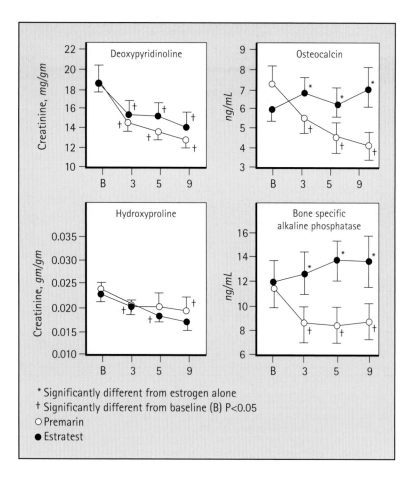

* Significantly different from estrogen alone
† Significantly different from baseline (B) P<0.05
○ Premarin
● Estratest

FIGURE 8-13.

Effects of conjugated equine estrogen or a combination of esterified estrogen on markers of bone turnover in women who have undergone oophorectomy. Low levels of testosterone in postmenopausal women are associated with increased rates of vertebral crush fracture. Testosterone is known to stimulate bone formation and is especially effective in increasing bone density in oophorectomized subjects when added to estrogen therapy. In a study in postmenopausal subjects, the markers of bone resorption, urinary deoxypyridinoline, and hydroxyproline, showed similar decreases with both oral estrogen and estrogen plus androgen, but markers of bone formation were significantly higher when androgen was added compared with estrogen alone.

Other antiresorptive treatments include vitamin D, bisphosphonates, progestins, and calcitonin. Another antiresorptive medication under current investigation is tibolone. Tibolone, a synthetic steroid and a derivative of 17-hydroxynorpregnenylone, has estrogenic, androgenic, and progestogenic properties. Tibolone prevents bone loss without inducing endometrial hyperplasia or causing vaginal bleeding.

Agents that enhance bone formation include anabolic steroids, parathyroid hormone, and sodium fluoride. Other preventative measures to prevent osteoporosis and fractures include preservation of ovaries, establishment of fall-proof living quarters, minimizing medications associated with bone loss or change in mental status, and promotion of healthy active lifestyles.

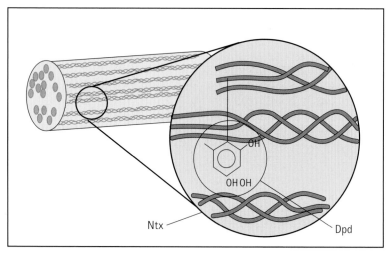

FIGURE 8-14.

Identification of site on bone collagen fibrils that are measured by urinary markers of bone resorption used for screening for osteoporosis. The use of noninvasive tests based on biochemical markers of bone turnover can be used in conjunction with bone densitometry to complement the screening of transitional and postmenopausal women and may improve treatment selection and compliance. The combined use of these tests is the first and best way to technically monitor the effectiveness of estrogen-replacement therapy. Although a positive therapeutic response is reassuring that bones are protected, it offers some additional evidence that other protective effects of estrogen may be happening. Certainly, if markers remain elevated and do not respond to therapy, it becomes important to reevaluate therapy and compliance, or to look for other complicating factors.

Markers of bone resorption can be used clinically to predict current and future bone mineral density (BMD) in postmenopausal women. The two most popular commercially available urinary immunoassays are Pyrilinks-D and Osteomark. Pyrilinks-D

measures free deoxypyridinoline (Dpd) crosslinks present only in type I collagen of bone. In women, levels over 7.4 nM Dpd/mM creatinine indicate high rates of bone resorption.

Osteomark provides a quantitative measure of the excretion of cross-linked N-teleopeptides (Ntx) of type I collagen. Within 3 months after initiation of antiresorptive therapy, Ntx values less than 35 BME or at least a 30% to 40% decrease from baseline indicates a therapeutic effect of therapy.

At least 25% of bone needs to be lost before osteoporosis is diagnosed by routine radiography. Quantitative computed tomography measures bone density in both the cortical and trabecular bone compartments (usually a lumbar vertebral body). The modern, upgraded version of dual photon absorptiometry is dual radiographic absorptiometry (DEXA) The reproducibility of measurements with DEXA is improved, examination times are reduced (2 minutes) and less radiation (1 to 3 mrem) is used. Ultrasonographic measurement of bone mass, based on transmission time through bone, presently lacks some of the sensitivity of other tests, but potentially would provide cost savings that would make widespread screening cost effective.

The World Health Organization has established cutoff values for low bone density and osteoporosis using bone mineral density data from a young adult reference group. Low bone density is calculated to be BMD between 1 and 2.5 SD below the reference group mean; in osteoporosis, the BMD is greater than 2.5 SD below the mean. A decrease of 1 SD in bone mass is associated with a 50% to 100% increase in fracture incidence. Optimal screening for bone density would include a routine BMD study in the early transitional or post menopause and a repeat study in the 60s. In women with normal BMD on estrogen-replacement therapy, a yearly check of urinary bone resorption markers evaluates the effectiveness of treatment and compliance. Women diagnosed with osteopenia or osteoporosis on DEXA or those that have had a significant bone loss compared with a previous study can be checked after 3 months of treatment for compliance with urinary markers.

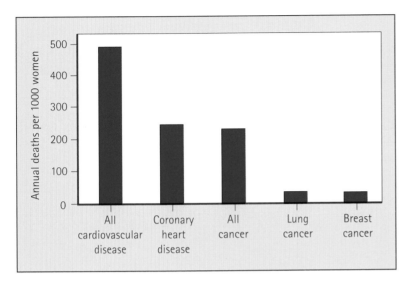

FIGURE 8-15.

Leading causes of death in women. Cardiovascular disease is the leading cause of death in women and men, significantly outweighing all other single causes.

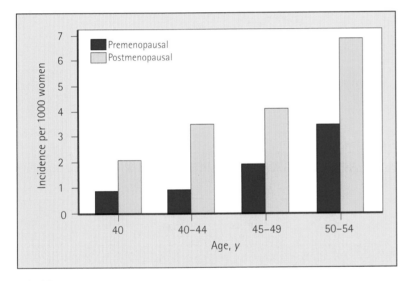

FIGURE 8-16.

Incidence of cardiovascular disease by menopausal status. As early as 1953, Wuerst *et al.* [2] observed that women were protected from coronary artery disease, and that this protection diminished in individuals over 60 years of age. A clear excep-

tion was women who had undergone bilateral oophorectomy, who had almost the same degree of coronary artery disease as men of the same age. The Framingham Study [5] and multiple other studies have confirmed that the age-adjusted risk of coronary heart disease among oophorectomized subjects up to age 55 is at least twofold greater than the risk for control subjects. There was a significant inverse association between coronary disease and estrogen therapy with doses of 0.3 mg (relative risk [RR], 0.4; CI, 0.29– 0.79) and 0.625 mg (RR, 0.35; CI, 0.25–0.50) daily conjugated estrogen, and this protection disappeared with higher doses. There is some evidence that surgical removal of the ovaries also increases the frequency of cerebrovascular disease.

Further links between estrogen deficiency and cardiovascular disease comes from a mounting number of studies showing a substantial reduction in risk of coronary artery disease associated with estrogen-replacement therapy. Cardiovascular disease, a disease in the past handled by general practitioners and internists, is now the focus of the gynecologist, who has both the opportunity to decrease or prevent cardiovascular disease by prescribing hormonal therapy or to increase the risk by performing oophorectomy. (*Adapted from* Gordon *et al.* [6].)

MECHANISMS OF CARDIOVASCULAR PROTECTION RELATED TO ESTROGEN

Direct vascular antiatherosclerotic effects	Direct vasodilation effects	Systemic effects
Inhibits deposition of LDL cholesterol and LDL byproducts in blood vessel walls	Decreases vascular tone	Decreases total and LDL cholesterol, and increases HDL cholesterol
Decreases lipoprotein-induced arterial smooth muscle proliferation	Modulates the release of vasoconstrictors and vasodilators by vascular endothelium, thereby decreasing vascular reactivity	Increases inotropic actions of the heart
Decrease foam cell formation in vessel wall	Modulates ionic channels in smooth muscle cell membranes of the vessels and cardiac cells	Improves glucose metabolism and decreases circulating insulin levels
Reduces arterial cholesterol ester influx and hydrolysis	Modulates the release of vasoactive substances and neurotransmitters including histamine, serotonin, and prostaglandins	Lowers blood pressure through vasodilation
Decreases elastin and collagen production and accumulation	Modulates vasoactive neurotransmitter release at presynaptic junctions; possibly decreases production or release of epinephrine and blocks neuronal uptake of norepinephrine	Reduces plasminogen activator inhibitor
Inhibits platelet aggregation		Decreases fibrogen
Increases prostacyclin production by endothelium and arterial smooth muscle cells	Increases vasodilating and antiplatelet aggregation factors in the endothelium, eg, nitric oxide and prostacyclin	
Decreases thromboxane A_2 formation	Increases vasodilation by nonendothelium-dependent factor	
Reduces oxidation of LDL cholesterol		

FIGURE 8-17.

Beneficial mechanisms of actions of estrogen. Scientific studies in animals and humans have reported these actions of estrogen that may relate to the cardioprotective action of estrogen.

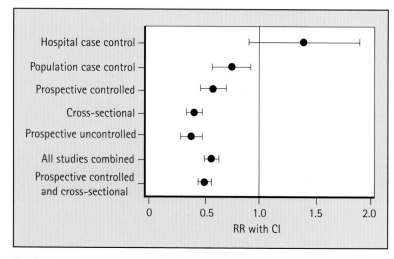

FIGURE 8-18.

Estrogen use and cardiovascular disease risk by study type. The hospital-based case-control studies were designed before it was widely appreciated that estrogens reduce the incidence of osteoporosis and fracture as well as a long list of other diseases. In these studies, prior estrogen use among women hospitalized for cardiovascular disease (CVD) was compared with that of women hospitalized for other reasons. Many of the women selected as control subjects were admitted for treatment of fractures. Such control subjects would be less likely to have taken estrogen than the general population. Thus, their inclusion in the study would likely reduce the protective effect of estrogen in reducing CVD.

One of the advantages of the population-based case-control studies is that they use healthy rather than hospitalized control subjects, which better represents the population from which the cases arose. The cross-sectional studies examined the extent of coronary artery disease among users and nonusers of postmenopausal estrogen replacement in women having coronary angiography. This study design avoids some of the methodologic problems of case-control studies, such as recall bias and control selection, because exposure status is determined prior to entry into the study and control subjects are the group of women who have no evidence of coronary artery stenosis after arteriography.

All but one of the 17 prospective studies have observed a protective effect of estrogen on CVD and mortality. In the only negative study, the Framingham study, the results were adjusted for high-density lipoprotein level, which is generally inappropriate. The Nurses Health Study is the largest prospective cohort to investigate estrogen use and heart disease. The study was established in 1976 and included 121,700 married female registered nurses aged 30 to 55 years who are asked to complete a mailed questionnaire every 2 years. In June, 1997, the most recent update was published in the *New England Journal of Medicine* [7]. After adjustment for confounding variables, current hormone users had a lower risk of death (0.63; 95% CI, 0.56–0.70) than women that had never taken hormones. The largest reduction of risk (49% decrease in death from all causes) occured in estrogen users with risk factors for cardiovascular disease, including obesity, smoking, parental history of premature myocardial infarction, high blood pressure, diabetes or high cholesterol levels.

PSYCHOLOGICAL AND COGNITIVE FUNCTIONING

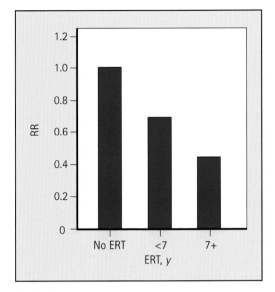

FIGURE 8-19.
Relative risk of Alzheimer's disease by years of estrogen-replacement therapy (ERT). Quality of life issues are becoming increasingly more important as life expectancy has increased. Prominent among complaints of post menopausal and perimenopausal women are changes in behavior, mood, memory, and sexual function. Often it is difficult to separate the role of sociocultural factors and environmental changes from a possible impact of declining sex steroids on these complaints. The increasing number of scientific studies that report the relationship between sex hormones and brain function provide a clearer understanding of these areas.

Administration of estrogen to postmenopausal women often improves mood, depression, memory, and extrapyramidal motor control.

Estrogen receptors are widely distributed throughout the central nervous system (CNS), with especially high concentrations in the hypothalamus and amygdala. Rodent studies document dramatic neuronal remodeling within the hypothalamus throughout the estrous cycle. Estrogen administration to ovariectomized rats stimulates regeneration of neurons within the arcuate nucleus. *In vivo* studies also show that estrogen stimulates neuronal growth and synaptogenesis. These and other studies give strong evidence that estrogen mediates its effects on the CNS through the stimulation of neurotrophic factors and plays an important role in the development of Alzheimer's disease. The important mechanism of action of estrogen is that it increases the rate of degradation of monoamine oxidase (MAS), the enzyme that catabolizes serotonin. Deficiency of MAS is thought to be one causal factor for development of depression.

One potentially important action of estrogen regarding memory function is the induction of choline acetyltransferase (CAT), the enzyme needed to synthesize acetylcholine. It is the cholinergic system that has been most closely associated with memory functions. It is also these cells that undergo the earliest and most pronounced degenerative changes seen in senile dementia of the Alzheimer's type. The deficiency of brain acetylcholine concentration is a hallmark of Alzheimer's disease. Estrogen also increases adrenergic function, also linked to cognitive thought.

There is compelling evidence that estrogen deficiency is a cause of Alzheimer's disease. The incidence of Alzheimer's disease increases in women after age 65, and is two to three times more common in women than men. Women who have had a myocardial infarct, considered an expression of estrogen deficiency, are five times more likely to develop dementia. Obese women, who have higher circulating estrogen levels, are less likely to get Alzheimer's disease (AD) than nonobese women. Current use of estrogen protects women from dementia. Interestingly, some protection afforded by estrogen for the prevention of hip fracture is attributed to CNS effects through better coordination and quicker response.

Alzheimer's disease has an enormous detrimental impact on the quality of life of the affected individual and his or her family. In a prospective case-control study of women living in a large retirement community, the use of ERT significantly reduced the risk of developing Alzheimer's disease. After 7 years of ERT use, the risk of developing Alzheimer's disease was 50% lower than for nonusers.

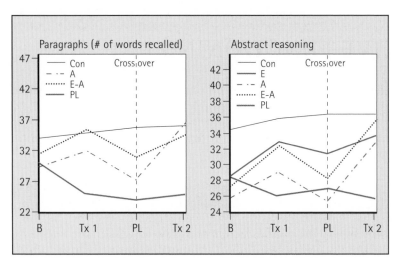

FIGURE 8-20.

Results of cognitive functioning tests. In a prospective crossover study, premenopausal women who were scheduled for a hysterectomy and bilateral salpingoophorectomy for benign disease were tested 1 month before surgery and again monthly for 3 months following surgery. Women undergoing just a hysterectomy were included as control subjects. Following TAH and BSO, women received either estrogen, androgen, or an estrogen–androgen combined preparation or placebo intramuscu-

larly once a month for 3 months. In both treatment phases, women who received placebo had higher depression scores when compared with those treated with any of the hormone groups. TAH—Total abdominal hysterectomy

Importantly, although a positive association between mood and sex hormones have been documented repeatedly, women are not clinically depressed. The women complained of "feeling blue" or had feelings of sadness. Mild levels of clinical depression often do improve with estrogen treatment, although a distinction between actual clinical depression and mild-to-moderate depression needs to be made.

In a similar study, those given estrogen postoperatively maintained their scores on several tests of memory and abstract reasoning, whereas the performance of oophorectomized, placebo-treated women decreased.

The integrity of tissues of the female reproductive tract is dependent on estrogen. Changes associated with urogenital atrophy adversely alter sexual function. However, sexual motivation or libido in women is linked to androgens and estrogens. Intramuscular or implant pellet studies as well as recent oral androgen–estrogen studies document enhancement of libido and sense of well-being in women following treatment. BSO—bilateral salpingoophorectomy; Con—control no oophorectomy; E—estrogen; A—androgen; E-A—estrogen-androgen; PL—placebo; TAH—Total abdominal hysterectomy. (*Adapted from* Sherwin [8].)

ESTROGEN–REPLACEMENT THERAPY AND RISK OF COLORECTAL CANCER

ERT use		RR (95% CI)
Fatal colon cancer, *n*=897	Ever used	0.71 (0.61–0.83)
	≥ 11 y	0.54 (0.39–0.76)
Incidence colon cancer		9/14 Decreased
		5/9 Significant decrease

FIGURE 8-21.

Estrogen-replacement therapy (ERT) and risk of colorectal cancer. A protective effect of ERT and oral contraceptive pills against colorectal cancer has been reported in several epidemiologic studies. In a large prospective study, 676,526 women were surveyed over a 7-year period. Relative risk of developing fatal colon cancer among current users of at least 11 years was only 0.45. The protection may be in part due to decreased bile synthesis and secretion associated with ERT. (*Adapted from* Calle *et al.* [9].)

ESTROGEN-REPLACEMENT THERAPY AND TOOTH LOSS

	RR of loss of 1 or more teeth (95% CI)	RR of edentia (95% CI)	RR of denture use (95% CI)
Current ERT	0.76 (C.72–0.80)	0.51 (0.37–0.70)	0.81 (0.64–0.94)
Post ERT	0.91 (0.85–0.96)	0.70 (0.56–0.88)	0.81 (0.67–0.97)

FIGURE 8-22.

Estrogen-replacement therapy (ERT) and tooth loss. Two studies report a significant reduction in tooth loss with current (relative risk, 0.76; CI, 0.72–0.80) or past ERT use (relative risk, 0.91; CI, 0.85–0.96). Current and past use of estrogen also resulted in significant reduced relative risk of edentia and denture use. (*Adapted from* [10,11].)

DISADVANTAGES OF ESTROGEN-REPLACEMENT THERAPY

META-ANALYSIS OF OVERALL RELATIVE RISK OF ESTROGEN-REPLACEMENT THERAPY AND BREAST CANCER

Study (year)	Studies, n	Summary RR (95% CI)
Armstrong (1988)	23	1.01 (0.95–1.08)
Dupont and Page (1991)	28	1.07 (NA)
Steinberg et al. (1991)	16	1.0 (NA)
Grady and Ernster (1991)	37	1.01 (0.98–1.06)
Sillero-Arenas (1992)	27	1.06 (1.00–1.12)
Colditz et al. (1993)	31	1.02 (0.93–1.12)

FIGURE 8-23.

Meta-analysis of overall relative risk of estrogen-replacement therapy (ERT) and breast cancer risk. The major issue that often dissuades women from taking ERT is its association with breast cancer. A real cause-and-effect relationship between ERT and breast cancer has not been proven due to the large number of confounding variables such as age, weight, type of menopause, family history of breast cancer, and social class. Meta-analyses suggest that overall incidence of breast cancer in estrogen users is not increased overall; however, long periods of treatment are associated with increased breast cancer rates. The studies reviewed in these meta-analyses primarily reflect the higher estrogen doses that were used 10 to 20 years ago.

META-ANALYSIS OF LONG-TERM ESTROGEN-REPLACEMENT THERAPY AND DIAGNOSIS OF BREAST CANCER

Study	Studies, n	Years of use	RR (95% CI)
Grady and Ernster	10	8+	1.25 (1.04–1.51)
Sillero-Arenas	9	12+	1.23 (1.07–1.41)
Steinberg	16	15+	1.3 (1.2–1.6)
Colditz et al.	5	15+	1.29 (1.04–1.60)

FIGURE 8-24.

Meta-analysis of long-term estrogen-replacement therapy (ERT) and breast cancer risk. Similar to the findings in Figure 8-26, these findings from the Nurses' Health Study found that although current hormone users had a lower overall risk of death than subjects who had never taken hormones, the benefit decreased with long-term use (after 10 years) because of an increase in mortality from breast cancer. However, mortality rates among women who use postmenopausal hormones is lower than among nonusers.

Research on low-dose ERT supports the belief that low doses offer the protection of estrogen yet minimizes or avoids any increase in breast cancer rates. Overall, however, the enormous health benefit from estrogens shown by studies of past doses of ERT indicate that approximately six deaths from heart disease are prevented for each incident case of breast cancer.

CONTRAINDICATIONS FOR ESTROGEN-REPLACEMENT THERAPY

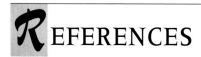

CONTRAINDICATIONS FOR ESTROGEN-REPLACEMENT THERAPY

Absolute contraindications

Known or suspected breast cancer except in appropriately selected women with very low risk of recurrence

Known or suspected estrogen-dependent neoplasia

Undiagnosed abnormal genital bleeding

Active thrombophlebitis or thromboembolic disease

Known or suspected pregnancy

Factors that make low-dose ERT or nonoral ERT preferable

Postoperative or confined to bed rest

Hepatic disease

Obesity

History of thrombophlebitis or thromboembolic disease

Mother or sister with premenopausal breast cancer

Unscheduled uterine bleeding

History of symptomatic leiomyomata or endometriosis

Fear of ERT

Elderly or petite

Side effects with standard ERT dose

Gastrointestinal absorption problems

FIGURE 8–25.

Absolute contraindications for estrogen-replacement therapy (ERT) and factors that make low-dose ERT or nonoral ERT preferable. Contraindications for ERT are uncommon. Endometrial cancer is no longer an absolute contraindication for ERT, although progestin-only treatment is often used until risk of recurrence is minimal. Transdermal therapy should be considered in women with a strong or current history of thromboembolic phenomena, gallbladder disease, liver disease, severe atherosclerotic vascular disease, or those confined to bed rest.

Women with a positive family history for breast cancer may use ERT. Use of ERT in women with a previously diagnosed breast cancer remains controversial and is under intense study. The ACOG Technical Bulletin 158, published in 1991, advised clinicians to consider ERT in women with a history of breast cancer who appear to be free from disease [5]. The most reasonable group to use ERT are those with the most favorable prognosis (least likely to have residual disease), which includes those with tumor size less than 1 cm, a nuclear grade of 1 (well-differentiated), ductal cancer *in situ*, and node negative cancer.

REFERENCES

1. Longcope C: Adrenal and gonadal androgen secretion in normal females. *Clin Endocrinol Metab* 1986, 15:213–228.

2. Brincat M, Moniz CF, Studd JWW, *et al.*: The long-term effects of the menopause and of administration of sex hormones on skin collagen and skin thickness. *Br J Obstet Gynecol* 1985, 92:256–259.

3. Wasnich RD, *et al.*: Osteoporosis. *Critique and Practicum* Honolulu: Banyan Press; 1989:179–213.

4. Paganini-Hill A, Ross RK, Gerkins VR, *et al.*: Menopausal estrogen therapy and hip fractures. *Ann Internal Med* 1981, 95:28–31.

5. Kannel WB, Hjortland MC, McNamara PM, Gordon T: Menopause and risk of cardiovascular disease. The Framingham Study. *Ann Intern Med* 1976, 85:447–452.

6. Gordon T, Kannel WB, Hjortland MC, *et al.*: Menopause and coronary heart disease. The Framingham Study. *Ann Intern Med* 1978, 89:157–161..

7. Grodstein F, Stampfer MJ, colditz GA, *et al.*: Postmenopausal hormone therapy and mortality. *N Engl J Med* 1997, 336:1769–1775.

8. Sherwin BB: Estrogen and/or androgen replacement therapy and cognitive functioning in surgically menopausal women. *Psychoneuroendocrinology* 1988, 13:345–357.

9. Calle EE, Miracle-McMahill HL, Thun MJ, *et al.*: Estrogen replacement therapy and risk of fatal colon cancer in a prospective cohort of postmenopausal women. *J Natl Cancer Inst* 1995, 87:517-523.

10. Grodstein F, Colditz GA, Stampfer MJ.: Postmenopausal hormone use and tooth loss: a prospective study *J Am Dent Assoc* 1996, 127:370–377.

11. Paganini-Hill A: The benefits of estrogen replacement therapy on oral health. The Leisure World cohort. *Arch Intern Med* 1995, 155:2325–2329.

SELECTED BIBLIOGRAPHY

Arnaud CD: Osteoporosis: using "bone markers" for diagnosis and monitoring. *Geriatrics* 1996, 51(Apr):24–30.

Colditz CA, Hankinson SE, Hunter DJ, *et al.*: The use of estrogens and progestins and the risk of breast cancer in postmenopausal women. *N Engl J Med* 1995, 332:1389.

Council on Scientific Affairs, American Medical Association: Intake of dietary calcium to reduce to incidence of osteoporosis-an update. *Acta Obstet Gynecol Scand* 1997, 76:189–199.

Cummings SR, Nevitt MC, Browner WS, *et al.*: Risk factors for hip fracture in white women. *N Engl J Med* 1995, 332:767–773.

Davis SR, McCloud P, Strauss BJ, Burger H: Testosterone enhances estradiol's effects on postmenopausal bone density and sexuality. *Maturitas* 1995, 21:227–236.

Davis SR, Burger HG: Androgens and the postmenopausal women. *J Clin Endocrinol Metab* 1996, 81:2759–2763.

Draper MW, Flowers DE, Huster WJ, *et al.*: A controlled trial of raloxifen HCl(LY139481): impact on bone turnover and serum lipid profile in healthy postmenopausal women. *J Bone Miner Res* 1996, 11(6):835–842.

Fernandez E, LaVecchia C, DAvanzo B, *et al.*: Oral contraceptives, hormone replacement therapy and the risk of colorectal cancer. *Br J Cancer* 1996, 73:1431–1435.

Genant HK, Lucas J, Weiss S, *et al.*: Low-dose esterified estrogen therapy. Effects on bone, plasma estradiol concentrations, endometrium and lipid levels. *Arch Inter Med* 1997, 157:2609–2615.

Henderson BE, Paganini-Hill A, Ross RK: Decreased mortality in users of estrogen replacement therapy. *Arch Intern Med* 1991, 151:75–78.

Honjo H, Ogino Y, Naitoh K, *et al.*: In vivo effect of estrone sulfate on the central nervous system-senile dementia (Alzheimer's Type). *J Steroid Biochem* 1989, 34:521–525.

Jick H, Derby L: The risk of hospitalization for idiopathic venous thromboembolism among users of postmenopausal estrogens. *Lancet* 1996, 348:981–983.

Junt K, Vessey M, McPherson K: Mortality in a cohort of long-term users of hormone replacement therapy: an updated analysis. *Br J Obstet Gynecol* 1990, 97:1080–1086.

Kasperk C, Fitzsimmons R, Strong D, *et al.*: Studies of the mechanism by which androgens enhance mitogenesis and differentiation in bone cells. *J Clin Endocrinol Metab* 1990, 71:1322–1329.

Kasperk C, Wergedal JE, Farley JR, *et al.*: Androgens directly stimulate proliferation of bone cells in vitro. *Endocrinology* 1989, 124:1576–1578.

Nachtigall LE: Enhancing patient compliance with hormone replacement therapy at menopause. *Obstet Gynecol* 1990, 75:77S–80S.

Nieves JW, Golden Al, Siris E, *et al.*: Teenage and current calcium intake are related to bone mineral density of the hip and forearm of women aged 30-39 years. *Am J Epidemiol* 1995, 141:342–351.

Notelovitz M: Osteoporosis, screening, prevention, and management. *Fertil Steril* 1993, 59:707–725.

Ohta H, Masuzawa T, Ikeda t, *et al.*: Which is more osteoporosis-inducing, menopause or oophorectomy? *Bone Miner* 1992, 19:273–285.

Paginini-Hill A: The benefits of estrogen replacement therapy on oral health, the Leisure World cohort. *Arch Inter Med* 1995, 155:2325–2329.

Paganini-Hill A, Henderson VW: Estrogen deficiency and risk of alzheimer's disease in women. *Am J Epidemiol* 1994, 140:256–261.

Persson L, Adami HO, Bergkvist L, *et al.*: Risk of endometrial cancer after treatment with oestrogens alone or in conjunction with progestogens. Results of a prospective study. *Br Med J* 1989, 298:147–151.

Persson I, Adami HO, Bergkvist L: Hormone replacement therapy and the risk of cancer in the breast and reproductive organs: a review of epidemiological data, In *HRT and Osteoporosis*. Edited by Drife JO, Studd JWW. London: Springer-Verlag; 1990:165–175.

Phillips SM, Sherwin BB: Effect of estrogen on memory function in surgically menopausal women. *Psychoneuroendocrinology 17* 1992, 5:485–495.

Raisz LG, Wiita B, Artis A, *et al.*: Comparison of the effects of estrogen alone and estrogen plus androgen on biochemical markers of bone formation and resorption in postmenopausal women. *J Clin Endocrinol Metab* 1995, 81:37–43.

Rosen CJ, Chestnut CH, Mallinak NJS: The Predicitive Value of Biochemical Markers of Bone Turnover for Bone Mineral Density in Early Postmenopausal Women Treated with Hormone Replacement or Calcium Supplementation. *J Clin Endocrinol Metab* 1997, 82:1904–1910.

Shoupe D, Brenner PF, Mishell DR. Menopause. In *Mishell's Textbook of Infertility, contraception and reproductive Endocrinology*. Editors Lobo RA, Mishell DR Jr., Paulson RJ, Shoupe D. Malden, MA: Blackwell Science edn 4; 1997.

Stampfer MJ, Grodstein F: Role of hormone replacement in cardiovascular disease. In *Treatment of the Postmenopausal Woman: Basic and Clinical Aspects*. Edited by Lobo RA. New York: Raven Press; 1994.

Steinberg K, Thacker SB, Smith SJ, *et al.*: A meta-analysis of the effect of estrogen replacement therapy on the risk of breast cancer. *JAMA* 1991, 265:1985–1990.

Steinberg KK, Thacker SB, Smith J, *et al.*: A meta-analysis of the effect of estrogen replacement therapy on the risk of breast cancer. *JAMA* 1991, 265:2985.

Toran-Allerand CD, Miranda RC, Bentham WDL, *et al.*: Estrogen receptors colocalize with low affinity nerve growth factor receptors in cholinergic neurons of the basal forebrain. *Pro Natl Acad Sci USA* 1992, 89:4668–4672.

Watts NB, Notelovitz M, Timmons MC, *et al.*: Comparison of oral estrogens and estrogens plus androgen on bone mineral density, menopausal symptoms, and lipid-lipoprotein profiles in surgical menopause. *Obstet Gynecol* 1995, 85:529–537.

The Writing Group for the PEPI Trial: Effects of estrogen on estrogen/progestin regimens on heart disease risk factors in postmenopausal women. The postmenopausal estrogen/progestin intervention trial. *JAMA* 1995, 273:199–208.

Diagnostic Evaluation of the Infertile Couple

CHAPTER

9

John E. Buster

In today's practice environment, diagnostic evaluation for infertility must be simple, inexpensive, and rapid. Physicians sophisticated in the treatment of infertile couples know to focus on a single goal: achieving pregnancy *economically* and *quickly*. *Economically* because infertility treatment takes place in a competitive, cost-containment environment. Procedures contributing modestly to outcome, such as routine diagnostic laparoscopy, are avoided because they are expensive. *Quickly* because patients have high expectations from today's technology. To an infertile couple wanting children, an expensive evaluation that renders a precise diagnosis, but delays effective therapy, is not satisfying—becoming pregnant is satisfying. Living with loss of privacy, disruption of spontaneous sexual habits, and feelings of reproductive failure is unacceptable.

The traditional definition of infertility, *ie*, 12 months of timely, unprotected intercourse without pregnancy, needs qualifica-tion. The 12-month rule must be carefully moderated when there is an adverse gynecologic history, when a woman's age exceeds 35 years, and when there are mitigating personal circumstances. A gynecologic history complicated by known tubal obstruction, active endometriosis, irregular menses or amenorrhea, should lead to an immediate investigation. Similarly, an older woman's age demands timely intervention because aggressive therapies become decreasingly effective as women pass their 35th year. Personal circumstances, however, are the final moderator. For some couples, a simple evaluation that identifies a difficult problem will lead to a decision not to have children. For most, however, a pregnancy is desired now—not a year from now.

For these reasons, the approach described in this chapter is results-oriented: identify and implement timely therapy and achieve pregnancy economically and quickly.

COUNSELING FOR INFERTILITY

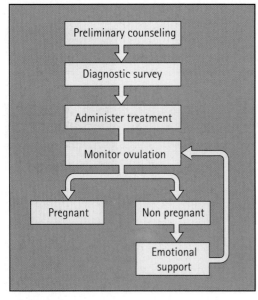

FIGURE 9-1.
Steps in the diagnostic evaluation of the infertile couple.

Preliminary Counseling

Identify simple problems that are inexpensive to treat
Counsel on deleterious effects of advanced maternal age
Counsel on fertility-impairing lifestyles
Establish realistic expectations

FIGURE 9-2.
Preliminary counseling. Careful consultation on simple problems, effects of maternal aging, and fertility-impairing lifestyles should be undertaken prior to beginning a formal diagnostic evaluation. Emotions may rise to crisis levels during the evaluation. Feelings of frustration, anger, powerlessness, isolation, and guilt are common. Loss of privacy, disruption of spontaneous sexual habits, and a felling of reproductive failure or inadequacy are frequent casues of depression, anxiety, and grief. Realistic expectations before treatment is essential to producing a satisfying outcome.

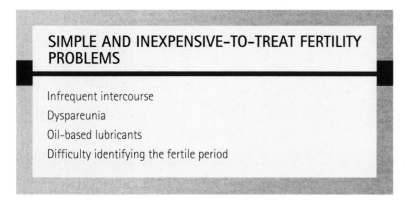

SIMPLE AND INEXPENSIVE-TO-TREAT FERTILITY PROBLEMS

Infrequent intercourse
Dyspareunia
Oil-based lubricants
Difficulty identifying the fertile period

FIGURE 9-3.
Simple and inexpensive-to-treat fertility problems. Infrequent intercourse may signal serious marital problems that should be resolved before engaging in treatment that may bring children into a troubled relationship. Dyspareunia may signal gynecologic disease or sexual dysfunction that needs attention. Oil-based lubricants may be spermatocidal and should be replaced with water-soluble agents. The fertile period, obvious to most individuals, may be a mystery to sophisticated people with no medical background. Simple explanation of urinary luteinizing hormone detection kits and basal body temperatures may be all that is needed to achieve pregnancy.

ADVANCED MATERNAL AGE

Decreases natural birth rates
Increases miscarriage rates
Prolongs time to achieve pregnancy
Impairs response to infertility treatment

FIGURE 9-4.
Advanced maternal age. The patient should be counseled on the deleterious effects of advancing maternal age. Reproductive performance decreases with increasing maternal age beyond 30. This concept is important to communicate in setting realistic expectations about treatment.

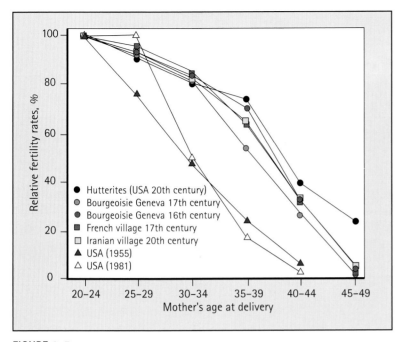

FIGURE 9-5.

Advanced maternal age and relative fertility rates. Advanced maternal age decreases natural fecundity. The data for this figure are collected from birth registry studies of closed, noncontracepting societies. Declining birth rates are observed as early as 30 to 35 years of age and are dramatic by age 40 [1]. Decreased fecundity is principally linked to oocyte aging [2]. Oocyte aging, in turn, is associated with increased aneuploidy, decreased fertilization, and increased miscarriages [3]. In the absence of gynecologic disease, a woman's most fertile years are between ages 15 and 30. After age 30, as age increases, fecundity decreases [4–9]. Increased prevalence of age-linked gynecologic maladies, endometriosis and fibroids, have an additional impact on oocyte aging. (*Adapted from* Maroulis [1]; with permission).

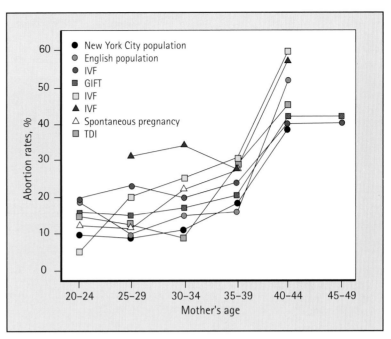

FIGURE 9-6.

Advanced maternal age and miscarriage rates. Miscarriage rates increase with advancing age: 10% below age 30, 18% in the late 30s, and soaring to 40% to 50% in the 40s. GIFT—gamete intrafallopian transfer; IVF—*in vitro* fertilization; TDI—Therapeutic donor insemination. (*Adapted from* Maroulis [1]; with permission).

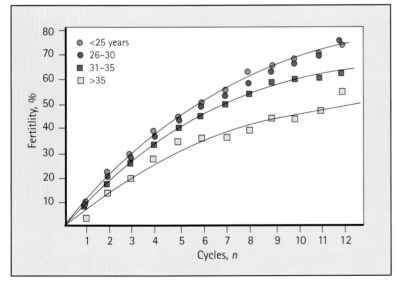

FIGURE 9-7.

Advanced maternal age and time to pregnancy. Advanced maternal age prolongs time to pregnancy. This is a study on spouses of azoospermic men from the French national donor insemination registry (Federation CECOS) [6]. These women, supposedly free of gynecologic diseases, demonstrated that diminishing fecundity, evident by age 30, is dramatic after 35 years. There were 371 women in the 25 years old and under group, 1079 in the 26 to 30 age group, 599 in the 31 to 35 age group, and 144 in the over 35 group. (*Adapted from* Schwartz and Mayaux [6]; with permission.)

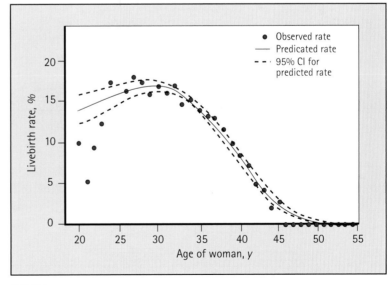

FIGURE 9-8.

Advanced maternal age and liveborn rates after one cycle of *in vitro* fertilization. Advanced maternal age impairs response to infertility treatment. Advancing maternal age adversely affects live birth rates from *in vitro* fertilization. This study of 36,961 *in vitro* fertilization cycles in the United Kingdom shows live birth rates plummeting between ages 35 and 40. (*Adapted from* Templeton *et al.* [9]; with permission.)

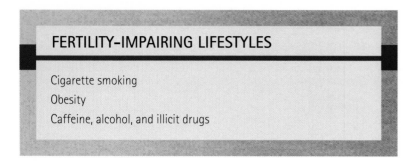

FIGURE 9-9.

Fertility-impairing lifestyles. Some physicians will not treat infertility patients who continue to smoke, are obese, abuse alcohol, or use illicit drugs.

FERTILITY-IMPAIRING LIFESTYLES

Cigarette smoking

Obesity

Caffeine, alcohol, and illicit drugs

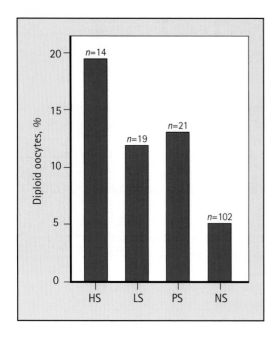

FIGURE 9-10.

Cigarette smoking. Cigarette smoking impairs reproductive efficiency. This is a cytogenetic study of 286 unfertilized oocytes recovered from 156 women undergoing follicle aspiration for *in vitro* fertilization. The nonsmoking (NS) group includes NS husbands; the passive smoking (PS) group includes NS wives; light smokers (LS) smoke less than 15 cigarettes per day; heavy smokers (HS) smoke more than 15 cigarettes per day. Oocytes from women who were heavy smokers showed a highly significant increase in oocyte diploidy, which is believed to result from failure to extrude the first polar body.

Smoking impairs cervical mucus production and alters tubal ciliary transport [10]. Early menopause, reduced spermatogenesis, and decreased sex steroid or estradiol production have been noted in individuals who use cigarettes [11]. Smoking also increases the risk of miscarriage, perinatal mortality, and low birth weight [11]. Smoking impairs fecundity in both women and men [12,13]. In a prospective study of women intending to conceive, 38% of nonsmokers conceived in the first cycle as compared with only 28% of women who smoke [12]. Life table analyses demonstrate a longer period of time to conception for smokers than non smokers. A delay of conception for more than 1 year is three to four times more likely in women who smoke [13,14]. Also, the greater the number of cigarettes smoked, the lower a woman's fertility rates [12–14]. Finally, data from an *in vitro* fertilization study suggest that smoking significantly reduces the chance of successful term pregnancy because of increased miscarriage rates [15]. When a couple is serious about becoming pregnant, both partners should stop smoking. (*Adapted from* Zenzes *et al.* [16]; with permission.)

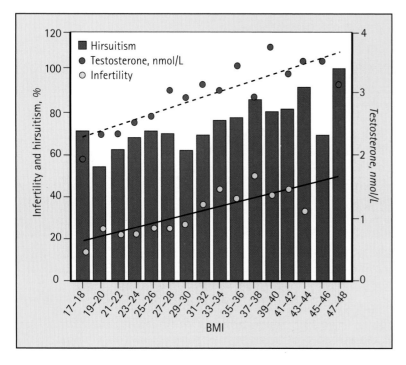

FIGURE 9-11.

Obesity and fertility. In this study of 1701 women diagnosed with polycystic ovarian syndrome (PCOS) by ultrasound, increasing body mass index (BMI) is significantly correlated with worsening hirsutism, rising testosterone concentrations, cycle disturbances, and infertility. Excess body fat impairs ovulation, interferes with ovulation-inducing drugs, and increases difficulty performing transvaginal oocyte retrieval for *in vitro* fertilization. There are no universally accepted guidelines; however, we ask overweight women in our *in vitro* fertilization program to maintain their weight below 130% of ideal body weight. Weight reduction reverses the endocrinopathy of PCOS. For some obese infertile women, weight reduction alone can lead to pregnancy [17,18]. (*Adapted from* Belen *et al.* [19]; with permission.)

CAFFEINE, ALCOHOL, AND ILLICIT DRUGS

Caffeine consumption in excess of 500 mg per day is associated with prolonged time to conception [20].

Alcohol and illicit drugs have been implicated as impairing fertility; however, their effects are difficult to prove in epidemiologic studies because of confounding variables [21].

Medical complications of alcohol and illicit drugs on pregnancy, however, are well documented; alcohol and illicit drugs should be prescribed during preconceptual counselling for infertile patients.

FIGURE 9-12.

Caffeine, alcohol, and illicit drugs. Patients should be counseled to moderate caffeine and alcohol consumption, and eliminate illicit drugs.

HUMAN REPRODUCTIVE INEFFICIENCY

Human reproduction is inefficient and wasteful. Even for young women in their reproductive prime, monthly fecundity is only 20% to 25% per month. Thus, in normal unions, mean cumulative probability of conception after 1 month of unprotected intercourse is only 25%; 70% by 6 months, and 90% by 1 year [4,6]

Some types of assisted reproductive technology (eg, *in vitro* fertilization) produce pregnancy rates that are only slightly more efficient than natural fecundity

FIGURE 9-13.

Human reproductive inefficiency. Patients need counsel regarding the time required for fertile couples to conceive. This counsel needs adjustment for maternal age, lifestyles, and infertility cause as it applies to that couple.

IAGNOSTIC TECHNIQUES

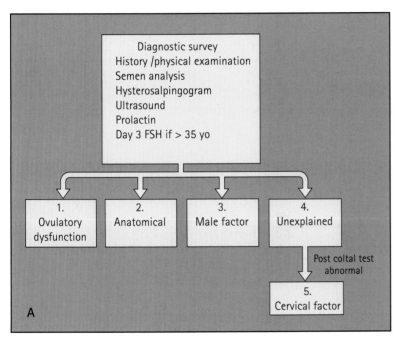

FIGURE 9-14.

Diagnostic survey. The diagnostic survey identifies optimal therapy. This algorithm segregates infertile patients into five nonspecific but treatment-oriented categories (**A**): 1) ovulatory dysfunction, 2) anatomic factor, 3) male factor infertility, 4) unexplained infertility, and 5) cervical factor. The survey begins with a medical history, physical examination of the woman, hysterosalpingogram (HSG), pelvic ultrasound, semen analysis, serum prolactin, and day 3 follicle-stimulating hormone (FSH) if the woman is older than 35 years of age.

(Continued on next page)

B. IDENTIFICATION OF OPTIMAL THERAPY FOR INFERTILITY

Category	Diagnostic criteria	Therapy
Ovulatory dysfunction	Oligo/amenorrhea	Ovulation induction or oocyte donation
Polycystic ovarian disease	FSH < 5 mIu/mL LH > 20 mIu/mL	Clomiphene or gonadotropins
Pituitary microadenoma	Prolactin > 20 mIu/mL	Bromyocryptine
Hypothalamic amenorrhea	FSH < 5 mIu/mL LH < 5 mIu/mL	Clomiphene or gonadotropins
Premature ovarian failure	FSH > 40 mIu/mL	Oocyte donation
Anatomic	Abnormal HSG/US Intrauterine adhesions Uterine anomalies Tubal obstruction Myomas; hydrosalpinges Endometriomas Ovarian neoplasm/cysts	In vitro fertilization
Male factor	Abnormal semen	IVF with ICSI Vas reanastamosis Varicocele ligation Medical therapy
Unexplained	Tests not informative	Empiric therapy COH + IUI
Cervical factor	Abnormal PCT/normal semen	Intrauterine Insemination

FIGURE 9-14. *(Continued)*

B, Diagnostic criteria and therapy for each category. *Ovulatory dysfunction* may be identified by its signature history of irregular or absent menses. A specific cause is identified by measuring serum prolactin, FSH (already obtained if >36 years of age),

FOUR OVULATORY DYSFUNCTIONS COMMONLY ASSOCIATED WITH INFERTILITY

Hyperprolactinemia is identified as a cause of amenorrhea/ oligomenorrhea by its association with elevated serum prolactin (>20 ng/mL). Bromocryptine is the treatment of this condition [22].

Premature ovarian failure is identified by a single elevated serum FSH > 40 mIU/mL [23]. However, any day 3 value > 25 mIU/mL signals high likelihood of low implantation rates, high miscarriage rates, and little likelihood of a viable pregnancy [24]. Oocyte donation is the treatment for POF as it responds poorly to ovulation induction [24].

Polycystic ovarian disease is identified on the basis of its characteristic oligomenorrhea and hyperestrogenism, with or without androgenization, associated with low or normal FSH, undulating and usually elevated LH, and normal serum prolactin. Clomiphene citrate or exogenous gonadotropins induce ovulation with high efficiency in PCOD [25].

Hypothalamic amenorrhea/oligomenorrhea is diagnosed on the basis of its association with hypoestrogenism, underweight, eating disorders, and anosmia. Clomiphene citrate or exogenous gonadotropins induce ovulation with high efficiency in this condition [26].

and adding a serum luteinizing hormone assay. These tests identify hyperprolactinemia, polycystic ovarian disease (PCOD), hypothalamic amenorrhea, and premature ovarian failure (POF). These conditions are treated specifically by ovulation induction or oocyte donation.

Anatomic factor is identified when the woman is previously diagnosed with a gynecologic disease, has an abnormal HSG, or has an abnormal ultrasound. These couples are treated by *in vitro* fertilization (IVF) vs. corrective surgery.

Male factor infertility is identified if the semen analysis is abnormal. These couples are managed by interventions involving the male partner. Such interventions may include correction of ejaculatory dysfunction, repair of obstructed ducts, varicocele ligation, or IVF with intracytoplasmic sperm injection (ICSI). (*see* chapters 11 and 13 for details of diagnosis and management of male factor infertility.)

Unexplained infertility is identified when no abnormality can be demonstrated. The couple is treated empirically. Empiric treatments include gonadotropin controlled ovarian hyperstimulation (COH) with intrauterine insemination (IUI), or *in vitro* fertilization.

Cervical factor is identified when the postcoital test (PCT) demonstrates mucous that is hostile to sperm when the male has a normal semen analysis. These couples are effectively treated by IUI.

FIGURE 9-15.

Four ovulatory dysfunctions commonly associated with infertility. Women with ovulatory dysfunction are identified by their history of amenorrhea or irregular menses. Some diagnoses require confirmation with 2 or 3 months of menstrual calendars and basal body temperatures. Conception fails to occur because timely ovulations are not present. The four most common ovulatory dysfunctions associated with infertility are 1) hyperprolactinemia, 2) premature ovarian failure (POF), 3) polycystic ovarian syndrome (PCOD) and 4) hypothalamic oligomenorrhea/amenorrhea. It is essential to identify these four diagnoses because their treatments are different (*see* Fig. 9-14). The distinctions can be made on the basis of history and measurements of serum prolactin, follicle-stimulating (FSH), and luteinizing hormone (LH).

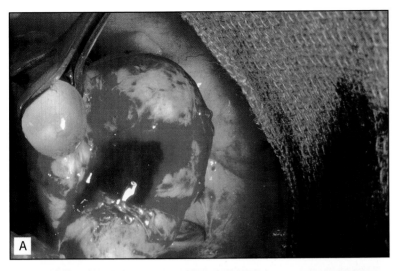

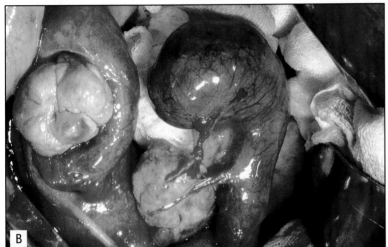

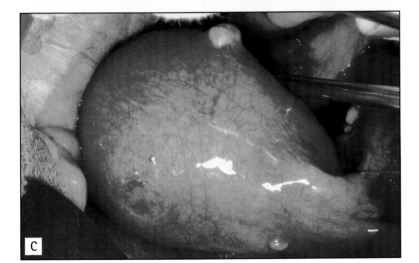

FIGURE 9–16.

Anatomic factors. Infertile women with anatomic infertility have complications of common gynecologic diseases. Patients with these conditions are satisfactorily diagnosed by hysterosalpingogram (HSG), pelvic ultrasound, occasionally by an office hysteroscopy, or frequently because they have an established history of gynecologic disease [27–30]. Although these examples are surgical photographs, diagnostic laparoscopy is not needed to identify these conditions in detail. Except for minimal cases, HSG and ultrasound identify them sufficiently well to enable selection of optimal fertility treatment. Information available from previous laparoscopies costs very little and should be reviewed.

A, Extensive endometriosis with adhesions around the fimbria, destruction of ovarian tissue (endometriomas), and peritoneal implants. Endometriosis this extensive probably interferes with pregnancy by its inflammatory response and mechanical impairment to gamete transport and fertilization.

B, Extensive pelvic inflammatory disease with bilateral tubal obstruction, hydrosalpinges, and tubovarian adhesions. Salpingitis, in addition to the distortion of anatomy visible here, also causes severe disruption to the lining of the oviducts. Even when tubes are rendered patent by salpingostomy or peritubal adhesiolysis, pregnancy rates are very low.

C, Uterine myomas. Myomas, particularly large examples such as these, greatly distort pelvic anatomy. It is not clear to what degree they impair fertility. Myomectomies leave extensive adhesions that are particularly troublesome if the tumors were removed from the back of the uterus. Myomas distorting the uterine cavity probably impair implantation and should be removed prior to *in vitro* fertilization. (*Courtesy of* L. Russell Malinak.)

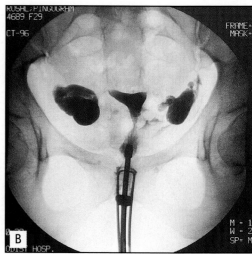

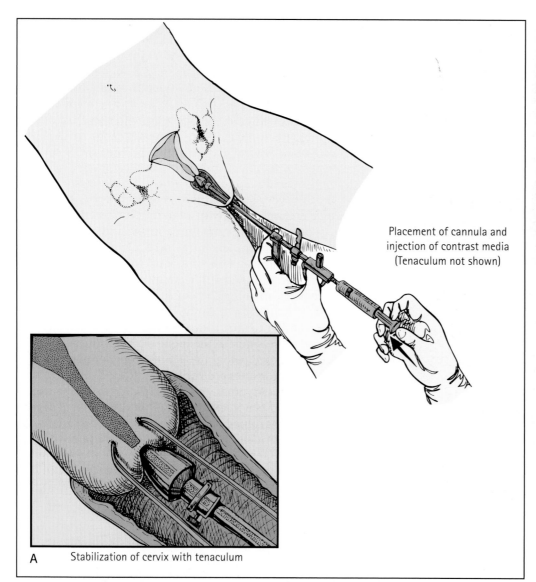

Placement of cannula and
injection of contrast media
(Tenaculum not shown)

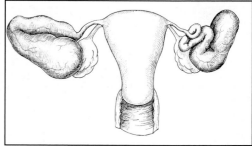

A Stabilization of cervix with tenaculum

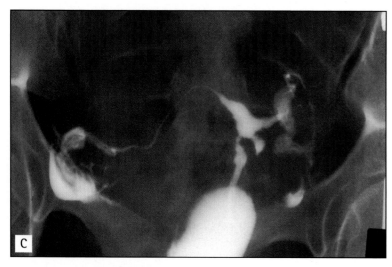

FIGURE 9–17.

Hysterosalpingography (HSG). The HSG provides information regarding the uterine cavity and fallopian tube patency. It is usually performed on cycle days 7 through 9, which for most women is the time between the cessation of menstrual blood flow and the expected occurrence of ovulation.

A, Technique of HSG. This drawing illustrates placement of the cannula and injection of radiographic contrast into the uterus. The cervix is cleansed with disinfectant. After stabilization of the cervix with a tenaculum, approximately 3 to 5 mL of radiopaque contrast is injected. To minimize cramping from this procedure, we routinely warm the radiographic contrast and inject it very slowly. The injected contrast allows visualization of the endocervical canal, uterine cavity, and both tubes. If the contrast, however, goes through one tube rapidly and fails to enter the other, the nonfilling tube is usually normal [31]. We first use water-soluble dye; then if both tubes are patent, we inject oil through the tubes for the possible therapeutic benefit, albeit controversial (an increased pregnancy rate appears to be more prevalent with the use of oil-soluble contrast media; randomized studies have confirmed this finding [31,32]). Assignment to the *anatomic factor* category is in order if the HSG shows evidence of tubal disease. We treat patients with obstructed tubes by *in vitro* fertilization (IVF) because induction of timely ovulations alone is unlikely to produce pregnancy.

B, Bilateral hydrosalpinges. This study demonstrates large, bilateral hydrosalpinges characteristic of pelvic inflammatory disease.

(Continued on next page)

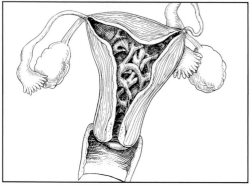

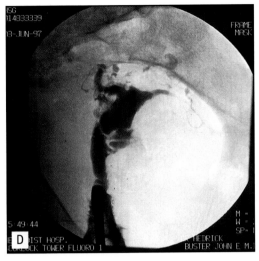

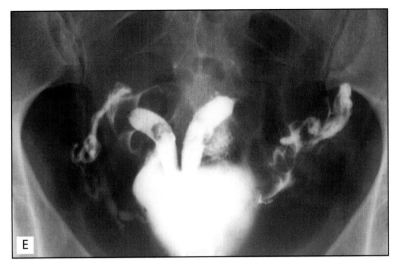

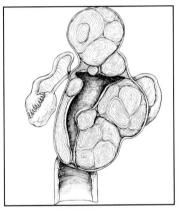

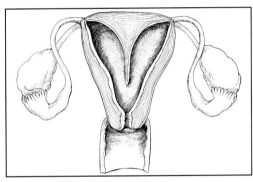

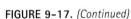

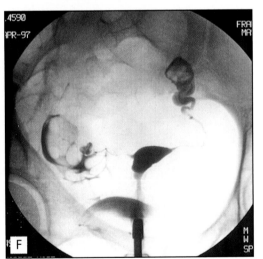

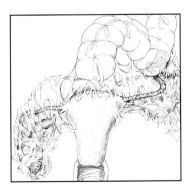

FIGURE 9-17. *(Continued)*
Hydrosalpinges are particularly troublesome when treating with IVF because they obstruct oocyte retrieval, become infected, are a site of ectopic pregnancy, and probably impair implantation because they discharge their inflammatory contents into the uterus after embryo transfer. It is probably best to remove them before IVF.

C, Intrauterine synechiae. This study demonstrates intrauterine synechiae in a patient with a history of retained placenta, postpartum hemorrhage, and fever followed by a dilatation and curettage. They were treated by hysteroscopic adhesiolysis, insertion of a foley catheter, and high-dose estrogens.

D, Submucous myoma. This study illustrates multiple large submucous myomas associated with menorrhagia in an infertility patient. It is not clear whether the myoma cause infertility; however, removal of them is appropriate prior to investing in a cycle of IVF because they may impair implantation.

E, Uterine septum. This study illustrates a uterine septum in a patient with unexplained infertility. The septum was resected hysteroscopically before undertaking a cycle of IVF.

F, Peritubal adhesions. This study illustrates loculation of contrast around the fimbria. Sensitivity of HSG in diagnosis of peritubal adhesions is not at the level of diagnostic laparoscopy [27]. Although some peritubal adhesions will be missed, they have little effect on conduct or outcome of IVF. (*C–E courtesy of* Peter R. Casson.)

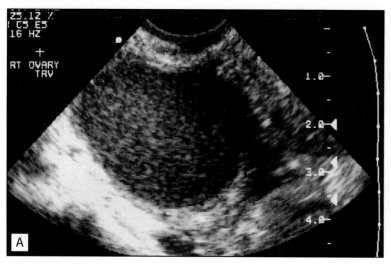

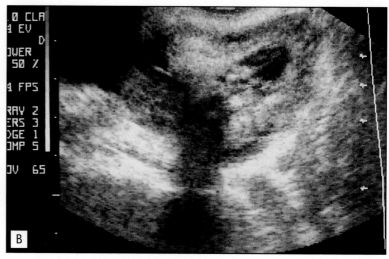

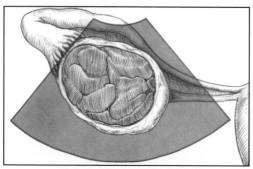

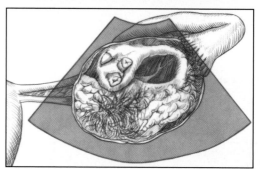

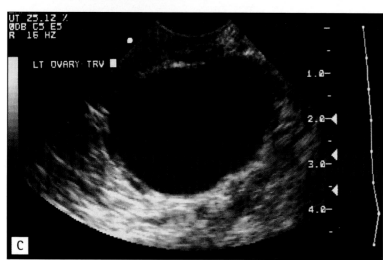

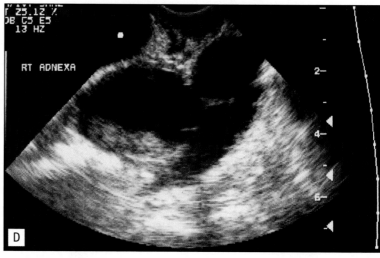

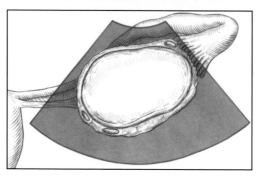

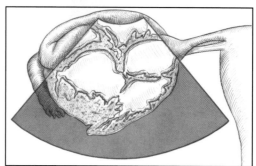

FIGURE 9–18.

Pelvic ultrasound. Vaginal ultrasound documents architecture of the ovaries and uterus. The presence of endometriomas, teratoma, ovarian cysts, hydrosalpinges, or myomas may affect conduct or outcome of *in vitro* fertilization (IVF).

A, Endometrioma. This example illustrates an endometrioma diagnosed in a patient wanting to begin IVF. The endometrioma was initially resected, but recurred, and was aspirated after a course of gonadotropin-releasing hormone agonist. The patient then underwent IVF and became pregnant. **B,** Teratoma. This example illustrates a patient with recurrent teratomas. The teratoma was resected prior to attempting IVF. **C,** Unilocular ovarian cyst. This patient had a persistent ovarian cyst associated with a failed stimulation for IVF. After aspiration, the patient was stimulated without complications and became pregnant. **D,** Hydrosalpinges.

(Continued on next page)

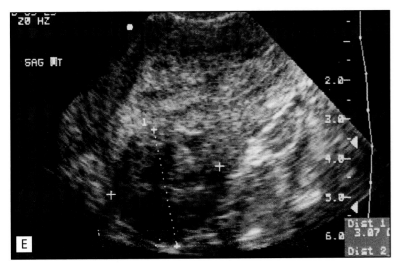

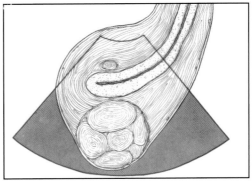

FIGURE 9-18. *(Continued)*

This patient underwent gonadotropin stimulation for IVF and had the hydrosalpinx penetrated during aspiration; she became febrile 1 day after aspiration and required embryo cryopreservation when she became ill and required intravenous antibiotics. **E**, Submucous myoma. This patient has an intramural myoma, which does not encroach the endometrial cavity as shown by hysterosalpinography. It is not clear whether this patient should undergo myomectomy.

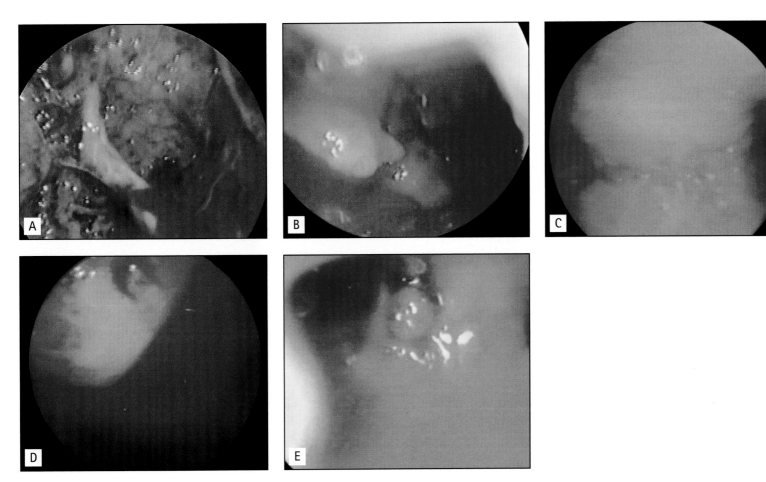

FIGURE 9-19.

Office hysteroscopy. Office hysteroscopy is complimentary to hystero-salpingography (HSG). Several reports show that patients with normal HSG have subsequent diagnostic hysteroscopy examinations that are also normal [29]. Hysteroscopy is best able to identify synechiae and polyps. Diagnostic, and some therapeutic, hysteroscopies are commonly performed in the office with intravenous nonsteroidal antin-flammatory drugs and a 1% xylocaine intracervical block. The procedure has an overall complication rate of about 2% [30]. With *in vitro* fertilization (IVF), it is essential with older women that the uterine cavity be documented as normal because it is believed that IVF failures are caused by problems with implantation. **A**, Intrauterine synechiae.

These intrauterine synechiae were identified in a patient with a history of a dilatation and curettage following a miscarriage. **B**, Endometrial polyps. These multiple endometrial polyps were identified in a nulliparous woman with a history of persistent intermenstrual bleeding and unexplained infertility. **C**, Intrauterine septum in an infertility patient. **D**, Submucous myoma. This patient's uterine cavity is distorted by multiple uterine myomas. It is not clear to what degree these myomas impair implantation. **E**, Retained products of conception. This patient had a history of irregular menses and a negative serum human chorionic gonadotropin level. Office hysteroscopy followed by curettage revealed degenerating trophoblasts. (*Courtesy of* David Zepeda.)

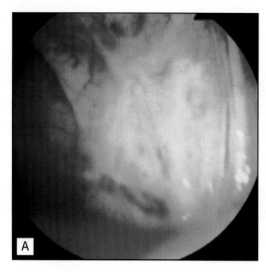 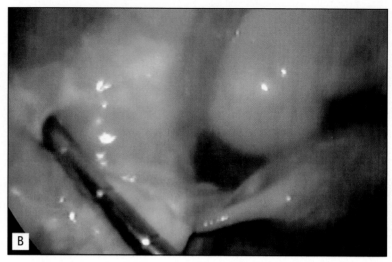

FIGURE 9-20.

Diagnostic laparoscopy. This traditional diagnostic test is becoming less necessary in infertility because most therapeutic decisions can be made on the basis of ultrasound and hysterosalpingography [33]. Reports from previous laparoscopies, however, should be reviewed.

A, Minimal endometriosis. This example of minimal endometriosis could only have been diagnosed by the direct visualization afforded by laparoscopy. If laparoscopy has been undertaken in an infertility patient, excision or destruction of even minimal endometriosis implants is prudent because of the increased spontaneous pregnancy rates from 18% to 31% over the 9 months of followup in this study [34]. This is a modest benefit, however. In light of the considerable costs of performing routine laparoscopy in all infertility patients and given the current success rates with *in vitro* fertilization (IVF), routine diagnostic laparoscopy on all infertility patients is really no longer justified.

B, Peritubal adhesions. Peritubal adhesions are best diagnosed by laparoscopy. These should certainly be lysed if they are seen in an infertility patient. They are frequently associated with endosalpingitis, however, and pregnancy rates following lysis of peritubal adhesions are disappointing when compared with IVF from a top clinic. A large number of screening laparoscopies must be undertaken to find the few favorable cases, and the expense is formidable [35]. (*Courtesy of L. Russell Malinak.*)

OTHER TYPES OF INFERTILITY

Semen Analysis Report

Woman's name:_____   MR #:_____
Man's name:_____   MR #:_____
Physician:_____   (ID #_____)   LAB #:_____

Collection Date:_____	Collection place:	[ ] On-Site [ ] Off-Site
Collection Time:_____	Collection method:	[ ] Masturbation [ ] SCD
Time Received:_____	Container Type:	[ ] Plastic cup [ ] Glass jar
Time Analyzed:_____	Specimen Collection:	[ ] Complete [ ] Incomplete
Days of Abstinence:_____		

Semen Parameters	Patient Value	Normal Ranges	Reference
Color		Whitish-Gray	1
Liquefaction		10-30 minutes	1
Viscosity		0–1+	1
pH		7.2–7.8	1
Agglutination		Absent	1
Red blood cells		0/hpf	1
Epithelial cells		Rare-Occasional/hpf	1
Volume		1.5–5.5 ml	1
Sperm count		>20 million/ml	1
Motility		>40%	1
Motile sperm concentration		>8 million/ml	1
Forward progression		>2	1
Morphology (Strict)		>14% Normal forms	2
Immature sperm		<4 million/ml	1
White blood cells		<1 million/ml	3
% Viable (non-motile)		%Viable (nonmotile) 5% Motile	1
Fructose test		Positive	1

Comments:

References   1. Keel and Webster, 1990   2. Kruger et al. 1986   3. WHO 3rd edition, 1992

Analysis evaluated by:_____   Lab Director:_____

Date/time report released:_____   Faxed to:_____

Form revised 7/30/96 AK

FIGURE 9-21.

Male factor infertility. These are normative values for our andrology laboratory. Couples with male factor have abnormal parameters on semen analysis. Diagnosis of male factor is not a reason to avoid evaluating the woman partner. (*see* chapter 11.) With the introduction of intracytoplasmic sperm injection (ICSI), strong collaboration between andrologist and reproductive endocrinologist has come to fruition. Highly effective therapies for even the most difficult male factor infertility cases are now available [36].

UNEXPLAINED INFERTILITY

Unexplained infertility is infertility of inapparent cause. About 15% of infertile couples have unexplained infertility [37].

When the basic evaluation has been normal, exotic tests are advised by some clinics in an effort to explain the infertility. These include the following:

Ultrasound evaluation of periovulatory events [38]

Tests for luteal phase deficiency [39]

Sperm antibody assays [40]

Routine antiphospholipid antibody screening [41]

Hamster egg penetration test [42]

in vitro human sperm activation test using frog oocytes.[43]

Although such studies are of academic interest and may occasionally result in a diagnosis, this is not satisfying because the finding is not directed into therapy documented as effective. IVF, even if not successful, can be diagnostic in the sense that it demonstrates nuances of sperm–oocyte interaction that would not otherwise be known.

Some couples with unexplained infertility may eventually conceive without treatment. Others may fail to reach their reproductive goals or, because of advancing age or disruption of their marriages, have no children. Empiric therapy increases cyclic fecundity and allows couples with unexplained infertility to conceive earlier than without therapy. In these cases, empiric therapies, such as COH with IUI and IVF which bypasses hitherto unknown barriers, can be effective. Although this is intellectually dissatisfying, empiric therapies do expedite conception and pregnancy. Therapy choice demands careful attention. Convenient, inexpensive office treatments, *eg*, empiric clomiphene citrate, empiric bromocriptine, and empiric IUI may prolong time to conception because they delay effective treatment. Further, empiric COH-IUI with gonadotrophins, while effective in younger women, is strikingly ineffective in women who are in their latter 30s.

FIGURE 9-22.

Unexplained Infertility. Treatment for unexplained infertility is empiric. Patients may not ever have the satisfaction of knowing the cause of their infertility. The dissatisfaction is short-lived when a properly selected couple conceives rapidly from a successful cycle of *in vitro* fertilization or controlled ovarian hyperstimulation (COH) with intrauterine insemination (IUI).

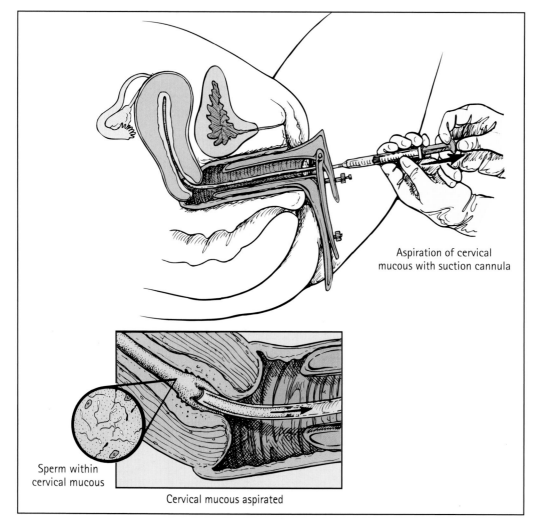

Aspiration of cervical mucous with suction cannula

Sperm within cervical mucous

Cervical mucous aspirated

FIGURE 9-23.

Cervical factor. Aspiration of cervical mucous using a suction cannula. We only perform the postcoital tests in patients whose infertility is otherwise unexplained. We schedule the procedure using home urinary luteinizing hormone (LH) tests. Patients are counseled to have intercourse on the night of positive urinary kit LH surge, and the examination is done the next morning. Cervical mucus is aspirated and examined for quantity, spinnbarkeit, fluidity, ferning, numbers of leukocytes, and sperm per high-powered field [44]. Leukocytes in the mucus suggest infection requiring culture and antibiotic therapy. Good-quality mucus with no sperm, all dead sperm, or a large proportion of shaking sperm (nonprogressive) in a couple with normal semen parameters suggests antisperm antibodies in either the male or female partner [45,46]. If the remainder of the infertility evaluation is normal, intrauterine insemination (without superovulatory drugs) with the husband's seminal plasma-free sperm is used to bypass the hostile cervical mucus [47]. Intrauterine insemination is successful in treating 30% to 40% of couples with uncomplicated cervical factor infertility [48].

$\mathcal{M}$ONITORING TECHNIQUES

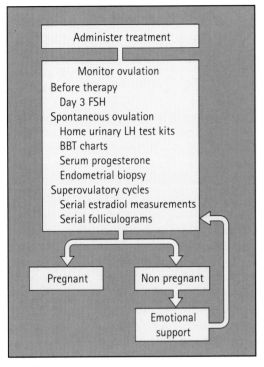

FIGURE 9–24.

Techniques to monitor ovulatory function before and during therapy. BBT—basal body temperature; FSH—follicle-stimulating hormone; LH—luteinizing hormone.

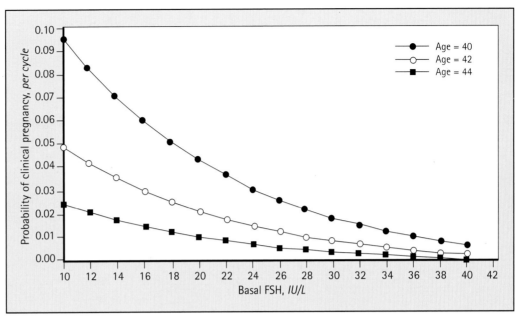

FIGURE 9–25.

Day 3 follicle-stimulating hormone (FSH) levels. This study of infertile women aged 40 and over undergoing ovulation induction depicts probability of pregnancy per cycle as a function of basal FSH and chronologic age. In women older than 40 years of age, cycle fecundity for controlled ovarian hyperstimulation with intrauterine insemination is very low, approximately 2% to 5% per cycle [49]. Pregnancy rates with *in vitro* fertilization (IVF) also decrease between ages 35 and 40 [9]. In couples who have the factors of advanced maternal age and unexplained infertility, an FSH drawn on day 3 of the menstrual cycle is helpful in counseling on fertility prognosis and options. Women with day 3 FSH higher than 25 mIU/mL have success rates with IVF or COH–IUI so low that the only viable alternative is donor oocytes [49,50]. If FSH is under 15 mIU/mL, the woman can proceed to COH–IUI or IVF [24,50]. Nevertheless, even with low FSH, couples should be warned that advanced maternal age seriously compromises response to empiric therapy. (*Adapted from* Pearlstone *et al.* [49]; with permission.)

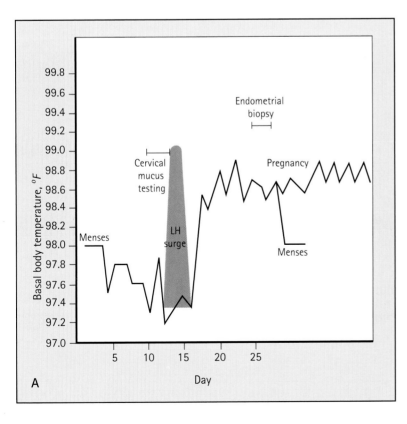

FIGURE 9–26.

Monitoring spontaneous cycles. Basal body temperature (BBT) charts, serum progesterone, and endometrial biopsy are methods of confirming ovulation clinically and monitoring luteal phase.

A, This BBT chart shows the signature thermal shift at midcycle. BBT charts can be used to obtain indirect confirmatory evidence of ovulation. The BBT record is biphasic in ovulatory cycles because of hypothalamic temperature–regulating response to a threshold of serum progesterone of about 4 ng/mL, which produces a 0.5° to 1°F increase in basal temperature [54]. A biphasic temperature chart with a sustained increased temperature of at least 0.4°F for 12 to 15 days is consistent with ovulation [39]. BBT charts are an inexpensive, retrospective means of ovulation detection. Many clinicians believe that appropriate use of the BBT chart, which costs almost nothing, can yield useful results. For some couples, the BBT has teaching value.

(*Continued on next page*)

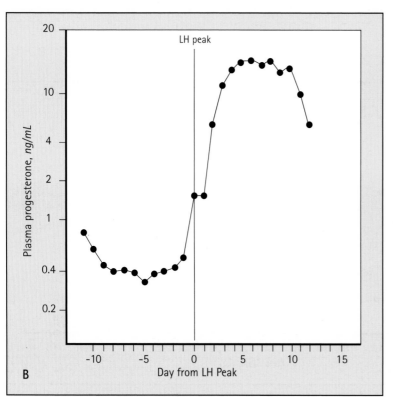

FIGURE 9-26. *(Continued)*

B, Luteal phase plasma progesterone concentrations. This figure depicts mean (SEM) serum progesterone concentrations over the menstrual cycle showing the rise occurring during the periovulatory period [55]. Although normal concentrations of progesterone in luteal phase have been known for over 25 years [55], the cutoff values that make or negate the diagnosis and predict pregnancy outcome are not clear. Concentrations in excess of 3 to 5 ng/mL is viewed as presumptive ovulation because of the correlation with secretory phase endometrial histology in 98% to 100% of cycles [56–59]. A serum progesterone level of less than 3 ng/mL follicular phase suggests anovulation [56–59]. Although progesterone measurements are a convenient way to document ovulation, they do not exclude or diagnose luteal phase defect [56–59]. Progesterone is secreted by the corpus luteum in a pulsatile fashion; attempts to dampen this variability by multiple samples have not been helpful in enhancing the utility of this test [56].

C, Endometrial biopsy. This figure depicts the performance of an endometrial aspiration using an office biopsy curette. A secretary phase endometrial biopsy performed during luteal phase signals presumptive ovulation, but the expense and discomfort of this approach is unacceptable for most [59]. The diagnosis of luteal phase defect (LPD) is still best made by endometrial biopsy because it is the gold standard—the only test that yields such a great deal of information [59]. Identification of this very contentious entity is no longer taken as seriously as it once was, because empiric therapies for unexplained infertility are very effective. LPD should still be considered as a possible cause in patients with recurrent miscarriage.

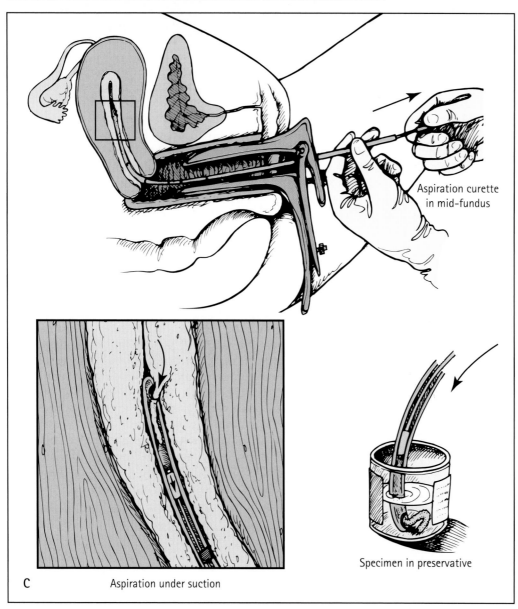

Aspiration curette in mid-fundus

Aspiration under suction

Specimen in preservative

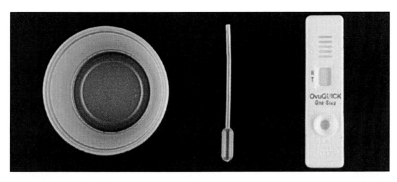

FIGURE 9-27.

Identifying spontaneous ovulation time. Home urinary luteinizing hormone (LH) kits are a convenient, relatively inexpensive method of identifying the time of spontaneous ovulation.They anticipante ovulation by 12 to 24 hours in approximately 90% of women [51]. In spontaneous ovarian cycles, follicular collapse and ovum release occur about 36 hours after inception of the LH surge, or about 24 hours after the LH peak [52]. We instruct our patient to test their first urine in the morning and have intercourse that night. The exact fertilizable life of the human sperm and oocytes is based on probability estimates and cannot be determined precisely in human cases. Best estimates are that sperm retain their ability to fertilize for 24 to 48 hours and that the human oocyte is fertilizable for 12 to 24 hours [53]. To maximize fertilization, it is best that sperm be present in the distal oviduct when the oocyte arrives so that fertilization can occur. These kits can also aid in timing of postcoital testing, inseminations, serum progesterone measurements, and timing of late luteal endometrial biopsies for analysis of corpus luteum function.

Ovuquick® (Quidel, Inc. San Diego, CA) is illustrated. A diposable pipette, plastic collection cup, and test device are provided. Five drops of urine are placed in the test well. After 3 to 5 minutes, the test is read. If both the control line (*bottom*) and test line (*top*) are positive, the LH surge has been detected. A positive control line and negative test line indicate negative test. Urinary LH kits cost between $25 and $60 per month.

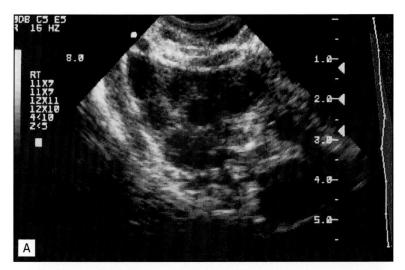

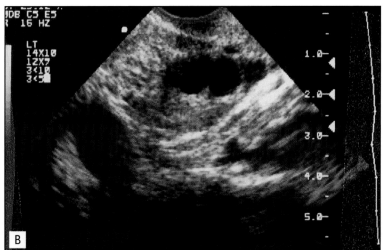

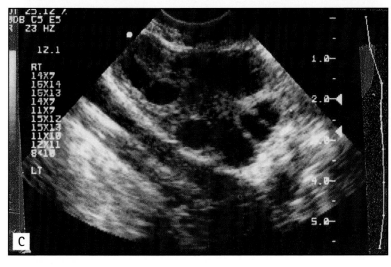

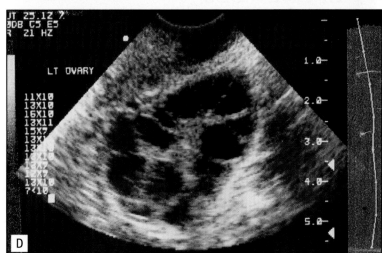

FIGURE 9-28.

Monitoring superovulatory cycles. Transvaginal ultrasound and serial serum estradiol are used together to monitor response to superovulatory drugs.

A–F, These folliculograms were obtained on the 6th, 8th and 9th day of a human menopausal gonadotropin–stimulated *in vitro* fertilization (IVF) cycle. Both right (**B,D,F**) and left (**A,C,E**) ovaries are shown. A baseline ultrasound was used to ascertain the quiescence (absence of follicles)of the ovary after downregulation with gonadotropin-releasing hormone agonist. Repeat examinations were obtained to ascertain response and to assist in the timing of the human chorionic gonadotropin dose and oocyte aspiration.

(Continued on next page)

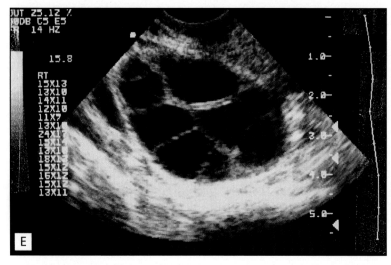

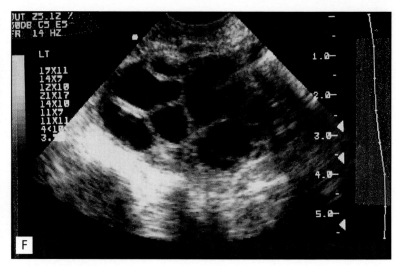

FIGURE 9-28. *(Continued)*

Serial estradiol measurements reflect the endocrine actively of developing follicles as they are stimulated by HMGs or follicle-stimulating hormone. On the first day of stimulation, estradiol concentrations should reflect a quiet ovary with a level of less than 50 pg/mL and should confirm a baseline folliculogram, which should show only very small follicles. Estradiol measurements are then used in combination with folliculograms to titrate dosing of superovulatory drugs. In an ideal stimulation, one follicle is seen on ultrasound for about every 200 pg/mL of serum estradiol [60]

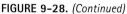

$\mathcal{A}$CKNOWLEDGMENTS

The author wishes to acknowledge Ms. Victoria Alderman for preparing the ultrasound and gynecologic anatomy illustrations.

$\mathcal{R}$EFERENCES

1. Maroulis GB: Effect of aging on fertility and pregnancy. *Sem Reprod Endocrinol* 1991, 9:165–175.

2. Sauer MV, Paulson RJ, Lobo RA: Reversing the natural decline human fertility: an extended clinical trial of oocyte donation to women of advanced reproductive age. *JAMA* 1992, 268:1275–1279.

3. Warburton D, Kline J, Stein Z, Strobino B: Cytogenetic abnormalities in spontaneous abortions of recognized conceptions. In *Perinatal Genetics: Diagnosis and Treatment*. Edited by Porter IH. New York: Academic Press; 1986:133-145.

4. Peek JC, Godfrey B, Matthews CD: Estimation of fertility and fecundity in women receiving artificial insemination by donor semen and in normal fertile women. *B J Obstet Gynecol* 1984, 91:1019–1024.

5. Shenfield F, Doyle P, Valentine A, *et al.*: Effects of age, gravidity and male infertility status on cumulative conception rates following artificial insemination with cryopreserved donor semen: analysis of 2998 cycles of treatment in one centre over 10 years. *Hum Reprod* 1993, 8:60–64.

6. Schwartz D, Mayaux MJ: Female fecundity as a function of age. *New Engl J Med* 1982, 306:404–406.

7. Stein ZA: A woman's age: Childbearing and childrearing. *Am J Epidemiol* 1985, 121:327–342.

8. Virro MR, Shewchuck AB: Pregnancy outcome in 242 conceptions after artificial insemination with donor sperm and effects of maternal age on the prognosis for successful pregnancy. *Am J Obstet Gynecol* 1984, 148:518–524.

9. Templeton A, Morris JH, Parslow W: Factors that affect outcome of in-vitro fertilization treatment. *Lancet* 1996, 348:1402–1406.

10. Feichtinger W: Environmental factors and fertility. *Hum Reprod* 1991, 6:1170–1175.

11. US Department of Health and Human Services: Female: pregnancy and pregnancy outcome. In *The Health Benefits of Smoking Cessation: A Report of the Surgeon General*. Washington DC: US Department of Health and Human Services; 1990:371–423 [Publication no. (CDC)90-8416].

12. Stillman RJ, Rosenberg MJ, Sachs BP: Smoking and reproduction. *Fertil Ster* 1986, 46:545–566.

13. Laurent SL, Thompson SJ, Addy C, *et al.*: An epidemiologic study of smoking and primary infertility in women. *Fertil Steril* 1992, 57:565–572.

14. Bolumar F, Olsen J, Boldsen J: Smoking reduces fecundity: a European multicenter study on infertility and subfecundity. The European Study Group on Infertility and Subfecundity. *Am J Epidemiol* 1996, 143:578–587.

15. Maximovich A, Beyler SA: Cigarette smoking at time of in vitro fertilization cycle initiation has negative effect on in vitro fertilization-embryo transfer success rate. *J Assist Reprod Genet* 1995, 12:75–77.

16. Zenzes MT, Wang P, Casper RF: Cigarette smoking may affect meiotic maturation of human oocytes. *Hum Reprod* 1995, 10:3213–3217.

17. Hollmann M, Runnebaum B, Gerhard I: Effects of weight loss on the hormonal profile in obese, infertile women. *Hum Reprod* 1996, 11:1884–1891.

18. Galletly C, Clark A, Tomlinson L, Blaney F: Improved pregnancy rates for obese, infertile women following a group treatment program: an open pilot study. *Gen Hosp Psychiatry* 1996, 18:192–195.

19. Balen AH, Conway GS, Kaltsas G, *et al.*: Polycystic ovary syndrome: the spectrum of the disorder in 1741 patients. *Hum Reprod* 1995, 10:2107–2111.

20. Bolumar F, Olsen J, Rebagliato M, Bisanti L: Caffeine intake and delayed conception: a European multicenter study on infertility and subfecundity. European Study Group on Infertility and Subfecundity. *Am J Epidemiol* 1997, 145:324–334.

21. Olsen J, Bolumar F, Boldsen J, Bisanti L: Does moderate alcohol intake reduce fecundability? A European multicenter study on infertility and subfecundity. European study Group on Infertility and Subfecundity. *Alcoho Clin Exp Res* 1997, 21:206–212.

22. Brenner SH, Lessing JB, Quagliarello J, Weiss G: Hyperpro- lactinemia and associated pituitary prolactinomas. *Obstet Gynecol* 1985, 65:661–664.

23. Rebar RW: Hypergonadotropic amenorrhea and premature ovarian failure: a review. *J Reprod Med* 1982, 27:179–186.

24. Toner JP, Philput C, Jones GS, Muasher SJ: Basal follicle stimulating hormone (FSH) level is a better predictor of in vitro fertilization (IVF) performance than age. *Fertil Steril* 1991, 55:784–791.

25. Chappel SC, Howles C: Reevaluation of the roles of luteinizing hormone and follicle-stimulating hormone in the ovulatory process. *Hum Reprod* 1991, 6:1206–1212.

26. Berga SL, Mortola JF, Suh GB, *et al.*: Neuroendocrine aberrations in women with functional hypothalamic amenorrhea. *J Clin Endocrinol Metab* 1989, 68:301–308.

27. Swart P, Mol BW, van der Veen F, *et al.*: The accuracy of hysterosalpingography in the diagnosis of tubal pathology: a meta- analysis. *Fertil Steril* 1995, 64:486–491.

28. Blumenfeld Z, Yoffe N, Bronshtein M: Transvaginal sonography in infertility and assisted reproduction. *Obstet Gynecol Surv* 1991, 46:36–49.

29. Fayez JA, Muti G, Schneider PJ: The diagnostic value of hysterosalpingram and hystetoscopy in infertility investigation. *Am J Obstet Gynecol* 1987, 156:558–560.

30. Brooks PG: Complications of operative hysteroscopy: how safe is it? *Clin Obstet Gynecol* 1992, 35(2):249–255.

31. Mackey RA, Glass RM, Olson LE, Vaidya RA: Pregnancy following hysterosalpingography with oil and water soluble dye. *Fertil Steril* 1971, 22:504–507.

32. Rasmussen F, Lindequist S, Larsen C, Justesen P: Therapeutic effect of hysterosalpingography: oil-versus water-soluble contrast media. A randomized prospective study. *Radiology* 1991, 179:75–78.

33. Opsahl MS, Miller B, Klein TA: The predictive value of hysteosalpingography for tubal and peritoneal infertility factors. *Fertil Steril* 1993, 60:444–448.

34. Marcoux S, Maheux R, Berube S: Laparoscopic surgery in infertile women with minimal or mild endometriosis: Canadian Collaborative Group on Endometriosis. *N Engl J Med* 1997, 337:217–222.

35. Schalff W, Massiakos D, Damewood M, Rock J: Neosalpingostomy for distal tubal obstruction: prognostic factors and impact of surgical techniques. *Fertil Steril* 1990, 54:984–990.

36. Tarlatzis BC: Report on the activities of the ESHRE task force on intracytoplasmic sperm injection: European Society of Human Reproduction and Embryology. *Hum Reprod* 1996, 4:160–185.

37. Ashushan A, Eisenberg VH, Schenker JH: Subfertility in the era of assisted reproduction: changes and consequences. *Fertil Steril* 1995, 64:459–469.

38. Stanger JD, Yovich JL: Failure of human oocyte release at ovulation. *Fertil Steril* 1984, 41:827–832.

39. Jordan J, Graig K, Clifton DK, Soules MR: Luteal phase deficit: the sensitivity and specificity of diagnostic methods in common clinical use. *Fertil Steril* 1994, 62:54–62.

40. Naz RK, Menge AC: Antisperm antibodies: origin, regulation, and sperm reactivity in human infertility. *Fertil Ster* 1994, 61:1001–1013.

41. Roussev RG, Kaider BD, Price DE, Coulam CB: Laboratory evaluation of women experiencing reproductive failure. *Am J Reprod Immunol* 1996, 5:415–420,

42. Honig SC, Thompson S, Lipshultz LI: Reassessment of male-factor infertility, including the varicocele, sperm penetration assay, semen analysis, and in vitro fertilization. *Cur Opin Obstet Gynecol* 1993, 5:245–251.

43. Brown DB, Nagamani M: Use of *Xenopus laevis* frog egg extract in diagnosing human male unexplained infertility. *Yale J Biol Med* 1992, 65:29–38.

44. World Health Organization: WHO laboratory manual for the examination of human semen and semen-cervical mucus interaction. New York: Cambridge University Press; 1987:1–20.

45. Moghissi KS, Sacco AG, Borin K: Immunologic infertility:I. Cervical mucus antibodies and post coital test. *Am J Obstet Gynecol* 1980, 136:941–950.

46. DeAlmerida M, Gazagne I, Jeulin C, *et al.*: In vitro processing of sperm with autoantibodies and in vitro fertilization results. *Hum Reprod* 1989, 4:49–53.

47. Confino E, Friberg J, Dudkeiwicz AB, Gleicher N: Intrauterine insemination with washed human spermatozoa. *Fertil Steril* 1986, 46:55–60.

48. te Velde ER, Van kooy RJ, Waterreus JJH: Intrauterine insemination of washed husband's spermatozoa: a controlled study. *Fertil Steril* 1989, 51:182–185.

49. Pearlstone AC, Fournet N, Gambone JC, *et al.*: Ovulation induction in women age 40 and older: the importance of basal folicle-stimulating hormone level and chronological age. *Fertil Steril* 1992, 58:674–679.

50. Burwinkel TH, Buster JE, Scoggan JL, Carson SA: Basal follicle stimulating hormone (FSH) predicts response to controlled ovarian hyperstimulation (COH)-intrauterine insemination (IUI) therapy. *J Assist Reprod Genet* 1994, 11:24–27.

51. Vermesh M, Kletzky OA, Davajan V, Israel R: Monitoring techniques to predict and detect ovulation. *Fertil Steril* 1987, 47:259–264.

52. World Health Organization Task Force on Methods for the Determination of the Fertile Period: Temporal relationships between ovulation and defined changes in the concentration of plasma estradiol-17 beta, luteinizing hormone, follicle-stimulating hormone, and progesterone. *Am J Obstet Gynecol* 1980, 138:383–390.

53. World Health Organization Task Force on Methods for the Determination of the Fertile Period: A prospective multicenter trial of the ovulation method of natural family planning: IV. The outcome of pregnancy. *Fertil Steril* 1984, 41:593-598.

54. Campbell KL: Methods of monitoring ovarian function and predicting ovulation: summary of a meeting. *Res Frontiers Fertil Regulation* (PARFR) 1985, 3:1–46.

55. Abraham GE, Odell WD, Swerdloff RS, Hopper K: Simultaneous radioimmunossay of plasma FSH, LH, progesterone, 17- hydroxprogesterone, and estradiol-17 beta during the menstrual cycle. *J Clin Endocrinol Metab* 1972, 34:312–318.

56. Jordan J, Craig K, Clifton DK, Soules MR: Luteal phase defect: the sensitivity and specificity of diagnostic methods in common clinical use. *Fertil Steril* 1994, 62:54–62.

57. Abdulla V, Diver MJ, Hipkin LJ, Davis JC: Plasma progesterone levels as an indicator of ovulation. *Br J Obstet Gynecol* 1983, 90:543–548.

58. Wathen NC, Perry L, Lilford RJ, Chard T: Interpretation of single progesterone measurement in diagnosis of anovulation and defective luteal phase: observations on analysis of the normal range. *BMJ* 1984, 288:7–9.

59. Jones GS: Luteal phase defect: a review of pathophysiology. *Curr Opin Obstet Gynecol* 1991, 3:641–648.

60. Kerin JF, Warnes GM: Monitoring of ovarian response to stimulation in in-vitro fertilization cycles. *Clin Obstet Gynecol* 1986, 29:158–170.

Ovulation Induction

Charles M. March

Ovulation induction accomplished either by pharmacologic agents or injury to the ovarian capsule has been restricted mainly to infertile women with oligomenorrhea or amenorrhea without ovarian failure. However, pharmacologic agents have been used effectively to treat women with presumed luteal phase defects, to induce the development of large numbers of follicles to facilitate recovery of multiple oocytes for assisted reproductive technologies, and to provide empiric therapy for couples with unexplained infertility [1]. This latter technique, called "superovulation," is often combined with intrauterine insemination with washed semen (these uses are discussed in other chapters in this volume).

In infertile women with oligomenorrhea (menses occurring at > 35-day intervals), it is not important to determine whether or not the cycles are ovulatory before beginning treatment. Ovulation should be induced monthly in order to increase the chance of conception. During one ovulatory cycle the chance of conception following midcycle intercourse is approximately 22%. Thus, all oligomenorrheic women who wish to conceive should be treated whether or not they occasionally ovulate spontaneously because these drugs will increase frequency of ovulation and, more importantly, will cause ovulation to occur at a consistently predictable time, thereby facilitating timed intercourse or inseminations.

AUSES AND EVALUATION OF FEMALE INFERTILITY

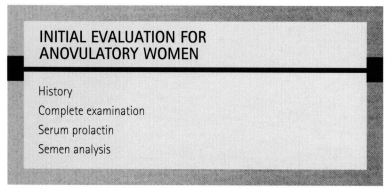

DIAGNOSED CAUSES OF FEMALE INFERTILITY

	Infertile women, %
Pelvic pathology	50
Ovulatory dysfunction	35
Cervical or uterine factors	15

FIGURE 10-1.

Diagnosed causes of female infertility. Infertility affects approximately 18% of couples [2]. Overall, the cause of infertility will be diagnosed in 90% of couples undergoing a complete investigation. Male and female factors only will be found equally in approximately one third of couples. Perhaps the most important group is the other one third in whom both male and female

TYPES OF OVULATORY DEFECTS

Luteal phase defects
Polycystic ovarian syndrome
Hypothalmic-pituitary dysfunction
Hypothalmic-pituitary failure
Premature ovarian failure

FIGURE 10-2.

Types of ovulatory defects. Women who are anovulatory may present with luteal phase defects, oligomenorrhea, or amenorrhea. Among women with oligomenorrhea, a diagnosis of polycystic ovarian syndrome or hypothalmic-pituitary dysfunction may be

INITIAL EVALUATION FOR ANOVULATORY WOMEN

History
Complete examination
Serum prolactin
Semen analysis

FIGURE 10-3.

Initial evaluation for anovulatory women. The initial evaluation for most anovulatory women is both brief and rapid. The history should be complete, and include a pelvic examination. The breast examination should be meticulous to elicit any inappropriate lactation. Studies should include a serum prolactin measurement

factors are identified. Among the female factors identified, the most common are pelvic factors, *eg*, tubal obstruction, adhesions, and endometriosis. The second most common factor, ovulatory defects, is diagnosed in approximately 35% of women [3]. The least common types of abnormality causing female infertility are cervical and uterine factors. Uterine factors are more likely to cause pregnancy loss rather than infertility, whereas cervical factors are more likely to cause infertility by impairing sperm transport. Many women will have more than one problem.

Except for those with premature ovarian failure, ovulation may be induced in almost all women. The pretreatment evaluation is usually simple. The established treatment protocols ensure safe, effective therapy. The newer agents may afford some advantages over earlier drugs. Teratogenicity has not been linked to these drugs. Careful monitoring will reduce the frequency of high-order multiple gestations. For some women in whom medical therapy fails, surgical treatment affords an effective alternative.

made. The amenorrhea may be primary or secondary. Amenorrheic women who have milder defects will have some ovarian function as evidenced by serum estradiol levels within the range of normal for the follicular phase of the cycle and with progesterone-induced withdrawal bleeding. Estrogen-deficient amenorrheic women have either hypothalamic-pituitary failure or ovarian failure. Women with ovarian failure have elevated levels of gonadotropins, with the follicle-stimulating hormone level being higher than that of luteinizing hormone and estradiol levels in the range expected for postmenopause (usually < 20 pg/mL). These individuals are not candidates for ovulation induction, although ovulation and even successful pregnancy have been reported on rare occasions. These women should be considered for ovum donation. Among normoestrogenic women, the work-up is minimal. Among amenorrheic women who are estrogen deficient, an extensive evaluation should be completed prior to ovulation induction to ensure that there is no contraindication for pregnancy.

and, if there is any history of thyroid disease or symptoms thereof, a serum thyroid-stimulating hormone (TSH) measurement. The older the woman, the more likely that a TSH measurement should be obtained—because the incidence of hypothyroidism rises with increasing age. For women who are close to 40 years of age, a serum follicle-stimulating hormone (FSH) and estradiol level should be obtained on day 3 of the cycle in order to obtain a measure of ovarian reserve. A semen analysis should be obtained from the woman's partner to rule out the presence of a significant male factor. If the semen analysis is not normal, multiple specimens should be analyzed over a few months' time to more completely evaluate the male factor. Mild degrees of reduced semen quality should not preclude treatment with ovulation-inducing agents, but should prompt the early investigation of the male factor by means of a postcoital test and evaluation by an andrologist. Treatment by intrauterine insemination with seperated spermatazoa should be performed while that investigation is being completed.

PHARMACOLOGIC TREATMENT AND CONTRAINDICATIONS

TREATMENT OF ANOVULATION

Clomiphene citrate

Bromocriptine

Human menopausal gonadotropins

Human menopausal FSH

Recombinant FSH

GnRH

Combinations

Surgery

FIGURE 10-4.

Treatment of anovulation. The agents used to treat anovulation include clomiphene citrate, bromocriptine, human menopausal gonadotropins, human menopausal follicle-stimulating hormone (FSH), highly purified human menopausal FSH, recombinant FSH, gonadotropin-releasing hormone (GnRH), and combinations thereof. Finally, surgical procedures have also come back into vogue. Each of these are addressed separately.

CONTRAINDICATIONS TO OVULATION-INDUCTION THERAPY

Drug allergy

Pregnancy

Ovarian cysts

FIGURE 10-5.

Contraindications to ovulation-induction therapy. These include drug allergy, pregnancy, and ovarian cysts. Ovarian cysts may enlarge during therapy. The magnitude of this risk and the seriousness of treating a woman with pre-existing ovarian enlargement is unknown. However, a pretreatment evaluation consisting of bimanual pelvic examination, ovarian ultrasound, and the review of the woman's prior treatment cycle or some combination of these prior to reinstituting therapy will assure the physician that there is neither ovarian enlargement nor pregnancy. Regarding clomiphene citrate, women who have had prior liver disease may be treated. However, it is important to verify that liver enzymes have returned to normal prior to therapy, and they should be monitored during clomiphene citrate treatment.

GRADUATED CLOMIPHENE CITRATE REGIMEN

50 mg/d × 5 d

100 mg/d × 5 d

150 mg/d × 5 d

200 mg/d × 5 d

250 mg/d × 5 d

250 mg/d × 5 d + 10,000 hCG

FIGURE 10-6.

Graduated clomiphene citrate regimen. This regimen begins with 50 mg/d for 5 days following a spontaneous or induced menses [4]. For women who have relatively short menstrual periods, treatment is begun on day 3 of the cycle. Similar rates of ovulation, luteal dysfunction, cycle fecundity, and abortion have been reported with starting dates between day 2 and day 5 of the cycle [5]. This starting date is especially important for women who have mild ovulatory defects such as luteal phase abnormalities. Because the dominant follicle is selected by day 5 of the cycle, it is important to begin therapy prior to this point so that the pharmacologic agent can override the woman's endogenous gonadotropin secretion. Ovulation usually occurs approximately 1 week after the last clomiphene citrate dose. This interval may range in some women from as early as 3 to as late as 12 days after the last tablet.

During the first treatment cycle, it is best if the woman records her basal body temperature daily in order to provide a record of the approximate date of ovulation as well as to provide presumptive evidence that ovulation has occurred. Menstruation will usually occur approximately 2 weeks after ovulation or about 3 weeks after the last tablet has been ingested. Because menses may occur secondary to decreased estradiol production without ovulation, it is important to document that ovulation has occurred in each treatment cycle. This may be accomplished either by reviewing a basal body temperature or by obtaining a serum progesterone concentration. To obtain the greatest amount of information, the serum progesterone level should be obtained about 1 week after ovulation. At this time the level should be at least 15 ng/mL [6]. If obtained several days prior to peak progesterone production or several days thereafter, any level in excess of 3 ng/mL will yield presumptive evidence of an ovulatory response; however, such evidence cannot be quantitated [7].

Measurement of urinary luteinizing hormone (LH) level to detect the day of the LH surge can also be used to predict the day of ovulation. These tests, using monoclonal antibody technology, are performed at home. The peak level of LH in urine usually occurs 1 day prior to ovulation; the results of these tests correlate well with the ovarian ultrasound findings. It is important to remember that these tests detect the presence of a large amount of LH in urine and do not guarantee that ovulation will follow. Secondly, during clomiphene citrate ingestion, large amounts of LH are released. Thus, urinary LH testing during or immediately after stopping clomiphene citrate can yield false-positive results. Therefore, 3 days should elapse between the last day of treatment with clomiphene citrate and the first day of urinary LH testing. If there is presumptive evidence of ovulation with a 50 mg/d regimen and if menses occur, the woman should be evaluated to rule out the presence of an ovarian cyst. If none is present, she should be treated with the same dose for the next cycle. If ovulation does not occur, menses are induced and 100 mg/d is prescribed for 5 days. If this dose results in ovulation, it should be maintained; if not, the dose should be increased again to 150 mg/d and subsequently in each successive treatment cycle by 50 mg/d increments. The maximum dose is 250 mg/d.

Some women will have significant follicular development as indicated by rising estradiol levels or increase in follicular size as monitored by ultrasound, but follicular rupture and ovulation do not occur. In these cases, ovulation may be induced by administering 10,000 units of human chorionic gonadotropin (hCG) to provide a surrogate LH surge. To identify the ideal day for hCG administration in these instances, ovarian ultrasound is used and hCG is administered when the largest follicle equals or exceeds 25 mm in maximal diameter. Other methods of monitoring follicular development prior to hCG administration are serum estradiol levels and the cervical scores [8]. Both of these have some value, but considerably less than ultrasound. If estradiol levels are measured, they should be greater than 300 pg/mL before hCG is given. If the cervical score is used, it should be 8 or greater at the time of hCG administration. The agent of choice for the pharmacologic induction of ovulation in most women is clomiphene citrate. Its half-life is between 5 and 7 days; because of this slow clearance, clomiphene citrate levels increase in serum over time following successive monthly treatment cycles [9]. Clomiphene citrate is safer and more effective than glucocorticoids for anovulatory women, and therefore corticosteroid therapy should be limited to those women with either congenital adrenal hyperplasia or adrenal androgen hyperfunction.

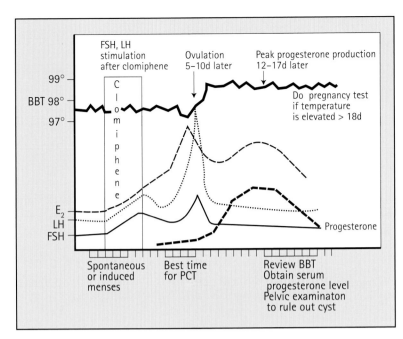

FIGURE 10-7.

Luteinizing hormone (LH), follicle-stimulating hormone (FSH), estradiol, and progesterone levels before, during, and after successful treatment with clomiphene citrate. Clomiphene citrate is a serum and acts by competing with estradiol for estrogen-binding sites in the hypothalamus and therefore prevents the normal negative feedback of endogenous estradiol. The result is a marked increase in the pulse frequency of gonadotropin-releasing hormone (GnRH) [10]. LH pulse frequency but not amplitude increases significantly during clomiphene citrate therapy. FSH pulse frequency increases, but less dramatically. In anovulatory women, GnRH pulse frequencies, at least as determined by measuring LH pulse frequencies, are decreased from normal during the follicular phase and in some women are absent. Some data suggest that clomiphene citrate may act directly on the pituitary, perhaps to increase the sensitivity to GnRH [11]. During drug therapy, serum levels of FSH, LH, and estradiol rise in those women who will have an ovulatory response. Although LH pulse frequency increases even if ovulation fails to occur, FSH and estradiol levels do not [12]. Thus, the rise in FSH level is the key to follicular development and subsequent ovulation. Following the 5 days of drug therapy, estradiol secretion increases and the rising endogenous estradiol levels produce a negative feedback action on the hypothalamic release of GnRH. Therefore, gonadotropin levels fall. The subsequent exponential rise in estradiol produced by the dominant follicle eventually has a positive feedback effect on the hypothalamus, resulting in a surge of gonadotropin output similar to that occurring in a spontaneous ovulatory cycle. Ovulation occurs 33 to 36 hours after the LH surge. Progesterone levels begin to rise immediately before ovulation and reach a peak 1 week following ovulation. BBT—basal body temperature; PCT—postcoital test.

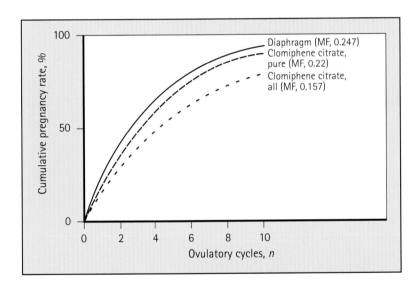

FIGURE 10-8.

Cumulative pregnancy rates in women undergoing ovulation induction compared with women discontinuing diaphragm use. Using the treatment regimen outlined previously, 85% of women will ovulate [4]. Approximately 50% will conceive. The incidence of ovulation is highest among women with oligomenorrhea and almost zero among estrogen-deficient amenorrheic women. Of all women who conceive, over 80% will do so within three ovulatory cycles and 95% will do so within six ovulatory cycles. Therefore, women whose histories or examinations indicate that other infertility factors are not likely to be present do not have any other infertility studies performed until they have ovulated three times with clomiphene citrate therapy. At this time, other studies such as a postcoital test, hysterosalpingogram (HSG), and laparoscopy will be performed. If the HSG is normal, laparoscopy is usually delayed until the sixth ovulatory cycle has been completed. Hammond and colleagues [13] demonstrated that the monthly fecundity (MF) rate was 22% for anovulatory women who had no other infertility factors and who ovulated when treated with clomiphene citrate. The cumulative pregnancy rate after 10 cycles of treatment was 97.5%. (*Adapted from* Hammond and coworkers. [13].)

OVULATION, CONCEPTION, AND DOSE OF CLOMIPHENE CITRATE

Daily dose, mg	Ovulation, %	Conception, %
50	52	53
100	22	21
150	12	10
200	7	10
250	5	6
250 + hCG	2	2

FIGURE 10-9.

Ovulation, conception, and dose of clomiphene citrate. Ovulation is most likely to occur at the 50- or 100-mg daily dose. However, 26% of all ovulations occur at doses above the package insert recommendation of no higher than 100 mg/d [4]. Similarly, 28% of the pregnancies occur at doses above those recommended by the package insert. The frequency of conception correlates with the frequency of ovulation irrespective of which dose is used. hCG—human chorionic gonadotropin.

COMBINATION REGIMEN OF CLOMIPHENE CITRATE AND DEXAMETHASONE

Criteria	Protocol
Anovulation with high-dose clomiphene	Dexamethasone, 0.5 mg/hs
DHEA-S > 2.8 µg/mL	Repeat DHEA-S measurement in 2 wk
	If normal
	Continue dexamethaone
	Induce menses
	Clomiphene at 250/mg × 5 d
	hCG when follicle mature

EXTENDED CLOMIPHENE CITRATE REGIMEN

Clomiphene, 250 mg/d × 8–10 d
hCG, 10,000 IU when follicle is mature

OVERALL RESULTS OF CLOMIPHENE CITRATE THERAPY

	Freqeuncy, %
Ovulation	
Oligomenorrhea	>90
Amenorrhea	67
Pregnancy (overall)	50
Pregnancy (no other infertility factors)	85
Twins	5
Spontaneous abortion	20
Side effects	15
Ectopic pregnancy	Slight increase
Teratogenicity	No increase

FIGURE 10–10.

Combination regimen of clomiphene citrate and dexamethasone. Anovulatory women in whom clomiphene citrate fails despite high doses and who have clinical and laboratory features of androgen excess may respond to a combination regimen of clomiphene citrate and dexamethasone. Those women whose dehydroepiandrosterone sulfate (DHEA-S) levels exceed 2.8 µg/mL are ideal candidates. Dexamethasone is prescribed using a daily dose of 0.5 mg nightly. After 2 weeks, the DHEA-S measurement is repeated to verify that it has decreased to within the normal range. If so, the nightly dexamethasone therapy is continued at the same dose and after another 2 weeks, progesterone in oil is administered to induce withdrawal bleeding. After withdrawal bleeding, clomiphene citrate, 250 mg/d, is prescribed for 5 days. The dexamethasone is continued and 10,000 U of human chorionic gonadotropin (hCG) is given after follicular maturation is demonstrated. Approximately 50% of the women with elevated DHEA-S levels will ovulate when treated with this combined regimen [14]. Dexamethasone is discontinued when pregnancy has been confirmed.

FIGURE 10–11.

Extended clomiphene citrate regimen. For women who are resistant to the 250 mg/d for 5 days dose, extended regimens with treatment durations of 8 to 10 days have been used [15]. Human chorionic gonadotropin (hCG) is administered after follicular maturation is adequate. The frequency of ovulation with these extended regimens is low. However, because clomiphene citrate therapy is easier and less expensive than is the use of gonadotropins, some women prefer extended regimens because other treatment options are not available to them.

FIGURE 10–12.

Overall results of clomiphene citrate therapy. More than 90% of women who have oligomenorrhea will ovulate with this treatment regimen. Among normoestrogenic amenorrheic women, approximately two thirds will ovulate. Estrogen-deficient women will not have a response. Of all women treated with clomiphene citrate, approximately 50% will conceive. However, among women who have no other infertility factors, 85% will conceive. The multiple gestation rate, nearly all twins, is 5%. Ovarian cyst formation will occur in about 5% of cycles. These cysts are functional in nature and will regress during the next 2 to 6 weeks, provided that no further ovarian stimulation is given. The spontaneous abortion rate of approximately 20% is not increased above the abortion rate in spontaneous conception cycles. There is a minimal increase in the rate of ectopic pregnancy [16]. Side effects occur in about 15% of cycles. These include headaches, hot flashes, mood swings, depression, and abdominal bloating. It is important that both partners understand that the emotional changes are related to drug therapy, not solely to the stress of infertility. In rare instances, the side effects are so severe that medication must be discontinued. At higher doses, usually only greater than of 150 mg/d, visual disturbances consisting of "flashing lights" can occur. This side effect usually does not mandate discontinuation of therapy, but obviously driving at night should cease. Following discontinuation of the medication, these visual disturbances will subside. There is no increase in congenital anomalies.

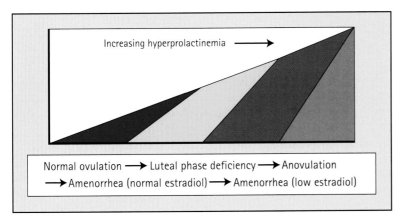

Increasing hyperprolactinemia →

Normal ovulation → Luteal phase deficiency → Anovulation → Amenorrhea (normal estradiol) → Amenorrhea (low estradiol)

FIGURE 10-13.

Ovulation and hyperprolactinemia. A second category of anovulatory or oligo-ovulatory women include is those with hyperprolactinemia. As a general rule, the higher the prolactin level, the greater the degree of disruption of ovulatory function. Thus, as prolactin levels rise, the ovulatory defect progresses from a luteal phase deficiency to oligo-ovulation to complete anovulation with normal estradiol levels. Finally, when prolactin levels are the highest or when hyperprolactinemia has been present for a long duration, the woman may become amenorrheic and estrogen deficient. Hyperprolactinemia hinders both gonadotropin-releasing hormone (GnRH) release and release of gonadotropins from the pituitary gland [17]. Thus, its primary effect is central, preventing ovarian stimulation.

RESULTS OF BROMOCRIPTINE THERAPY FOR HYPERPROLACTINEMIA

Women, n	Suppression of prolactin to normal, %	Return of menses, %	Ovulation, %
286	80	84	82

FIGURE 10-14.

Results of bromocriptine therapy for hyperprolactinemia. Multiple studies have demonstrated the efficacy of bromocriptine in reducing prolactin levels to normal. Thus, gonadotropin-releasing hormone (GnRH) pulse frequency and subsequently gonadotropin pulse frequency are restored. Unlike clomiphene citrate, there is no direct stimulatory effect. Because the excessive prolactin levels are inhibited, normal ovulatory function and menses resume [18,19]. Thus, multiple gestation rates are the same as those that occur in spontaneous ovulatory cycles. The efficacy of bromocriptine to restore ovulatory function seems to be similar whether the woman has pituitary lactotroph hyperplasia, a pituitary microadenoma, or even a macroadenoma [20]. Although the work-up of women with hyperprolactinemia will usually include an imaging study to identify those who may have a micro- or macroadenoma, induction of ovulation and pregnancy for infertile women with bromocriptine is safe for those who have a microadenoma [21]. Although it is important to individualize the management of infertile women who have a macroadenoma, most can expect to have a successful pregnancy without complications from tumor expansion. If these symptoms do occur, management may be by induction of labor or the use of glucocorticoids to reduce swelling around the enlarging gland. Rarely is surgical intervention necessary in pregnancy. (*Adapted from* Vance and coworkers [19].)

OUTCOME OF BROMOCRIPTINE-RELATED PREGNANCIES

	Frequency, n/n(%)
Spontaneous abortion	620/6239 (9.9)
Prematurity	519/4139 (12.5)
Multiple pregnancy	89/5031 (1.7)
Congenital malformation	998/5213 (1.8)

FIGURE 10-15.

Outcome of bromocriptine-related pregnancies. Rates of prematurity, multiple gestation, and congenital malformations are based on available details in each category (total pregnancies, 6339). Although multiple studies have demonstrated a slight increase in the frequency of multiple gestations, virtually all of those multiple pregnancies occurred during combination therapy with bromocriptine and another agent (either clomiphene citrate or gonadotropins).[22]

COMBINATION TREATMENT WITH BROMOCRIPTINE AND CLOMIPHENE CITRATE

Criteria

    Estrogen levels within normal range for follicular phase and anovulation persists

Regimen

    Continue bromocriptine

    Induce withdrawal bleeding

    Begin clomiphene citrate

RESULTS OF BROMOCRIPTINE THERAPY

	Frequency, %
Ovulation	90
Pregnancy (overall)	50
Pregnancy (no other cause)	80
Twinning	No increase
Spontaneous abortion	20
Persistent side effects	25
Teratogenicity	No increase

FIGURE 10–16.

Combination treatment with bromocriptine and clomiphene citrate. The efficacy of bromocriptine in reducing prolactin levels to normal is not dependent on the woman's estrogen status. However, some estrogen-deficient women will have a reduction of their prolactin levels to normal or almost normal, but will remain anovulatory. If the woman's estrogen levels have been restored partially (*ie*, within the range of normal for the follicular phase of the cycle), the woman is a candidate for treatment with combined bromocriptine and clomiphene citrate. In these instances, bromocriptine therapy is continued, withdrawal bleeding is induced by the administration of progesterone in oil, and clomiphene citrate therapy is prescribed as it would be for any anovulatory woman. In all instances, bromocriptine is discontinued when the diagnosis of pregnancy is made.

FIGURE 10–17.

Results of bromocriptine therapy. Bromocriptine can be expected to induce ovulation in 90% of hyperprolactinemic women. About one half of these women will conceive. However, as is true with clomiphene citrate, the pregnancy rate is approximately 80% among couples in whom hyperprolactinemia and anovulation is the only cause of infertility. There is no increase in the frequency of multiple gestations nor is there a rise in the rate of spontaneous abortion. Persistent side effects such as nausea, dizziness, and nasal congestion persist in about 25% of women. For some women who are bothered by severe gastrointestinal side effects, bromocriptine administered vaginally will cause fewer gastrointestinal side effects. There is no evidence of an increase in teratogenicity when bromocriptine is used to induce ovulation and pregnancy occurs. The newer dopamine receptor agonist, cabergoline, has similar effects but may have a lower rate of gastrointestinal side effects. The dose is 0.25 mg twice weekly.

GONADOTROPIN

GONADOTROPIN OR GONADOTROPIN-RELEASING HORMONE PRETREATMENT PROCEDURES

FSH, LH, estradiol, prolactin measurement

Graduated clomiphene regimen (unless estrogen deficient)

Semen analysis

Hysterosalpingogram or hysteroscopy

Laparoscopy

FIGURE 10–18.

Gonadotropin or gonadotropin-releasing hormone (GnRH) pretreatment procedures. The main indication for injectable ovulation-inducing drugs is anovulatory infertility. In some women this therapy will be considered because the drugs of primary choice failed. In other women, severe side effects of the primary drug of choice will mandate conversion to injectable agents. Finally, in a subset of women, injectable fertility drugs will be the first drug of choice. Because the cost, inconvenience, and complexity of using these agents is considerable, more pretreatment procedures are necessary to ensure that the outcome will be successful. Measurement of serum gonadotropin, estradiol, and prolactin levels are important as is obtaining either a hysterosalpingogram or hysteroscopy to verify that the uterine contour is without defects. Laparoscopy is also necessary prior to treatment to rule out a significant pelvic factor. Ideal women are those in whom oral agents have failed or those who have suffered significant side effects. The final category is those women who are amenorrheic and estrogen deficient with a normal prolactin level and who do not have premature ovarian failure. Treatment regimens for all gonadotropins are similar whether equal amounts of urinary follicle-stimulating hormone (FSH) and luteinizing hormone (LH), or urinary FSH only or highly purified urinary FSH are used, because outcomes are similar irrespective of the presence of LH. Only the last of these drugs is given subcutaneously rather than intramuscularly. The recombinant FSH products are also given subcutaneously. The subcutaneous route of administration is preferred by women because of less discomfort. Although no data are available to demonstrate "toxicity" from the urinary preparations, highly purified FSH has only 1% of "nonspecific" urinary proteins and none are present in the recombinant products.

GONADOTROPIN PROTOCOL

Individualized graduated dose

Baseline estradiol and real-time ultrasound scan

Estradiol and scan every 3–4 d until estradiol level increased

Ultrasound scan every 2 d until follicle 12–14 mm

Cervical score and postcoital test

Ultrasound scan every day until follicle ≥18 mm

10,000 IU hCG 24 h after last gonadotropin dose

FIGURE 10-19.

Gonadotropin protocol. Following the work-up as outlined previously, the woman has a baseline estradiol and a real-time ultrasound examination of her ovaries to rule out the presence of generalized ovarian enlargement or ovarian cyst formation. She is begun on an individualized graduated dose of gonadotropins, usually starting at 150 U/d. Serum estradiol levels and ovarian scanning are repeated in 3 to 5 days. If the estradiol level is unchanged, the dose of gonadotropins is increased by 50% and the estradiol level is measured 3 days later. If the estradiol remains similar to the baseline level, this sequence of increasing the dose by 50% and measuring the estradiol level every 3 days is continued until the estradiol level doubles. At this time, the woman has an ultrasound scan every 2 days until the leading follicle is between 12 and 14 mm in its largest diameter. At this time the woman has a postcoital test and is scanned daily until the largest follicle equals or exceeds 18 mm in diameter. Then ovulation is induced with a single dose of 10,000 U of human chorionic gonadotropin (hCG).

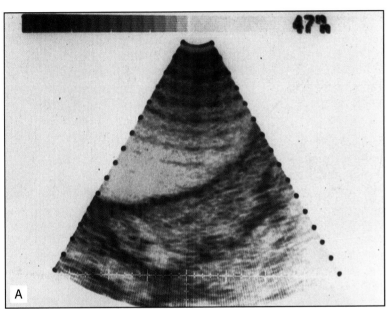

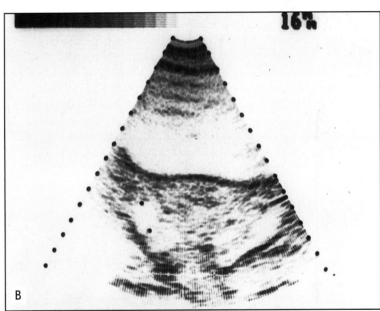

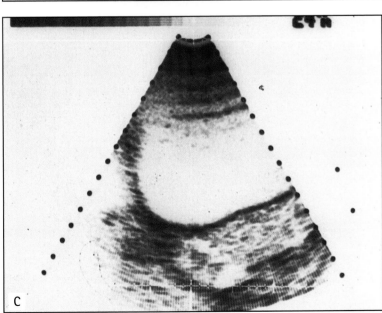

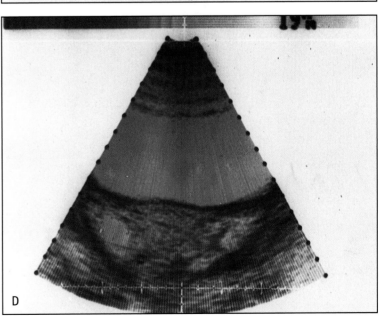

FIGURE 10-20.

Ultrasound scans showing progressive rise in serum estradiol levels and enlargement of dominant follicle during treatment with gonadotropins. **A**, Serum estradiol, 229 pg/mL; follicle size, 11 by 12 mm. **B**, Serum estradiol , 379 pg/mL; follicle size, 13 by 15 mm. **C**, Serum estradiol , 505 pg/mL; follicle size, 16 by 18 mm. **D**, Serum estradiol, 890 pg/mL; follicle size, 17 by 19 mm.

RESULTS OF ULTRASOUND MONITORING OF HUMAN MENOPAUSAL GONADOTROPIN THERAPY

Menstrual Pattern	Women, n	Pregnancies, n(%)
Without ultrasonography		
Oligomenorrhea	15	7 (46.7)
Amenorrhea	26	15 (57.7)
Total	41	22 (53.7)
With ultrasonography		
Oligomenorrhea	97	69 (71.1)
Amenorrhea	14	11 (78.6)
Total	111	80 (72.1) (P<0.05)

FIGURE 10-21.

Results of ultrasound monitoring of human menopausal gonadotropin (hMG) therapy. Since ultrasonography has been used to monitor hMG therapy, the pregnancy rate in our center has increased significantly among normoestrogenic women [23]. At the same time, the mean estradiol level reached at the time of human chorionic gonadotropin (hCG) administration is twice the mean level reached when hCG was administered in the years before the use of ovarian scanning, when only serum estradiol levels were used to judge response. Thus, it is likely that in the past many women received hCG before a mature preovulatory follicle developed. Among normoestrogenic women, such as those with polycystic ovarian syndrome or oligomenorrhea, two or more follicles reach maturity in 70% of treatment cycles. Because all follicles, both large and small, contribute to the total serum estradiol concentration, it is difficult to be certain that even one follicle is mature even if the estradiol level is approximately 1000 pg/mL Conversely, if the estradiol level equals or exceeds 2000 pg/mL, the physician cannot be certain that an excessive number of mature follicles are present. Although the mean estradiol level at the time when at least one mature follicle is identified by ultrasonography is more than 1600 pg/mL among normoestrogenic women, levels can be between 600 and 3000 pg/mL. Monitoring follicular development by frequent ultrasonographic studies is mandatory to gauge the response to hMG.

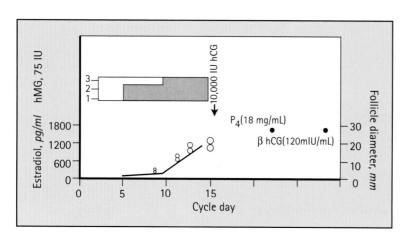

FIGURE 10-22.

Inducing ovulation with human menopausal gonadotropin (hMG) and human chorionic gonadotropin (hCG).Stepwise increase in the dose of gonadotropins from 150 IU/d to 225 IU/d results in a progressive rise in the serum estradiol concentration to 1150 pg/mL and the development of two mature follicles. One week after hCG administration, the progesterone (P_4) level is 18 ng/mL and after one more week the BhCG level is 120 mIU/mL.

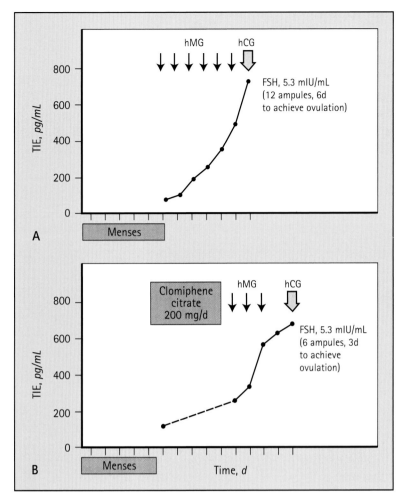

FIGURE 10-23.

Effect of clomiphene citrate pretreatment on total immunoreactive estrogens (TIE) and human menopausal gonadotropin (hMG) requirements in a woman with a normal serum follicle-stimulating hormone (FSH) level and intramuscular progesterone–induced menses. **A,** hMG dose and duration requirements without clomiphene pretreatment. **B,** Effect induced by clomiphene citrate pretreatment. Some women who are normoestrogenic may benefit from combined therapy with clomiphene citrate and gonadotropins [24]. Normoestrogenic women who do not have an ovulatory response with clomiphene citrate frequently will achieve partial follicular maturation as indicated by rising estradiol levels and increases in follicular diameter. However, complete maturation of the oocyte does not occur. In these women, treatment with sequential clomiphene citrate before gonadotropin use is advantageous. The protocol includes beginning clomiphene citrate at a daily dose of 200 mg/d for 5 days. On day 6 of treatment, gonadotropin therapy is begun and continued as outlined previously. The duration of therapy and the overall gonadotropin dose needed are reduced composed with use of hCG alone.

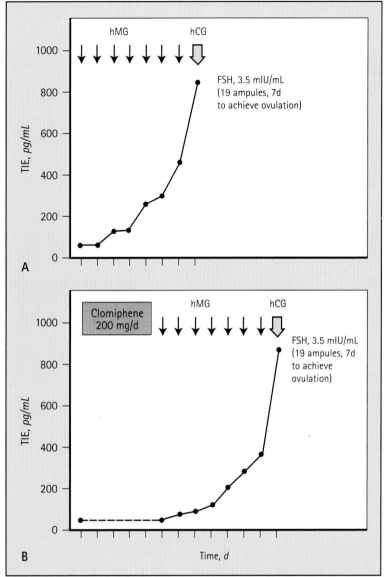

FIGURE 10-24.

Clomiphene pretreatment. Effect of clomiphene citrate pretreatment on total immunoreactive estrogens (TIE) and human menopausal gonadotropin (hMG) requirements in a woman with a low serum follicle-stimulating hormone (FSH) level in whom intramuscular administration of progesterone did not induce menses. **A,** hMG dose and duration of therapy without clomiphene pretreatment. **B,** Effect induced by clomiphene citrate pretreatment. Among estrogen-deficient women, clomiphene citrate pretreatment does not alter estradiol levels; thus gonadotropin requirements are unchanged compared with hMG alone. [24].

EFFECT OF CLOMIPHENE ON HUMAN MENOPAUSAL GONADOTROPIN DOSAGE IN TWO ANOVULATORY AMENORRHEIC POPULATIONS

	Normal estrogen levels	Estrogen deficient, low FSH
Progesterone-induced menses	Yes	No
Serum estradiol, pg/mL	52–121	7–40
FSH, mIU/mL	5.3–6.8	1.5–3.5
LH, mIU/mL	9.8–60	2.2–12.0
hMG only, ampules/days	19.8/7.6	53.0/9.8
CC + hMG, ampules/days	8.3/3.7	51.9/8.0
	P<0.01	Not significant

FIGURE 10-25.

Effect of clomiphene citrate (CC) on human menopausal gonadotropin (hMG) dosage in two anovulatory amenorrheic populations. There are two populations of anovulatory amenorrheic women: those who are estrogen deficient and have low follicle-stimulating hormone (FSH) levels and variable levels of luteinizing hormone (LH), and those with normal estrogen levels. Women in the former group need significantly more gonadotropins in order to induce follicular maturation in contrast to their normoestrogenic counterparts. Among those estrogen-deficient women, clomiphene citrate pretreatment results in no change in the gonadotropin requirements. In contrast, normoestrogenic women who have normal FSH levels will have a 50% reduction in their gonadotropin requirements when they are pretreated. The duration of therapy is decreased as is cost [24].

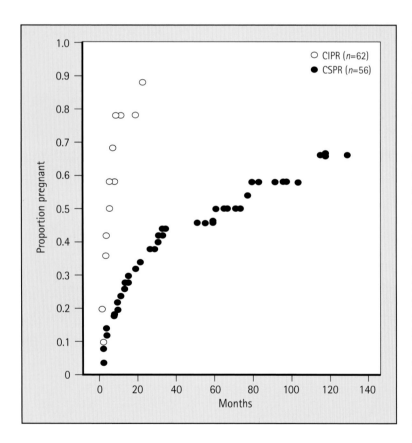

FIGURE 10-26.

Induced pregnancy life-table curves. Life-table curves for cumulative pregnancy rate *(open dots)* in patients treated with human menopausal gonadotropin (hMG) (n=62) and cumulative spontaneous pregnancy rate *(closed dots)* (n=56) [25]. Gonadotropin therapy is both complex and expensive. When efficacy was assessed by life-table analysis, pregnancy rates of 58.5% and 77.2% at 6 and 12 months, respectively, were reported. Gonadotropins can be expected to induce ovulation in virtually all anovulatory women who do not have ovarian failure. With careful monitoring, the pregnancy rate should be approximately 70%. The multiple gestation rate should be below 10% and the great majority of these should be twins. These results can be achieved only with meticulous monitoring. The abortion rate is higher than that which occurs in spontaneous cycles. About 8% of treatment cycles result in transient ovarian enlargement. Therefore, following menses, ultrasound is necessary to rule out the presence of ovarian enlargement before beginning another treatment cycle. The very serious complication of the ovarian hyperstimulation syndrome should be extremely rare (see Fig. 10-34). There is no evidence that gonadotropins are teratogenic. The overall effects of all gonadotropin preparations are almost identical. Except for women who are amenorrheic and estrogen deficient and have almost no luteinizing hormone (LH), these products may be used interchangeably. For those women who have a marked LH deficiency, the use of gonadotropins that have both follicle-stimulating hormone (FSH) and LH is desirable.

ROLES OF GONADOTROPIN-RELEASING HORMONE IN WOMEN WHO ARE ANOVULATORY WITHOUT PITUITARY FAILURE

Initiate follicular development

Complete follicular maturation

Stimulate ovum release

Maintain corpus luteum

FIGURE 10-27.

Roles of gonadotropin-releasing hormone (GnRH) in women who are anovulatory without pituitary failure. GnRH may be used to begin or complete follicular maturation, provide a surrogate luteinizing hormone surge, maintain the corpus luteum, or it may be the sole ovulatory agent used to perform all of these functions. GnRH is administered via a pump that delivers medication in an hourly pulse. A small, fine catheter delivers the medication either intravenously or subcutaneously.

Various dosages, frequencies, and routes of administration have been used. The doses of intravenous administration vary between 1 and 20 µg per pulse, with pulse intervals of 60 to 180 minutes administered via a pump. The dose depends primarily on the route of administration. Intravenous administration is less costly because lower doses are used.

RESULTS OF SUBCUTANEOUS GONADOTROPIN-RELEASING HORMONE THERAPY FROM SEVERAL STUDIES

GnRH, µg/pulse	Interval, min	Cycles, n	Ovulation, n(%)	Pregnancy, n(%)
2–25	90–240	620	440 (71)	148 (24)

FIGURE 10-28.

Results of subcutaneous gonadotropin-releasing hormone (GnRH) therapy from several studies. Most women will respond to doses of 75 µg/kg intravenously or 300 µg/kg subcutaneously. The pulse interval should be 60 to 120 minutes. Monitoring by serum estradiol determinations and ultrasound scans of the ovaries is necessary to reduce the frequency of multiple pregnancy and ovarian enlargement. If GnRH is discontinued after ovulation, human chorionic gonadotropin (1000 to 2500 IU) should be given every 3 to 4 days to maintain the corpus luteum.

Subcutaneous administration is more convenient and results in a monthly fecundity of about 24% [26]. Reid and colleagues demonstrated that subcutaneous GnRH treatment can lead to irregular absorption patterns that cause a luteinizing hormone–follicle-stimulating hormone response typical of that seen in women with polycystic ovary syndrome [27]. In addition, some women in whom subcutaneous therapy fails do respond to intravenous administration.

RESULTS OF INTRAVENOUS GONADOTROPIN-RELEASING HORMONE THERAPY FROM SEVERAL STUDIES

µg/pulse	Interval, min	Cycles, n	Ovulation, n(%)	Pregnancy, n(%)
1–30	62–180	724	626 (88)	157 (22)

FIGURE 10-29.

Results of intravenous gonadotropin-releasing hormone (GnRH) therapy from several studies. Women with severe hypothalamic amenorrhea may require high doses of GnRH to initiate and maintain oocyte maturation. In this group of women, intravenous doses up to 20 µg of GnRH every 90 minutes have been used. Women with hypothalamic amenorrhea or other ovulatory defects not associated with androgen excess are more likely to ovulate and to conceive than are those with polycystic ovarian disease [28,29].

Intravenous therapy is somewhat less convenient, but is

cheaper than subcutaneous therapy. The hormonal response to intravenous GnRH is more reproducible and uniform and results in a higher rate of ovulation compared with subcutaneous administration [26]. However, fecundity and pregnancy rates are identical. The decision on the route of administration probably depends on issues of convenience rather than efficacy. GnRH appears to have little or no advantages over gonadotropin therapy. Moreover, it is only suitable for women whose defect is a hypothalamic one. Obviously, women with pituitary failure will not respond to GnRH.

OVULATION INDUCTION IN WOMEN WITH POLYCYSTIC OVARY SYNDROME

PULSATILE GONADOTROPIN-RELEASING HORMONE OVULATION INDUCTION IN WOMEN WITH POLYCYSTIC OVARY SYNDROME

Optimal ovulatory and pregnancy rates are achieved when pulsatile GnRH is administered to hypogonadotropic women

Pulsatile GnRH is often ineffective in PCOS

GnRH analogue can induce a reversible hypogonadotropic state in PCOS

FIGURE 10–30.

Pulsatile gonadotropin-releasing hormone (GnRH) ovulation induction in women with polycystic ovary syndrome (PCOS). As is true of gonadotropin therapy, some women with PCOS do not respond well to any of the injectable agents. In these women, initial therapy with a GnRH analogue that will produce a hypoestrogenic state analogous to that of hypothalamic amenorrhea results in a higher pregnancy rate. Although this therapy is more expensive because of the cost of the GnRH analogue and the higher gonadotropin requirements, it does result in a higher pregnancy rate.

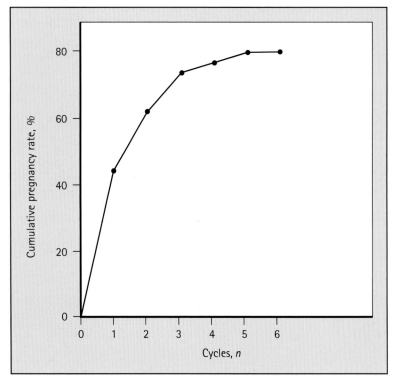

FIGURE 10–31.

Cumulative pregnancy rates in women with polycystic ovary syndrome receiving combined gonadotropin-releasing hormone (GnRH) agonist and human menopausal gonadotropin (hMG) therapy [30].

RESULTS OF THERAPY FOR POLYCYSTIC OVARY SYNDROME USING COMBINED GONADOTROPINS AND DEXAMETHASONE (N=27)

	hMG–hCG	hMG–dexamethaxone
Cycles, n	220	56
Cycles per woman, n	8.14	2
Average dose of hMG	25	18 (P <0.01)
Ovulation (cycles), n(%)	89 (40 %)	38 (67 %)
Ovulation (women), n(%)	18 (67 %)	22 (81 %)
Pregnancies, n(%)	0	20 (74 %)
Abortions, n(%)	0	5 (25 %)

FIGURE 10-32.

Results of therapy for polycystic ovary syndrome using combined gonadotropins and dexamethasone. As mentioned previously, dexamethasone therapy may improve the efficacy of clomiphene citrate for hyperandrogenic women. The same is true with those women who have hyperandrogenism and who are treated with gonadotropins. Evron and colleagues [31] reported a marked increase in the frequency of ovulation when combined therapy was used. Pregnancies occurred only among women who received both drugs.

OVULATION INDUCTION IN AMENORRHEIC WOMEN

DRUGS OF CHOICE FOR INDUCING OVULATION IN AMENORRHEIC WOMEN

Estradiol level	Prolactin level	Drug of choice
Normal	Normal	Clomiphene citrate
Normal	Elevated	Clomiphene/bromo-criptine
Low	Elevated	Bromocriptine (cabergoline)
Low	Normal	Gonadotropins/GnRH

FIGURE 10-33.

Drugs of choice for inducing ovulation induction in amenorrheic women. The ideal agent for inducing ovulation, clomiphene citrate, may be used in all women who have oligomenorrhea. Among amenorrheic women who are normoestrogenic, clomiphene citrate would be the treatment of choice for women who have normal prolactin levels.

Among normoestrogenic amenorrheic women who have high prolactin levels, either bromocriptine or clomiphene citrate may be used. In a normoestrogenic setting, clomiphene citrate would be likely to induce ovulation irrespective of the hyperprolactinemia [32]. The advantages of clomiphene citrate are fewer side effects and more clinical experience. Proponents of bromocriptine would argue that this drug specifically corrects the endocrinopathy and does not increase the frequency of multiple gestations. These advantages must be weighed against its higher cost and higher frequency of side effects.

For estrogen-deficient amenorrheic women, the prolactin level is important. Women who are hyperprolactinemic should be treated with bromocriptine. The injectable therapy, whether it is gonadotropin-releasing hormone (GnRH), combined follicle-stimulating hormone–luteinizing hormone, or FSH only is reserved for amenorrheic women who do not have ovarian failure and whose prolactin levels are normal. Any of these drugs would also be used for women who cannot tolerate the primary drug of choice or who do not respond to that agent. Using the agents available, ovulation may be induced safely in virtually all anovulatory women, and a very high rate of successful pregnancy can be expected.

RESULTS OF OVARIAN HYPERSTIMULATION

CLASSIFICATION, DIAGNOSIS, AND TREATMENT OF OVARIAN HYPERSTIMULATION SYNDROME

Classification	Diagnosis	Therapy
Mild		
Before hCG		
Laboratory:	Estradiol ≥3000 pg/mL; ≥4 mature or ≥20 immature follicles	Withhold hCG ? Indomethacin ? Intravenous albumin
After hCG		
Subclinical:	Ovarian diameter, 5–6 cm	Observation and bedrest
Clinical:	Ovarian enlargement of 6–10 cm plus abdominal pain, distention, and weight gain	Observation and bedrest
Moderate	Ovarian enlargement ≥ 10 cm and/or ascites, nausea, vomiting	Serial CBC and pelvic ultrasound. Measure electrolytes. Measure weight daily
Severe	Moderate plus clinical evidence of ascites and/ or hydrothorax; serum creatinine 1.2–1.9 mg/dL Hematocrit 45%–54%	Above plus hospitalize Measure girth daily Control fluid balance Possibly paracentesis Possibly thoracentesis
Critical	Severe plus hematocrit ≥ 55%, hypovolemia, hypercoagualability, hypotension, oliguria, serum creatinine ≥ 2.0 mg/dL; creatinine clearance <50 mL/min; adult respiratory distress syndrome	As for severe, plus mannitol. Fluid resuscitation

FIGURE 10–34.

Classification, diagnosis, and treatment of ovarian hyperstimulation syndrome (OHSS). Although OHSS with marked ovarian enlargement (>10 cm), ascites, pleural effusions, hemoconcentration, hypercoagulability, and oliguria should occur in less than 0.1% of properly monitored treatment cycles, milder examples occur more often [32]. The diag- nosis should be made early and appropriate measures instituted to reduce morbidity. Continued luteal phase support by exoge- nous human chorionic gonadotropin (hCG) and the further ovarian stimulation by endogenous hCG produced during a pregnancy increase the severity of this complication. Progressive worsening of early OHSS during early pregnancy until the corpus luteum regresses is not a rare event [34]. Although ovarian hyperstimu- lation occurs more commonly during gonadotropin or gonadotropin-releasing hormone (GnRH) treatment than with clomiphene citrate, the latter drug has been associated with the syndrome.

Prevention of this complication is accom- plished by withholding hCG if the serum estradiol level is above 3000 pg/mL and if more than four mature follicles or more than a total of 20 follicles are identified by ultrasonography [34–36]. Large numbers of small (< 9 mm) preovulatory follicles carry an especially poor prognosis [35]. If hCG is administered, indomethacin, 100 mg thrice daily, may ameliorate the symp- toms. The incidence of ovarian hyper- stimulation has also been reported to be higher in women with polycystic ovary syndrome who had premature luteinizing hormone increases during human follicle- stimulating hormone (FSH) treatment [37]. Discontinuation of human FSH treatment or alternate-day therapy, following which estradiol levels declined slightly, was able to decrease the frequency of this complica- tion. Tulandi and colleagues [38] reported that the pregnancy rate was three times higher among women who developed ovarian hyperstimulation compared with those who did not.

OVARIAN GROWTH FACTORS THAT MAY INFLUENCE STEROIDOGENESIS

Epidermal growth factor

Transforming growth factor-α

Transforming growth factor-β

Insulin-like growth factor-1

Tumor necrosis factor

Fibroblast growth factor

Platelet-derived growth factor

FIGURE 10-35.

Ovarian growth factors that may influence steroidogenesis. Several ovarian growth factors have been identified over the past decade. Insulin-like growth factor-1 (IGF-1) has been studied

extensively as a potential stimulator of follicular growth. IGF-1 synthesis by the liver and perhaps the ovary is stimulated by growth hormone [39]. IGF-1 has been shown to augment follicle-stimulating hormone (FSH)-stimulated ovarian steroidogenesis. The addition of growth hormone reduced both the number of ampules of hMG and of days of hMG administration required to achieve ovulation.

If growth hormone itself is the augmenter, a more physiologic treatment than growth hormone adjuvant therapy might be cotreatment with growth hormone releasing factor (GRF) and exogenous gonadotropins. In a study using combined GRF and human menopausal gonadotropin (hMG) for stimulation of follicular growth in *in vitro* fertilization cycles, Hugues and colleagues [40] showed that combined therapy was superior in terms of plasma estradiol levels, yield of oocytes, and follicular fluid IGF-1 levels.

These results show that growth factors other than FSH are probably involved in FSH-stimulated follicular growth. These factors, which may be paracrine or ovarian origin, may be deficient in some women. Further work is required to establish which growth factors are involved in human ovarian folliculogenesis.

OVULATION AND PREGNANCY RATES AFTER ELECTROCAUTERY AND LASER TREATMENT OF POLYCYSTIC OVARIES

Method and women, n	Ovulation, %	Pregnancy, %	Study
Electrocautery			
35	92	69	Gjønnaess (1984)
6	83	67	Greenblatt and Casper (1987)
14	64	36	v.d. Weiden *et al.* (1989)
21	81	52	Armar *et al.* (1990)
29	71	52	Abdel Gadir (1990)
7	71	57	Gürgan *et al.* (1991)
10	70		Kovacs *et al.* (1991)
22		86	Armar and Lachelin (1993)
104	76	70	Naether *et al.* (1993)
10	70		Tirtinen *et al.* (1993)
Laser vaporization			
85	53	56	Daniell and Miller (1989)
19	80	37	Keckstein *et al.* (1990)
10	70		Gürgan *et al.* (1991)
Wedge resection			
8	65	0	Huber *et al.* (1988)
12	83	58	Koijima *et al.* (1989)

FIGURE 10-36.

Ovulation and pregnancy rates after electrocautery and laser treatment of polycystic ovaries. Ovulatory cycles induced after wedge resection are often transient, and the previous anovulatory pattern is usually resumed. Peritubal and periovarian adhesions occur frequently after ovarian wedge resection, thereby introducing another cause for infertility [41]. Therefore, ovarian wedge resection should not be performed.

Modifications of ovarian wedge resection that have been advocated include multiple punch biopsy, coagulation of the multiple surface cysts in women with polycystic ovaries, laser ablation of these cysts, and ovarian puncture and coagulation using a unipolar needle. Between four and 20 sites per ovary have been treated in different series [42–44]. In one series, the overall rate of ovulation was 92%; of those women whose only identifiable cause of infertility was polycystic ovary syndrome, 116 of 138 (84%) conceived [44]. However, adhesions have been reported after this procedure [42] as has ovarian atrophy [45]. Overall, laparoscopic treatment of polycystic ovaries appears to yield high rates of ovulation and pregnancy. Compared with gonadotropin therapy, there is a low rate of multiple gestation and abortion. However, more data are needed, including comparative studies and more stringent woman selection. Perhaps transvaginal aspiration of the tiny subcapsular cysts will prove to be equally efficacious and without the attendant surgical and anesthetic risks [46]. (*Adapted from* Gjønnaess [47]; with permission.)

INCIDENCE OF OVARIAN CANCER

Incidence, %	New cases per year, n	Five-year survival, %
1.4	25,000	40

FIGURE 10-37.

Incidence of ovarian cancer. Ovarian cancer occurs in 1.4% of women and is the most fatal among all gynecologic malignancies, having a 5-year survival rate of about 40%. This disease has gained more notoriety recently because of a possible association with the use of "fertility drugs" [48–51].

REPRODUCTIVE FACTORS IN PROTECTION AGAINST OR RISK OF OVARIAN CANCER

Protective factors	Increased risk factors
Pregnancy	Infertility
Lactation	Incessant ovulation
Oral contraceptives	

FIGURE 10-38.

Reproductive factors which are considered to increase or decrease risk of ovarian cancer. The number of pregnancies and abortions, duration of breast feeding, infertility, and age of menopause have all been associated with changes in the risk of ovarian cancer. Depending on the number of pregnancies, nulligravidas have been shown to have between 1.3 and 2.5 times the risk of those who had conceived previously [52,53]. The risk of ovarian cancer among infertile women is considered to be between 1.8 and 6.5 times that of parous and nulliparous control subjects [54–56].

The most striking evidence of a protective benefit is from the use of oral contraceptives. Estimates of a protective effect range between 20% and 70% [57,58]. Because the frequency of ovarian cancer rises dramatically with the onset of menopause and because levels of follicle-stimulating hormone and to a lesser extent luteinizing hormone increase markedly after menopause, investigators have questioned whether or not gonadotropins contribute to the development of ovarian cancer [59,60].

Incessant ovulation as a cause of ovarian carcinoma was proposed originally by Fathalla [61]. The greater risk of malignancy in never-pregnant women, the greater frequency of ovarian inclusion cysts in those with repetitive ovulation and those with cancer, and the greater exposure of the surface epithelium to mitogens among those who ovulate repetitively all suggest a link. The protection afforded by pregnancy, by breast feeding, and by oral contraceptive use strengthens the theory of a link between ovulation and cancer.

The review article by Whittemore and colleagues [48] identified 12 nulligravidas and eight parous women who had invasive epithelial ovarian cancer who had used "fertility drugs." Type, duration of treatment, outcome, and so on were not reported. Rossing and colleagues [51] reported four invasive epithelial cancers, five borderline ovarian tumors, and two granulosa cell tumors in 3837 infertile women. Nine of these women had taken clomiphene citrate. The relative risk of ovarian tumors with the use of this drug for more than 1 year was 2.3 times higher than that among infertile women who had not used the drug. The authors concluded that the prolonged use of clomiphene citrate may increase the risk of ovarian neoplasms. The short duration of use in some women, the inclusion of other than epithelial tumors, and the brief treatment-to-diagnosis interval make interpretation of the data impossible. The distinction between an association and a causal effect is critical because an association can occur by chance and does not necessarily indicate a causal link. To prove a causal relation, large collaborative multicenter studies are needed. Until such studies are carried out, the results of these two studies cannot be used to demonstrate that a true causal relation exists between the use of ovulation-inducing agents and an increased risk of developing ovarian cancer.

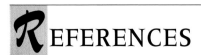EFERENCES

1. Dobson WC, Whitesides DB, Hughes CL, *et al.*: Superovulation with intrauterine insemination for infertility: a possible alternative to gamete intrafallopian transfer and in vitro fertilization. *Fertil Steril* 1987, 48:441–445.

2. Zinamen MJ, Clergy ED, Brown CC, *et al.*: Estimate of human fertility and pregnancy loss. *Fertil Steril* 1996, 65:505–509.

3. Speroff L, Glass RH, Kase NG: Investigation of the infertile couple. In *Clinical Gynecologic Endocrinology and Infertility*, edn 4. Baltimore: Williams & Wilkins; 1989:513–546.

4. Gysler M, March CM, Mishell DR Jr., *et al.*: A decade's experience with an individualized clomiphene treatment regimen including its effect on the postcoital test. *Fertil Steril* 1982, 37:161–167.

5. Wu CH, Winkel CA: The effect of therapy initiation day on clomiphene therapy. *Fertil Steril* 1989, 52:564–568.

6. Hull MGR, Savage PE, Bromham DR, *et al.*: The value of a single serum progesterone measurement in the midluteal phase as a criterion of a potentially fertile cycle ("ovulation") derived from treated and untreated conception cycles. *Fertil Steril* 1982, 37:355–360.

7. Israel R, Mishell DR Jr., Stone SC, *et al.*: Single luteal phase serum progesterone assay as an indicator of ovulation. *Am J Obstet Gynecol* 1972, 112:1043–1046.

8. Insler V, Melmed H, Eichenbrenner I, *et al.*: The cervical score: a simple semiquantitative method for monitoring of the menstrual cycle. *Int J Gynecol Obstet* 1972, 10:233–228.

9. Mikkelson TJ, Kroboth PD, Cameron WJ, *et al.*: Single dose pharmacokinetics of clomiphene citrate in normal volunteers. *Fertil Steril* 1986, 46:392–396.

10. Kerin JF, Liu JH, Phillipou G, *et al.*: Evidence for a hypothalamic site of action of clomiphene citrate in women. *J Clin Endocrinol Metab* 1985, 61:265–268.

11. Adashi EY: Clomiphene citrate: mechanism(s) and site(s) of action: a hypothesis revisited. *Fertil Steril* 1984, 42:331–344.

12. Sir T, Alba F, Denoto L, Rossmanith W: Clomiphene citrate and LH pulsatility in PCO syndrome. *Horm Metab Res* 1989, 21:583.

13. Hammond MG, Halme JR, Talbert LM: Factors affecting the pregnancy rate in clomiphene citrate induction of ovulation. *Obstet Gynecol* 1983, 62:196–202.

14. Lobo RA, Paul W, March CM, *et al.*: Clomiphene and dexamethasone in women unresponsive to clomiphene alone. *Obstet Gynecol* 1982, 60:497.

15. Lobo RA, Granger LR, Davajan V, *et al.*: An extended regimen of clomiphene citrate in women unresponsive to standard therapy. *Fertil Steril* 1982, 37:762.

16. Marchbanks PA, Coulam CB, Annegers JF: An association between clomiphene citrate and ectopic pregnancy: a preliminary report. *Fertil Steril* 1985, 44:268–270.

17. Klibanski A, Beitins IZ, Merriam GR, *et al.*: Gonadotropin and prolactin pulsations in hyperprolactinemic women before and during bromocriptine therapy. *J Clin Endocrinol Metab* 1984, 58:1141–1147.

18. Molitch ME, Reichlin S: Hyperprolactinemic disorders. *Dis Mon* 1982, 28:1–58.

19. Vance ML, Evans WS, Thorner MO: Bromocriptine. *Ann Intern Med* 1984, 100:78–91.

20. MacLeod RM, Lehmeyer JE: Suppression of pituitary tumor cell growth and function by ergot alkaloids. *Cancer Res* 1973, 33:849–855.

21. Kletzky OA, Marrs RP, Davajan V: Management of women with hyperprolactinemia and normal or abnormal tomograms. *Am J Obstet Gynecol* 1983, 147:528–532.

22. Krupp P, Monka C, Richter: The safety aspects of infertility treatment. Presented at the Second World Congree of Gynecology and Obstetrics, Rio de Janeiro, 1988.

23. March CM: Improved pregnancy rate with monitoring of gonadotropin therapy by three modalities. *Am J Obstet Gynecol* 1987, 156:1473–1479.

24. March CM, Tredway DR, Mishell DR Jr.: Effect of clomiphene citrate upon amount and duration of human menopausal gonadotropin therapy. *Am J Obstet Gynecol* 1976, 125:699–704.

25. Lam SY, Baker G, Pepperell R, *et al.*: Treatment-independent pregnancies after cessation of gonadotropin ovulation induction in women with oligomenorrhea and anovulatory menses. *Fertil Steril* 1988, 50:26–30.

26. March CM: Induction of ovulation. In *Infertility, Contraception & Reproductive Endocrinology*, edn 4. Edited by Mishell DR Jr., Lobo RA, Paulson R, Shoupe D. Cambridge, MA: Blackwell Scientific Publications; 1997: 507–535.

27. Reid RL, Leopold GR, Yen SSC: Induction of ovulation and pregnancy with pulsatile luteinizing hormone-releasing factor: dosage and mode of delivery. *Fertil Steril* 1981, 36:553–559.

28. Berg FD, Hinrichsen MJ: Cumulative pregnancy rates in women treated by pulsatile administration of GnRH. In *The Brain and Female Reproductive Function*. Edited by Genazzani AR. Park Ridge, NJ: Parthenon Publishing; 1987:533–536.

29. Homberg R, Eshel A, Armar NA, *et al.*: One hundred pregnancies after treatment with pulsatile luteinizing hormone releasing hormone to induce ovulation. *BMJ* 1989, 298:809–812.

30. Fleming R, Haxton MJ, Hamilton MPR, *et al.*: Combined gonado-tropin-releasing hormone analog and exogenous gonadotropins for ovulation induction for infertile women: efficacy related to ovarian function assessment. *Am J Obstet Gynecol* 1988, 159:376–381.

31. Evron S, Navot D, Laufer N, *et al.*: Induction of ovulation with combined human gonadotropins and dexamethasone in women with polycystic ovarian disease. *Fertil Steril* 1983, 40:183–186.

32. March CM, Davajan V, Mishell DR Jr.: Ovulation induction in amenorrheic women. *Obstet Gynecol* 1979, 53:8–11.

33. Golan A, Ron-EI R, Herman A, *et al.*: Ovarian hyperstimulation syndrome: an update review. *Obstet Gynecol Surv* 1989, 44:430–440.

34. McClure N, Leya J, Radawauska E, *et al.*: Luteal phase support and severe ovarian hyperstimulation syndrome. *Hum Reprod* 1992, 7:758–764.

35. Blankstein J, Shalev J, Saadon T, *et al.*: Ovarian hyperstimulation syndrome: prediction by number and size of preovulatory follicles. *Fertil Steril* 1987, 47:597–602.

36. Haning RV Jr., Austin CW, Carlson IH, *et al.*: Plasma estradiol is superior to ultrasound and urinary estradiol glucuronide as a predictor of ovarian hyperstimulation during induction of ovulation with menotropins. *Fertil Steril* 1983, 40:31–36.

37. Mizunuma H, Andoh K, Yamada K, *et al.*: Prediction and prevention of ovarian hyperstimulation by monitoring endogenous luteinizing hormone release during purified follicle-stimulating hormone therapy. *Fertil Steril* 1992, 58:46–50.

38. Tulandi T, McInnes RA, Arrovet GH: Ovarian hyperstimulation syndrome following ovulation induction with human menopausal gonadotropin. *Int J Fertil* 1984, 29:113–117.

39. Adashi EY, Resnick C, Hernandez ER, *et al.*: Rodent studies on the potential relevance of insulin-like growth factor (IGF-1) to ovarian physiology. In *Growth Factors and the Ovary*. Edited by Hirshfield AN. New York: Plenum; 1989:95–106.

40. Hugues JN, Torresani T, Herve F, *et al.*: Interest of growth hormone-releasing hormone administration for improvement of ovarian responsiveness to gonadotropins in poor responder women. *Fertil Steril* 1991, 55:945–951.

41. Buttram VC, Vaquero C: Post-ovarian wedge resection adhesive disease. *Fertil Steril* 1975, 26:874–876.

42. Greenblatt E, Casper RF: Endocrine changes after laparoscopic ovarian cautery in polycystic ovarian syndrome. *Am J Obstet Gynecol* 1987, 156:279–285.

43. Daniell JF, Miller W: Polycystic ovaries treated by laparoscopic laser vaporization. *Fertil Steril* 1989, 51:232–236.

44. Gjønnaess H: The course and outcome of pregnancy after ovarian electrocautery in women with polycystic ovarian syndrome: the influence of body-weight. *Br J Obstet Gynaecol* 1989, 96:714–719.

45. Dabirashaafi H: Complications of laparoscopic ovarian cauterization. *Fertil Steril* 1989, 52:878–879.

46. Myo Y, Toda T, Tanikawa M, *et al.*: Transvaginal ultrasound-guided follicular aspiration in the management of anovulatory infertility associated with polycystic ovaries. *Fertil Steril* 1991, 56:1060–1065.

47. Gjønnaess H: Ovarian electrocautery in the treatment of women with polycystic ovary syndrome (PCOS). Factors affecting the result. *Acta Obstet Gynecol Scand* 1994, 73:407-412.

48. Whittemore AS, Harris R, Intyre J, *et al.*: Characteristics relating to ovarian cancer risk: collaborative analysis of 12 US case-control studies. I. Methods. *Am J Epidemiol* 1992, 136:1175–1183.

49. Whittemore AS, Harris R, Intyre J, *et al.*: Characteristics relating to ovarian cancer risk: collaborative analysis of 12 US case control-studies. IV. The pathogenesis of epithelial ovarian cancer. *Am J Epidemiol* 1992, 136:1212–1220.

50. Harris R, Whittemore AS, Itnyre J, *et al.*: Characteristics relating to ovarian cancer risk: collaborative analysis of 12 US case-control studies. III. Epithelial tumors of low malignant potential in white women. *Am J Epidemiol* 1992, 136:1204–1211.

51. Rossing MA, Dalin JR, Weiss NS, Moore DE, *et al.*: Ovarian tumors in a cohort of infertile women. *N Engl J Med* 1994, 331:771–776.

52. Cramer DW, Hutchinson GB, Welch WR, *et al.*: Determinants of ovarian cancer risk: I. Reproductive experience and family history. *J Natl Cancer Inst* 1983, 71:711–716.

53. Demopoulos RI, Seltzer V, Dubin N, et al.: The association of parity and marital status with the development of ovarian carcinoma: clinical implications. *Obstet Gynecol* 1979, 54: 150-155.

54. Negri E, Franceschi S, Tzonou A, *et al.*: Pooled analysis of 3 European case-control studies: I. Reproductive factors and risk of epithelial cancer. *Int J Cancer* 1991, 49:50–56.

55. Ron E, Lunenfeld B, Menczer J, *et al.*: Cancer incidence in a cohort of infertile women. *Am J Epidemiol* 1987, 125:780–790.

56. Whittemore AS, Wu ML, Paffenbarger RS, *et al.*: Epithelial ovarian cancer and the ability to conceive. *Cancer Res* 1989, 49:4047–4052.

57. Cramer DW, Hutchinson GB, Welch WR, *et al.*: Factors affecting the association of oral contraceptives and ovarian cancer. *N Engl J Med* 1982, 307:1047–1051.

58. Rosenblatt KA, Thomas DB, Noonan EA, *et al.*: High-dose and low-dose combined oral contraceptives: protection against epithelial ovarian cancer and the length of the protective effect. *Eur J Cancer* 1992, 28:1872–1876.

59. Monroe SE, Menon KMJ: Changes in reproductive hormone secretion during the climacteric and postmenopausal periods. *Clin Obstet Gynecol* 1977, 20:113–122.

60. Stouffer RL, Grodin MS, Davis JR, *et al.*: Investigation of binding sites for follicle-stimulating hormone and chorionic gonadotropin in human ovarian cancers. *J Clin Endocrinol Metab* 1984, 59:441–446.

61. Fathalla MR: Incessant ovulation: a factor in ovarian neoplasia? *Lancet* 1971, 11:163.

Diagnostic Evaluation of Male Infertility

CHAPTER

11

Rebecca Z. Sokol

Male factor infertility is a heterogeneous disorder. According to the experience at most infertility centers, the majority of subfertile men do not have an identifiable cause of their infertility. As a result, no specific treatment for the idiopathic category of male infertility has been developed. However, there are specific treatment regimens for those men who present with a clearly definable disorder. The task of the andrologist is to evaluate the male partner of a couple presenting with infertility and determine the specific treatment for each candidate. The history, physical examination, and semen analysis are the cornerstones of that evaluation. Additional sperm function testing, endocrine evaluation, testicular biopsy and imaging studies are requested as indicated. Based on the data collected, the cause of infertility can be assigned to four major diagnostic categories: 1) anatomic defects, 2) hypogonadotropic hypogonadism, 3) hypergonadotropic hypogonadism, and 4) idiopathic infertility. Once the correct diagnosis is made, the appropriate treatment plan can be initiated.

COMPONENTS OF THE MALE REPRODUCTIVE SYSTEM

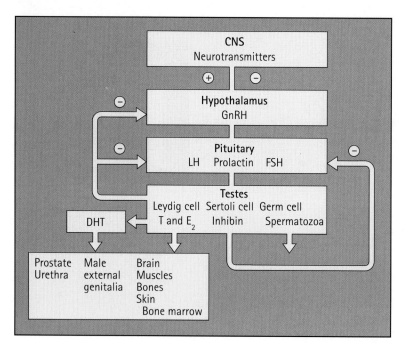

FIGURE 11-1.

The male reproductive axis. The hypothalamic-pituitary axis is a closely integrated system. Testicular function is regulated by a series of closed-loop feedback systems involving the higher centers in the central nervous system (CNS), the hypothalamus, the pituitary, and the testicular endocrine and germinal compartments. Extrahypothalamic neurotransmitters regulate gonadotropin-releasing hormone (GnRH) synthesis and release from the hypothalamus. GnRH stimulates the synthesis and secretion of luteinizing hormone (LH) and follicle-stimulating hormone (FSH) from the pituitary gland. These gonadotropins stimulate testicular steroid secretion (testosterone and estradiol E_2) from the Leydig cells. The Sertoli cells in the testis secrete the peptide inhibin. Spermatogenesis takes place in the seminiferous tubules of the testis. Control and coordination of testicular function occurs via feedback signals, both positive and negative, exerted by the hormones secreted at each level of the hypothalamic-pituitary axis. DHT—dihydrotestosterone.

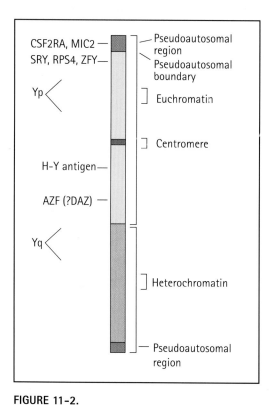

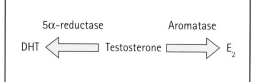

FIGURE 11-3.

Testosterone metabolism. Testosterone is converted to dihydrotestosterone (DHT) by 5alpha-reductase. In the male fetus, testosterone is responsible for the development of the epididymis, vas deferens, seminal vesicles, and ejaculatory duct. DHT stimulates the development of the male external genitalia, urethra, and prostate. Testosterone also is aromatized to estradiol (E_2) in the peripheral tissues. The normal circulating testosterone-to-estradiol ratio in the adult man is 9:1.

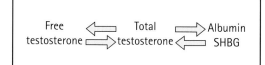

FIGURE 11-4.

Total and free testosterone metabolism. Testosterone circulates bound to sex hormone–binding globulin (SHBG) or albumin (98%; known as "total testosterone") and in a free form (2%). It is the free form of testosterone that enters into the androgen-sensitive cells.

FIGURE 11-2.

The human Y chromosome. The human Y chromosome is made up of the euchromatic and the heterochromatic regions. The *SRY* genes located on the Y_p region must be present and functional for the gonad to become a testis. The *AZF* gene (azoospermic factors) is located in euchromatic Y_q region. The *DAZ* (deleted in azoospermia) gene may be synonymous with *AZF*. (*Adapted from* Jaffe and Oates [1].)

CONDITIONS THAT ALTER SEX HORMONE–BINDING GLOBULIN LEVELS

Conditions that decrease SHBG level	Conditions that increase SHBG levels
Hypothyroidism	Hyperthryroidism
Androgen therapy	Pregnancy
Corticosteroid therapy	Estrogen therapy
Obesity	Cirrhosis
Acromegaly	

FIGURE 11–5.

Conditions that alter sex hormone–binding globulin (SHBG) level. A change in the amount of available SHBG alters the degree of tissue entry of testosterone. Specific medical conditions will either increase or decrease SHBG levels.

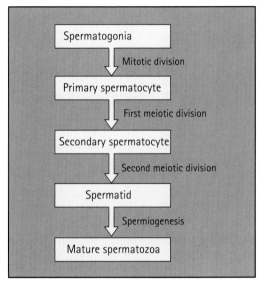

FIGURE 11–6.

Stages of human spermatogenesis. Spermatogenesis is the orderly process during which spermatogonia evolve into mature spermatozoa. In humans, the process covers a 72-day period.

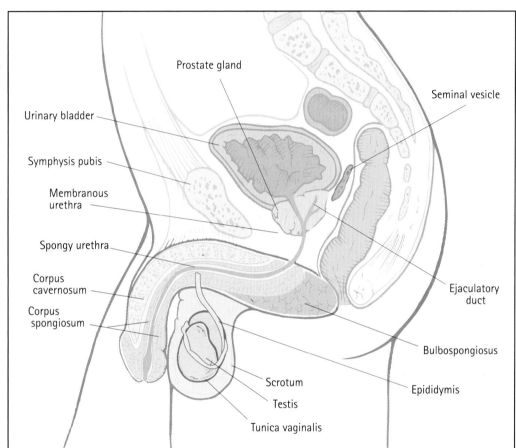

FIGURE 11–7.

Anatomy of male genitalia. Spermatozoa move from the testicle into the epididymis where they are rendered motile and fertile. In humans, this process occurs in approximately 10 days. During ejaculation, the spermatozoa move through the vas deferens and out the ejaculatory duct. The seminal vesicles provide the seminal plasma with fructose and the prostate provides zinc, citrate, spermine, and acid phosphatases and proteases that are important in the liquefaction of semen.

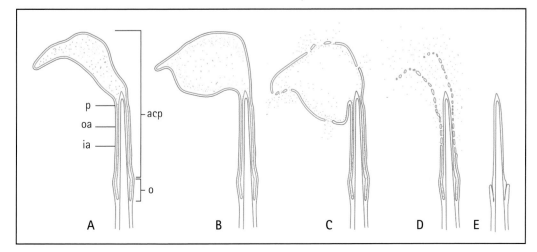

FIGURE 11–8.

Acrosome reaction. To fertilize an ovum, spermatozoa must first undergo capacitation and the acrosome reaction. During the acrosome reaction (**A** and **B**), the outer acrosomal membrane and the plasma membrane of the spermatozooan undergo fusion and vesiculation. This process results in the release of acrosomal enzymes (**C–E**).

*E*VALUATION

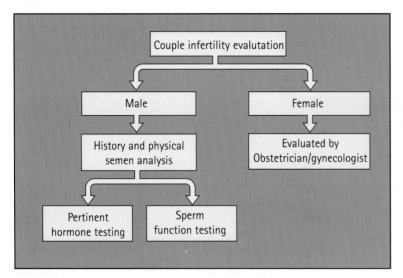

FIGURE 11–9.

Basic evaluation of the man presenting with infertility. The cornerstone of the work-up is the history, physical examination, and semen analysis. Infertility is a presenting complaint of a couple; thus the man's physician should stay in close communication with the woman's physician.

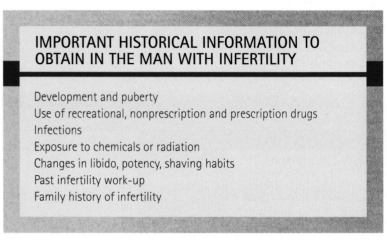

IMPORTANT HISTORICAL INFORMATION TO OBTAIN IN THE MAN WITH INFERTILITY

Development and puberty
Use of recreational, nonprescription and prescription drugs
Infections
Exposure to chemicals or radiation
Changes in libido, potency, shaving habits
Past infertility work-up
Family history of infertility

FIGURE 11–10.

The history. A careful history is necessary to uncover any underlying medical or endocrine disease. Important historical information to obtain includes a detailed account of the patient's developmental and fertility history; past and present illnesses and surgeries; use of alcohol, recreational drugs, and prescription medication; environmental or occupational toxicant exposure; and family history of infertility or other endocrine disorders.

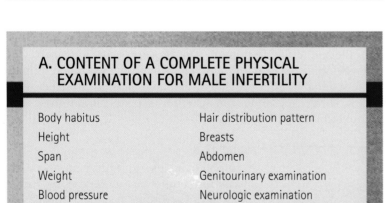

SYMPTOMS OF ANDROGEN DEFICIENCY

Fatigue	Osteopenia
Depression	Increased fracture rate
Impotence	Infertility
Muscle weakness	

FIGURE 11–11.

Symptoms of androgen deficiency. A small subset of men presenting with infertility will have androgen deficiency. Presenting symptoms are often insidious in onset and therefore can be difficult to detect.

A. CONTENT OF A COMPLETE PHYSICAL EXAMINATION FOR MALE INFERTILITY

Body habitus	Hair distribution pattern
Height	Breasts
Span	Abdomen
Weight	Genitourinary examination
Blood pressure	Neurologic examination
Skin	

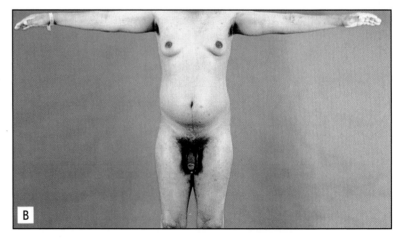

FIGURE 11–12.

The physical examination. **A,** Components of a complete physical examination. This examination is necessary to uncover any underlying medical conditions, as well as hypogonadism. **B,** Physical characteristics of male infertility. The genitalia and secondary sexual characteristics are evaluated to determine if sexual development is normal. Hepatomegaly may suggest alcoholic liver disease or other disorders associated with abnormal steroid metabolism. Gynecomastia is frequently associated with hypogonadism or an imbalance in the testosterone-to-estradiol ratio.

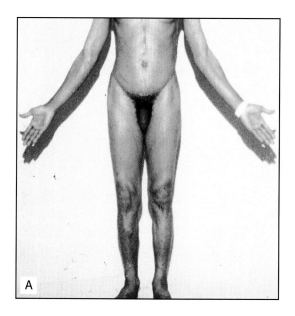
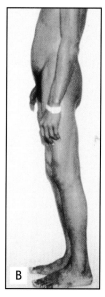

FIGURE 11-13.

Eunuchoid proportions. Leydig cell failure that occurs prior to puberty will disrupt normal sexual maturation, resulting in the failure of androgen-induced closure of the epiphyses of the long bones. Eunuchoidism is defined as an arm span more than 2 inches longer than the height, and a lower body segment (pubic area to heel) more than 2 inches longer than the upper body segment (crown to pubic area).

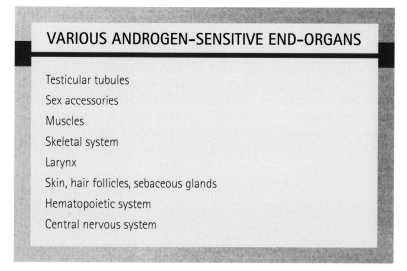

VARIOUS ANDROGEN-SENSITIVE END-ORGANS

Testicular tubules

Sex accessories

Muscles

Skeletal system

Larynx

Skin, hair follicles, sebaceous glands

Hematopoietic system

Central nervous system

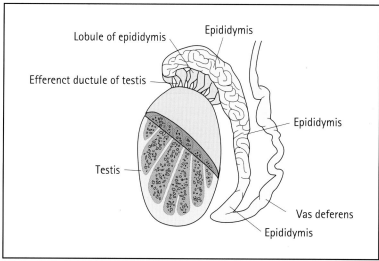

FIGURE 11-14.

Androgen-sensitive end-organs. The physician pays close attention to those organ systems that are responsive to androgen. These systems include the skin and hair follicles, the bones, and the genitourinary system.

FIGURE 11-15.

Anatomy of the scrotum. During examination, the scrotal contents are carefully palpated for the presence of the vas deferens and epididymis, and for varicocele. Thickening or irregularities in the epididymis suggest a past infection or possible obstruction. A small percentage of infertile men will have congenital absence of the vas, a condition associated with cystic fibrosis. The testes are palpated for position, shape, consistency, masses, and size.

FIGURE 11-16.

The orchidometer. Testicular volume is measured with an orchidometer or calipers. Adult testicular volume ranges from 15 to 25 cm^3. Most of the testicular volume is derived from the germ cells. Thus, a small testicular volume suggests inadequate sperm production.

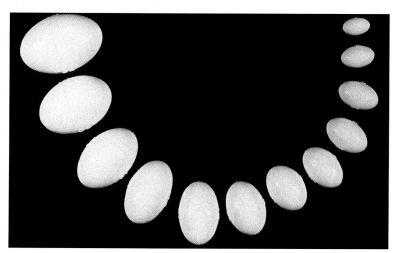

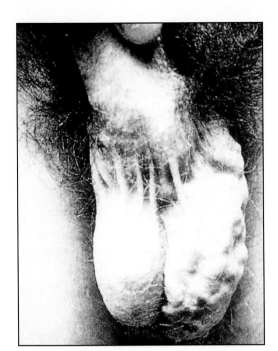

FIGURE 11-17.

Varicocele. A varicocele is a dilatation of the scrotal portion of the pampiniform plexus–internal spermatic venous system that drains the testicle. Whereas a large varicocele similar to the one seen in this picture is easy to identify, a small varicocele may be noted only when the patient performs a Valsalva maneuver, or by examining the patient first in the supine and then the standing position. A nonpalpable varicocele (identified only by radiologic or ultrasonographic techniques) is not clinically relevant.

CLINICAL ASPECTS OF VARICOCELE

8%–22% of normal men have varicoceles

21% to 39% of men undergoing infertility evaluations have varicoceles

90% of palpable varicoceles are left-sided

Size of varicocele may not correlate with severity of oligospermia

FIGURE 11-18.

Clinical aspects of varicocele. The varicocele was first implicated as a cause of male factor infertility in the 1950s, when the observation was made that the incidence of varicocele was higher in men presenting with a history of infertility than in the general population. Anatomically, the varicocele is more common on the left side because the venous system drains into the renal vein rather than directly into the inferior vena cava.

FIGURE 11-19.

Semen analysis. The semen analysis is traditionally the most important tool in the investigation of male infertility. However, there is marked variability in sperm density, motility, and morphology among multiple semen samples from an individual man. Collection of three to six samples over 2 to 3 months increases the reliability of the mean values calculated. Standardization of abstinence time also improves the reliability of the interpretation of the results.

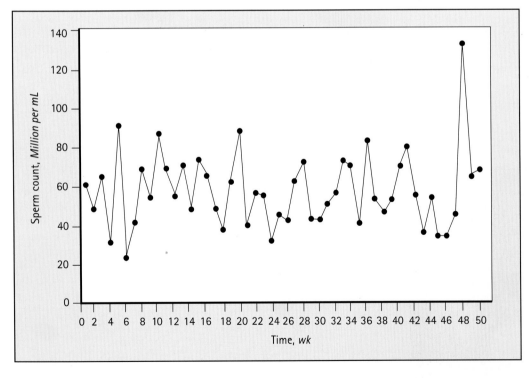

NORMAL SEMEN VALUES

Volume: >2mL

pH: 7.2–7.8

Sperm concentration: >20 million sperm/mL

Motility: >50% with forward progression

Normal morphology: > 30% per WHO standards

> 14% per "strict morphology" standards

FIGURE 11–20.

Normal parameters in semen analysis. Semen samples are collected into a wide-mouthed sterile jar following 2 to 5 days of abstention. Initial evaluation of the sample should take place within 60 minutes of collection. The standards recommended by the World Health Organization (WHO) are shown, along with recently proposed alternative standards. This "strict morphology" format suggests 14% as the lower limit of normal for morphology.

SPERM FUNCTION TESTS

Computer-assisted semen analysis

In vitro cervical mucus penetration test

Zona-free hamster ova–*in vitro* sperm penetration assay

Hemizona assay

Hypo-osmotic swelling test

Acrosome assessment tests

FIGURE 11–21.

Sperm function tests. Because the semen analysis does not definitively predict fertility potential, several sperm function tests were developed. In general, these assays test different steps in the biologic cascade that the spermatozoon must pass through before fertilization takes place. No single test definitively predicts fertility.

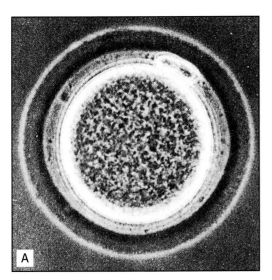
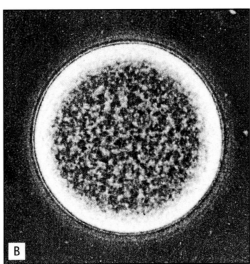
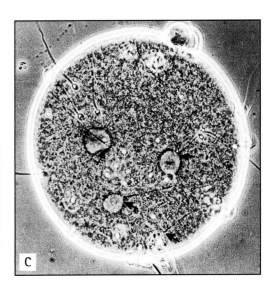

FIGURE 11–22.

The sperm penetration assay (SPA). The SPA assesses the ability of capacitated sperm populations to penetrate into zona-free hamster ova. The incubated egg is gently compressed between a slide and a coverslip and is viewed in phase contrast (**A** and **B**). Swollen sperm heads appear as large, clear areas associated with a sperm tail (**C**).

TESTS OF HYPOTHALAMIC–PITUITARY–TESTICULAR FUNCTION

Serum LH and FSH

Serum testosterone

Serum estradiol

Serum prolactin

FIGURE 11–23.

Endocrine function evaluation. Evaluation of the endocrine status of the reproductive hormonal axis requires the measurement of serum luteinizing hormone (LH), follicle-stimulating hormone (FSH), and testosterone. If clinically indicated, estradiol and prolactin levels also are measured. Gonadotropin-releasing hormone (GnRH) and human chorionic gonadotropin stimulation testing is performed in selected patients.

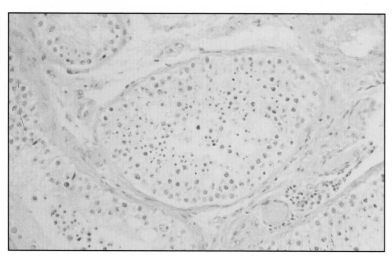

FIGURE 11–24.

Normal spermatogenesis as revealed by testicular biopsy. For the infertile patient who presents with azoospermia, normal-size testes, and normal reproductive hormone levels, testicular biopsy will differentiate between obstruction of the vas deferens or epididymis and spermatogenic arrest.

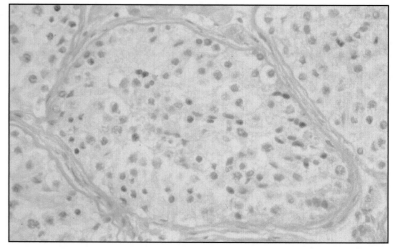

FIGURE 11–25.

Spermatogenic arrest. Spermatogenic arrest is the failure of immature spermatozoa to develop into mature spermatozoa. Note the absence of any sperm elements with tails in this testicular biopsy sample.

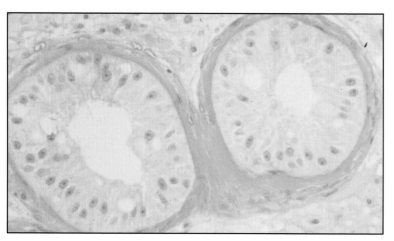

FIGURE 11–26.

Sertoli–cell only syndrome. A new indication for testicular biopsy is to determine if the testicle contains any sperm forms that might be aspirated and used in an intracytoplasmic sperm injection procedure. Note the absence of any sperm elements and the abundance of Sertoli cells in this testicular biopsy sample.

DIFFERENTIAL DIAGNOSIS AND TREATMENT

DIFFERENTIAL DIAGNOSIS OF MALE INFERTILITY

Anatomic defects
Endocrine dysfunction
    Hypogonadotropic hypogonadism
    Hypergonadotropic hypogonadism
    Irreversible germ cell failure
    Testosterone resistance
Idiopathic infertility

FIGURE 11–27.

Differential diagnosis. Based on the history, physical examination, hormone evaluation, and semen analysis, causes of infertility can be placed into three major diagnostic categories: anatomic defects, endocrine dysfunction, and idiopathic infertility.

ANATOMIC DEFECTS THAT CONTRIBUTE TO MALE INFERTILITY

Congenital absence of the vas
Obstruction of the vas deferens
Obstruction of the epididymis

FIGURE 11–28.

Anatomic defects. The causes of obstructive azoospermia include congenital absence of vas deferens, vasectomy, inadvertent ligation or transection of the vas during herniorrhaphy or pelvic surgery, and epididymal obstruction. Abnormality of the ejaculatory duct is a rare cause of obstruction. Disruption of the innervation of the vasa deferentia and bladder neck may result in retrograde ejaculation.

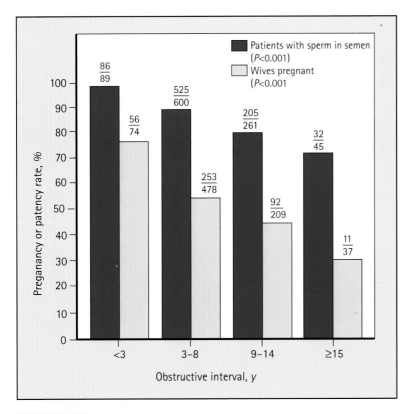

FIGURE 11-29.

Vasectomy reversal. Patency and pregnancy rates following vasectomy reversal. The numerator equals the number of patients achieving patency or pregnancy; the denominator equals the total number of patients in each group. There is an inverse correlation of patency and pregnancy rate with obstruction interval. (*Adapted from* Belker and coworkers [2]; with permission.)

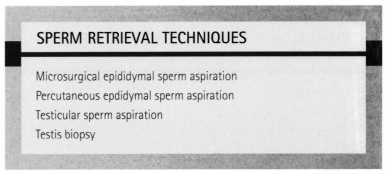

SPERM RETRIEVAL TECHNIQUES

Microsurgical epididymal sperm aspiration
Percutaneous epdidymal sperm aspiration
Testicular sperm aspiration
Testis biopsy

FIGURE 11-30.

Sperm retrieval techniques. Alternative, less invasive sperm harvesting techniques have recently been described in lieu of vasectomy reversal, or as the primary treatment for congenital absence of the vas and severe retrograde ejaculation as well as nonobstructive azoospermia. In each instance, the harvested sperm are subsequently prepared for an intracytoplasmic sperm injection (ICSI) procedure. Recovery of spermatozoa from men diagnosed with obstructive azoospermia using one of these above techniques can lead to the development of viable embryos and a reported 50% pregnancy rate. Success in the patient with nonobstructive azoospermia is lower. Testicular sperm aspiration from men with tubular sclerosis, Sertoli cell–only syndrome, or severe maturation arrest is less likely to yield viable spermatozoa for ICSI. For the patient with nonobstructive azoospermia, testicular histopathology is the strongest predictor of successful testicular sperm recovery, suggesting that a diagnostic testicular biopsy should be considered prior to the ICSI procedure.

CLINICAL SIGNS OF HYPOGONADOTROPIC HYPOGONADISM

Low testosterone
Low LH and FSH
Variable response to stimulation testing
Variable sperm concentration

FIGURE 11-31.

Clinical signs of hypogonadotropic hypogonadism. This disorder is caused by a deficiency in luteinizing hormone (LH) and follicle-stimulating hormone (FSH) secretion, resulting in a failure to stimulate the testes to produce testosterone and spermatogenesis. The differential diagnosis includes pituitary tumor, Kallmann's syndrome, idiopathic infertility, and secondary to infiltrative diseases such as sarcoidosis, tuberculosis, and hemochromatosis. Usually, prolactin-secreting pituitary tumors in men are large at the time of discovery. Presenting complaints include visual field defects and impotence.

TREATMENT OF HYPOGONADOTROPIC HYPOGONADISM

Initial treatment
   hCG: 1500–3000 IU 2–3 × weekly for 6–8 mo
To restore fertility
   hMG: 37–150 IU, 2–3 × weekly in addition to hCG therapy

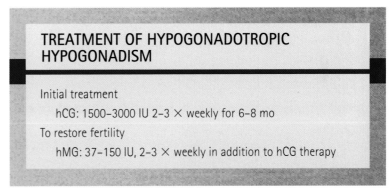

FIGURE 11-32.

Treatment of hypogonadotropic hypogonadism. In general, pituitary tumors are treated surgically. Postoperative patients and all other patients with this diagnosis are primarily treated with gonadotropin-replacement therapy: either human chorionic gonadotropin (hCG) or human menopausal gonadotropin (hMG) to restore spermatogenesis if fertility is the goal. Patients not interested in fertility are treated with androgen-replacement therapy.

CLINICAL SIGNS OF HYPERGONADOTROPIC HYPOGONADISM

Low testosterone

Elevated LH and FSH

No reponse to hCG Test

Oligospermia or azoospermia

FIGURE 11-33.

Clinical signs of hypergonadotropic hypogonadism. Men with this condition have primary testicular failure. The classic presentation is one of elevated gonadotropins with decreased testosterone values and severe oligospermia or azoospermia. Klinefelter's syndrome is the most common cause. A subset of men present with normal luteinizing hormone (LH) and testosterone values, but have elevated follicle-stimulating hormone (FSH) levels and oligospermia. In these cases the abnormality is localized to the germ cells in the testes. HCG—human chorionic gonadotropin.

SIDE EFFECTS OF TESTOSTERONE THERAPY

Edema and weight gain

Hot flashes and headaches

Hypertension

Gynecomastia

Increased alterations in libido and potency

Azoospermia

Increased prostate size

Liver toxicity

Changes in cholesterol and lipid levels

FIGURE 11-35.

Side effects of testosterone therapy. Several potential side effects can occur following either form of testosterone-replacement therapy. Skin irritation has been reported with certain forms of patch therapy.

CLINICAL SIGNS OF IDIOPATHIC INFERTILITY

History of infertility

Normal LH, FSH, testosterone values

Oligospermia

TESTOSTERONE REPLACEMENT THERAPY

Long-acting testosterone ester (200 mg intramuscular q. 2 wk)

Transdermal patch (daily)

FIGURE 11-34.

Testosterone replacement therapy. Patients with hypogonadotropic hypogonadism who are not interested in fertility and patients with primary testicular failure with androgen deficiency are prescribed testosterone. The traditional replacement dose is a bimonthly injection of esterified testosterone. An alternative administration method is the transdermal patch.

CLINICAL DEFINITION OF ANDROGEN RESISTANCE

Serum testosterone elevated or normal

Serum LH elevated

Serum FSH normal

Serum estradiol elevated

LH suppression by androgen impaired

FIGURE 11-36.

Clinical signs of androgen resistance. A small number of infertile men will be diagnosed with incomplete testosterone resistance. These men may present with normal external male genitalia or varying degrees of gynecomastia, hypospadius, and infertility. Men with deficiency of 5alpha-reductase also exhibit partial androgen resistance. No hormonal therapies are available to treat these men. FSH—follicle-stimulating hormone; LH—luteinizing hormone.

FIGURE 11-37.

Clinical signs of idiopathic infertility. The majority of infertile men have idiopathic infertility, for which there are no treatments except ICSI. FSH—follicle-stimulating hormone; LH—luteinizing hormone.

EFFECTS OF VARICOCELE REPAIR ON PREGNANCY RATES

Study	Year	Pregnancy rate after surgery, %	Pregnancy rate with no surgery, %
Nilsson	1979	8	18
Baker	1985	47	45
Vermeulen	1986	24	56
Nieshlag	1995	26	27
Madgar	1995	70	10

FIGURE 11–38.

Effects of varicocele repair on pregnancy rates. Animal studies suggest that varicoceles damage the testes. Prospective controlled clinical studies report no improvement in pregnancy rates with varicocele ligation. One crossover study does suggest improvement in pregnancy rates.

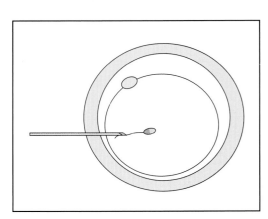

FIGURE 11–39.

Intracytoplasmic sperm injection (ICSI). The advent of ICSI in combination with *in vitro* fertilization has revolutionized the treatment of male factor infertility. Although the procedure does not provide a therapeutic intervention that cures the disorder, it offers an avenue for successful pregnancy. Large studies report a 25% to 35% pregnancy rate.

*R*EFERENCES

1. Jaffe T, Oates RD: *Infertility in the Male*. St. Louis: Mosby; 1997:280.

2. Belker AM, Thomas AJ, Fuchs EF, *et al.*: Results of 1469 microsurgical vasectomy reversals by the Vasovasostomy Study Group. *J Urol* 1991, 145:505.

*S*UGGESTED BIBLIOGRAPHY

Aitken J: Diagnostic value of the hamster oocyte penetration assay. *Int J Androl* 1984, 7:273.

Barraclough CA: The role of catecholamines in the regulation of pituitary LH and FSH secretion. *Endo Rev* 1982, 3:91.

Baum J, Langenin R, D'Costta M, *et al.*: Serum pituitary and steroid hormone levels in the adult male: one value is as good as the mean of three. *Fertil Steril* 1988, 49:123.

Clermont Y: The cycle of seminiferous epithelium in man. *Am J Anat* 1986, 112:35.

Cunningham GR, Cordero E, Thornby JI: Testosterone replacement with transdermal therapeutic systems. *JAMA* 1989, 261:2525.

Eddy EM: The spermatozoon. In *The Physiology of Reproduction*. New York: Raven Press; 1988: 27.

Glazner CMA, Kelly NJ, Weir MJA, *et al.*: The diagnosis of male infertility: prospective time-specific study of conception rates related to seminal analysis and post coital sperm-mucus penetration and survival in otherwise unexplained infertility. *Hum Reprod* 1987, 2:665.

Howards SS: Varicocele. *Infertility and Reproductive Medicine Clinics of North America* 1992, 3:429–441.

Jarow JP: Role of ultrasonography in the evaluation of the infertile male. *Semin Urol* 1994, 12:274.

Kalra SP, Kalra PS: Neural regulation of luteinizing hormone secretion in the rat. *Endo Rev* 1983, 4:311.

Kruger TF, Acosta AA, Simmons KF, *et al.*: New method of evaluating sperm morphology with predictive value for human in vitro fertilization. *Urology* 1987, 30:248.

MacLeod J: Human male infertility. *Obstet Gynecol Surv* 1971, 12:325.

McCullagh DR: Dual endocrine activity of the testes. *Science* 1932, 76:19.

Palermo GD, Cohen J, Alikani M, *et al.*: Intracytoplasmic sperm injection: a novel treatment for all forms of male factor infertility. *Fertil Steril* 1995, 63:1231–1240.

Partridge WM: Transport of protein-bound hormones into tissues in vivo. *Endo Rev* 1981, 2:103.

Rogers BJ: The sperm penetration assay: its usefulness reevaluated. *Fertil Steril* 1985, 43:821.

Rogers BJ, Van Capmen A, Ueno M, *et al.*: Analysis of human spermatozoa fertilizing ability using zona-free ova. *Fertil Steril* 1979, 32:664.

Rudak E: Interspecific fertilization. In *Bioregulators of Reproduction*. New York: New York Academic; 1981:167.

Santen RJ, Bardin CW: Episodic luteinizing hormone secretion in man: pulse analysis, clinical interpretation, physiologic metabolism. *J Clin Invest* 1973, 52:2617.

Schrader SM, Turner TW, Breitenstein MJ, Simon SD: Longitudinal study of semen quality of unexposed workers. *Reprod Toxicol* 1988, 2:183.

Sherins RJ, Brightwell D, Sternthal PM: Longitudinal analysis of semen of fertile and infertile men. In *New Concepts of the Testis in Normal and Infertile Men: Morphology, Physiology and Pathology*. Edited by Troen P, Nankin H. New York: Raven Press; 1977:473.

Sokol RZ: Male factor in infertility. In *Infertility, Contraception and Reproductive Endocrinology*. Edited by Lobo RA, Mishell DR Jr., Paulson RJ. Malden, MA: Blackwell Science; 1997;P547–P566.

Sokol RZ: Medical endocrine therapy of male factor infertility. *Infertility and Reproductive Medicine Clinics of North America* 1992, 3:389.

Van Steirteghem A, Joris H, Liu J, *et al.*: Evolution of intracytoplasmic injection (ICSI) results. *Fertil Steril* 1994, 62:S83.

World Health Organization: *WHO Laboratory Manual for the Examination of Human Semen and Semen Cervical Mucus Interaction*. Cambridge, UK: Cambridge University Press; 1987 and 1993.

Yanagimachi R, Chang MC: Fertilization of hamster eggs in vitro. *Nature* 1963, 200:281.

Treatment of Unexplained Infertility

John Collins

Despite numerous advances in the diagnostic assessment of infertility, the problem of unexplained infertility, first described by Southam in 1960, remains unsolved. The problem is that an up-to-date, sophisticated evaluation of semen, ovulation, and genital tract competence cannot disclose many of the possible defects in the complex process leading to conception. Thus, incomplete understanding of the prerequisites for conception and limited clinical tools for diagnosis present a challenge for both biologic and clinical research.

Infertility is unexplained in approximately 20% of infertile couples. The proportion with unexplained infertility varies with female partner age, in part because declining fertility in older female partners is not necessarily associated with abnormal diagnostic test results. The untreated prognosis with unexplained infertility is better than it is with other infertility diagnoses. The likelihood of conception without treatment is 23% in the first year after diagnosis, and 35% during follow-up to 3 years. Older female partners have lower pregnancy rates, an effect that is significant with longer duration of infertility.

In the absence of a known cause, there can be no specific therapy for unexplained infertility. Nevertheless, advances in treatment technology provide a range of empiric therapy options. The rationale for empiric therapy depends on recruiting multiple follicles or bringing the oocytes and spermatozoa into proximity. Judging from the results of randomized clinical trials, bromocriptine does not appear to be effective; clomiphene citrate, intrauterine insemination of prepared semen, and controlled ovarian stimulation with gonadotropin show each have significant benefits. *In vitro* fertilization has not been tested within the diagnostic category of unexplained infertility in a trial protocol that made use of an untreated comparison group.

Knowledge of the benefits, adverse effects, and costs of treatment can provide useful support for shared decision making. Such support will help to ensure that each treatment plan meets the preferences of the individual couple.

CLINICAL DIAGNOSIS OF INFERTILITY

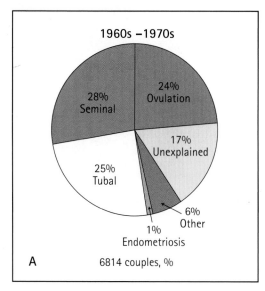

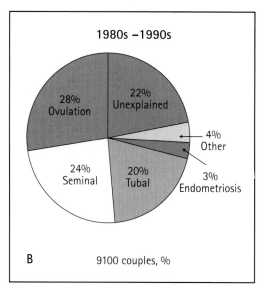

FIGURE 12-1.

Distribution of diagnoses for infertility. The distribution of diagnostic assignments for infertility from large published reports in the past 40 years show that unexplained infertility was the diagnostic assignment for 17% of couples prior to 1980 (**A**), and 22% of couples since 1980 (**B**). Diagnostic assignment refers to the primary clinical diagnosis. Despite advances in the diagnostic assessment of infertility, approximately one fifth of couples have infertility that remains unexplained after a standard work-up.

Because of the complexity of fertilization and implantation, standard tests are limited. Standard testing can evaluate tubal patency, but cannot evaluate numerous tubal transport and membrane functions; also, the tests provide no assessment of the role of the fallopian tube in harboring the fertilized oocyte for 3 or 4 days. Moreover, the most sophisticated semen analysis cannot define the fertilizing capacity of the given ejaculate. No test in clinical use can determine whether the sperm can endure storage in the cervix, undergo transportation to the site of fertilization, or achieve the reactions that are necessary for penetration of the oocyte membrane. Further, although it is known that endometrial receptivity during the implantation window is crucial to successful conception, no histologic or biochemical assessment of endometrial responses has been reliably associated with conception.

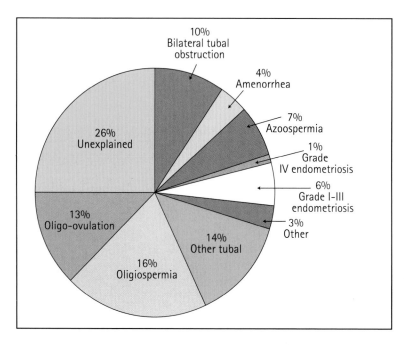

FIGURE 12-2.

Diagnostic assignment and cause of infertility. Does a diagnostic assignment such as oligospermia or oligo-ovulation mean that the infertility has been explained? This figure shows the distribution of diagnostic assignments among 2198 couples enrolled in the Canadian infertility evaluation study [1]. Twenty-six percent of the couples had unexplained infertility. A further 22% of couples had a clear explanation for their infertility, in the form of bilateral tubal obstruction, prolonged amenorrhea, azoospermia, or grade 4 endometriosis. For the remainder, various degrees of anovulation, oligospermia, tubal adhesions, and unilateral obstruction may represent coincidental findings, rather than the true underlying cause of the infertility.

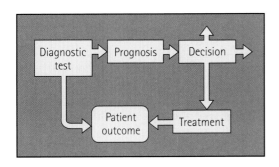

FIGURE 12-3.

Outline of the clinical approach to unexplained infertility. This figure outlines the clinical process comprising decisions shared between physician and patient, guided by the judgment and experience of the physician, and the preferences and characteristics of the patient. In the course of medical practice, the clinician offers advice about diagnostic tests, intuitively or explicitly calculates a prognosis once a diagnosis has been made, considers a range of treatment options to be offered, and makes judgments about the balance between the benefits and the costs and adverse effects of each treatment option. As the figure shows, the value of diagnostic tests and the effectiveness of treatment are best judged on the patient outcome, and the outcome of greatest interest to the patient in the case of infertility is the birth of a healthy child. This algorithm underlies the approach to unexplained infertility.

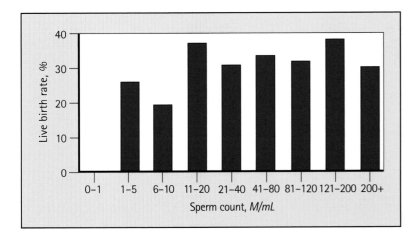

FIGURE 12-4.

Sperm count and live birth rate without treatment. Are the standard diagnostic tests accurate when judged according to the correlation with the outcome of interest? This figure shows the frequency of live birth conceptions, arranged according to sperm concentration among infertile couples with normal female partners. Semen analysis is clearly an important diagnostic test, because it is needed to detect the small proportion of men with azoospermia or virtual azoospermia in whom no pregnancy can be expected without treatment. For the remaining categories of sperm density, a correlation with live birth does not exist. Clearly, however, there is a need for tests of sperm function and fertilizing capacity that may explain the infertility. (*Data from* Collins *et al.* [1].)

VALIDITY OF THE POSTCOITAL TEST FOR INFERTILITY

Postcoital Test Result	No Conception, *n*	Conception, *n*	Total, *n*
Abnormal	194	127	321
Normal	160	228	388
Total	354	355	709

Negative predictive value: 228/388 = 59%; positive predictive value: 194/321 = 60%; abnormal frequency: 321/709 = 45%.

FIGURE 12-5.

Validity of the postcoital test for infertility. Whether the postcoital test provides information about sperm function has been debated for many decades. This figure summarizes the correlation between postcoital test results and conception from a diagnostic test meta-analysis [2]. Few tests have generated more controversy than the postcoital test, although no one disputes whether cervical malfunction could be a cause of infertility. The disagreement concerns whether the postcoital test is a test that accurately defines normal and abnormal cervical function. As the table shows, the negative and positive predictive values are only marginally better than a chance association (50%). Also, nearly half of the tests reported in the clinical literature are abnormal. Thus, although it may be weakly correlated with pregnancy, the test as reported has too many abnormal results and should not be used.

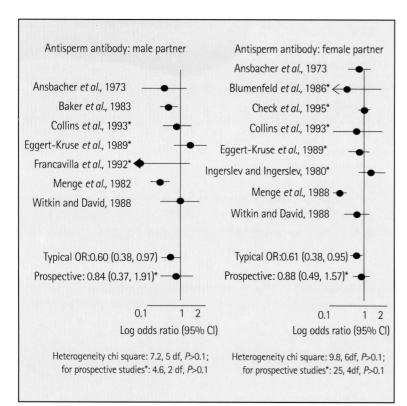

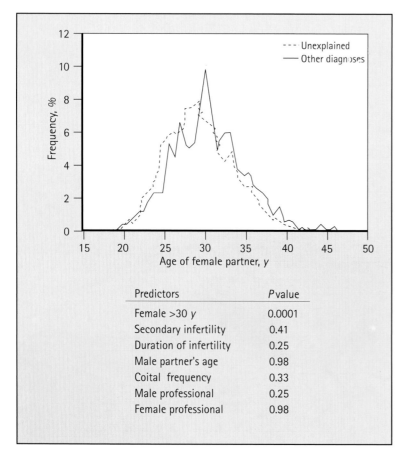

FIGURE 12-6.

Evaluation of antisperm antibody. A further question that arises in the diagnostic assessment of infertility is the evaluation of antisperm antibody in the male or female partner. This figure summarizes the results of studies in which antisperm antibody presence in serum was correlated with the occurrence of conception during follow-up. Prospective studies are shown in *blue*. Summary analysis of the prospective studies of antisperm antibody in male partner serum shows that there is a 16% reduction of the likelihood of conception and this result is not significant. Similarly, with antisperm antibody presence in female partner serum there is a nonsignificant 12% reduction in conception. A small percentage of antibody-positive male partners may have extensive antibody attachment to the surface of sperm in the ejaculate. Further research is needed to determine the significance of this finding. Therefore, measurement of circulating antisperm antibodies in male and female patients should not be performed. OR—odds ratio.

CLINICAL PREDICTORS

FIGURE 12-7.

Distribution of age of female partners with unexplained infertility versus other diagnoses. Age of the female partner is a significant predictor of the likelihood of a couple having unexplained infertility, compared with any other infertility diagnosis. The figure shows that the distribution of the age of female partners with unexplained infertility (*blue*) is slightly but more significantly advanced than the age distribution with other diagnoses (*yellow*). In the accompanying table, the results of a logistic regression indicate that among the potential factors that might lead to unexplained infertility, female age over 30 years is the only significant predictor. A couple in which the female partner is aged 30 years or more is 1.7-fold more likely (95% CI 1.3–1.9) to have unexplained infertility than in a younger woman.

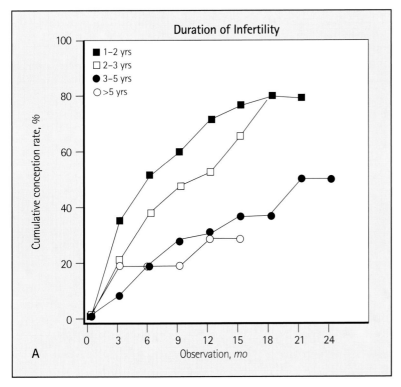

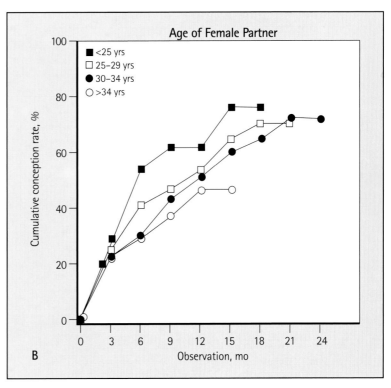

FIGURE 12-8.

Prognostic factors that contribute to the likelihood of conception among couples with unexplained infertility. These figures show that a superior cumulative conception rate during the first 2 years (**A**) of follow-up is correlated with shorter duration of the infertility, and younger female partners (**B**). (*Adapted from* Hull *et al.* [3].)

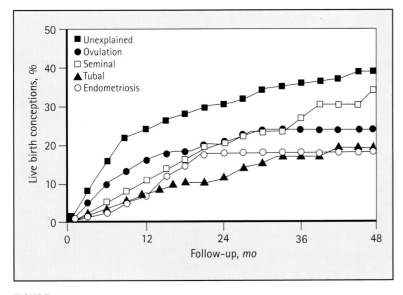

FIGURE 12-9

Frequency of live birth conceptions occurring without treatment. This figure shows the likelihood of live birth conceptions independently of treatment during 4 years of follow-up. The prognosis with unexplained infertility is 23% at 12 months, 30% at 2 years, and 33% at 3 years duration of follow-up. The average duration of infertility for the couples in this study was 42 months.

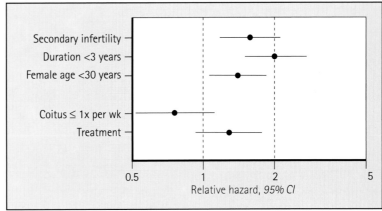

FIGURE 12-10.

Predictor model for live birth conception. This figure shows the results of a proportional hazards analysis evaluating the association between clinical variables and time to conception, once again considering only live birth conceptions [2]. The proportional hazards analysis shows that the relative likelihood of conception is significantly higher for couples with unexplained infertility if there is a history of a prior pregnancy in this partnership, a duration of infertility less than 3 years, or the female partner's age is less than 30 years. Coital frequency once or less per week was associated with a nonsignificant reduction in the likelihood of conception. The overall impact of treatment was not significant, implying that the contribution of the other clinical variables is independent of treatment.

A. PROGNOSIS FOR LIVE BIRTH CONCEPTION AFTER DIAGNOSIS

Months, n	Live Births, %
3	7
6	13.8
12	22.6
24	29.7
36	33.3

B. EFFECT OF PROGNOSTIC FACTORS ON UNEXPLAINED FERTILITY

Prediction Model	Multiplication Factor
Secondary infertility	1.6
Duration <3 y	2.0
Female age <30 y	1.4

FIGURE 12-11.

Application of the predictor model to unexplained fertility. From the proportional hazards analysis shown in Figure 12-10, the significant prognostic factors comprise a prediction score or model that can be applied to calculate the prognosis for individual couples. For most couples, the period of interest is the next year, when the prognosis for a conception leading to live birth is 23%. **A**, Prognosis of live birth conception after diagnosis. **B**, Effect of prognostic factors.

As an example, consider a couple with a female partner of 35 years of age who have 42 months duration of primary infertility. The average prognosis would be 23% for this couple. Considering a couple in which the female partner is 28 years of age, with only 2.5 years duration of primary unexplained infertility, the prognosis would be 63% (22.6 × 2.0 × 1.4). (*Adapted from* Collins *et al.* [1].)

UNEXPLAINED INFERTILITY OUTCOMES

Outcome		Couples, n	Percent of conceptions, n=123	Percent of untreated couples, n=381
Pregnancy		123	32	0
	Live birth	84	22	68
	Abortion	21	6	17
	Premature	6	2	5
	Perinatal loss	6	2	5
	Ectopic	6	2	5
Continued follow-up		127	33	
Lost to follow-up		94	25	
Resolved		29	8	
Adopted		8	2	

FIGURE 12-12.

Unexplained infertility outcomes. Among this reported group of couples with unexplained infertility, 181 received treatment. For the remaining 381 couples, there were 123 (32%) conceptions, of which 84 (22% of 381) were live births. A total of 127 couples continued under follow-up, and many of these would be expected to receive treatment after the completion of the study. Only 2% of the total were successful at adopting.

Treatment Decisions

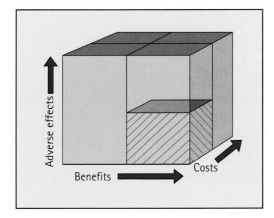

FIGURE 12-13.

Treatment decision process for unexplained infertility. In considering treatment options, the physician makes judgments based on benefits, costs, and adverse effects of each treatment option. The preferred treatment would have the highest possible effect on live birth outcome, with the lowest proportion of adverse effects, at the least cost.

The balance between these considerations is particularly important with respect to the treatment of unexplained infertility, because lacking a known cause and a specific therapy, any treatment under consideration must be empiric. The rationale for such therapy in general is to increase the availability and the proximity of gametes. Ovulation induction agents such as clomiphene and gonadotropins tend to increase the number of mature follicles available for fertilization; intrauterine insemination of prepared sperm and *in vitro* fertilization techniques bring gametes into proximity.

Treatment Results

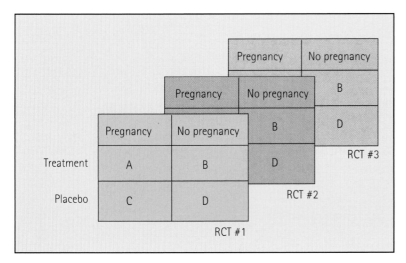

FIGURE 12-14.

Meta-analysis of treatment results. Many of the studies on the effectiveness of treatment of unexplained infertility are relatively small. Also, there is variability among the results of the reported studies. Thus it is necessary to draw on a group of statistical procedures (meta-analysis) to combine the results of studies. In this figure, the 2 × 2 tables express the results of treatment compared with a placebo. The treatment effect is most simply expressed as an odds ratio (OR), calculated as *AD/BC*. The outcome from three hypothetical studies would be derived from the average of the logs of the individual ORs. In each case, the individual OR would be weighted by the inverse of its variance, which can be derived from the confidence interval (CI). Thus, the typical OR gives more weight to the individual estimates, which are most precise and generally come from the larger sample sizes. A 95% CI can be estimated from the variance of the estimate of the typical OR. The results are frequently displayed as an "OR tree" (*see* Figs. 12-15 to 12-17). RCT—randomized clinical trial.

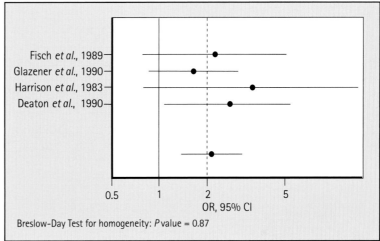

FIGURE 12-15.

Results of clomiphene citrate treatment for unexplained fertility. Clomiphene citrate was introduced as an ovulation induction agent in the 1960s. Its use as an empiric therapy for unexplained infertility began in the 1970s, but it was not until the 1980s that its effectiveness was subjected to experimental proof [7–10]. Once again, the trials were relatively small, and only one was associated with a significant result [19]. Nevertheless, the typical odds ratio (OR) was 2.1 (95% CI 1.3–3.3. The trials ranged in duration from 3 to 6 months, and the overall effectiveness was similar despite differences in dosage and cointerventions. For the average couple with unexplained infertility, the untreated prognosis for live birth conceptions is 7% at 3 months and 14% at 6 months (*see* Fig. 12-11); therefore, the expected effect of clomiphene therapy would be 14% and 28% (× 2.1) respectively. There is no proven value in providing such empiric therapy for longer than 6 months.

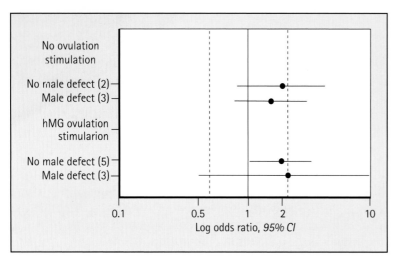

FIGURE 12-16.

Intrauterine insemination (IUI) versus timed intercourse (TI). The rationale for the use of IUI for unexplained infertility is to place spermatozoa in closer juxtaposition with the oocyte, in the hope that some unidentified defect in sperm transport will be overcome. A variety of studies have evaluated this outcome, but only two studies provide information that is specific to couples with unexplained infertility [11, 12]. Additional studies included couples who also received human menopausal gonadotropin (hMG) ovulation stimulation, and those with a seminal disorder. The treatment effect of IUI is also approximately two-fold higher (typical odds ratio, 1.8; 95% CI, 0.8–4.2). This result, however, is not significant. Although the evidence is not conclusive, IUI alone seems to provide a promising but unproven benefit among couples with unexplained infertility. Better evidence on this point is necessary, because IUI is a reasonably safe therapy.

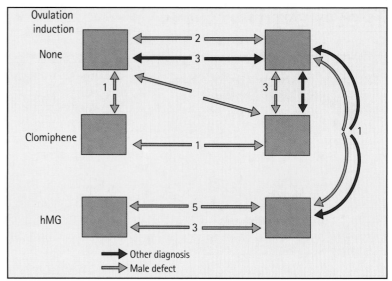

FIGURE 12-17.

Various approaches for treatment of unexplained infertility. To address the effect of gonadotropin ovulation induction with or without intrauterine insemination, a novel approach to meta-analysis was required. Given that the individual trials of gonadotropin therapy did not include a placebo, a search was conducted for all trials that included one arm in which intrauterine insemination was the standard or experimental therapy [7, 11–22]. The analysis then took into account the basic intervention (intrauterine insemination versus timed intercourse), cointerventions (clomiphene or gonadotropins), and the presence of a World Health Organization– defined male defect or other diagnosis. This figure indicates the variety of comparisons taken in the thirteen trials that met these criteria, and the number of intergroup comparisons at each level [35]. hMG—human menopausal gonadotropin.

FFECTIVENESS OF TREATMENT

TIMED INTERCOURSE VERSUS INTRAUTERINE INSEMINATION		
	Pregnancy per Number of Cycles (%)	
Ovulation Stimulation	Timed intercourse	Intrauterine insemination
None	25/963 (3)	61/1102 (6)
Clomiphene	5/54 (9)	27/249 (11)
hMG	21/331 (6)	90/625 (14)

FIGURE 12-18.

Results of cycles of timed intercourse versus intrauterine insemination reported in 13 randomized clinical trials, according to the presence or absence of ovulation stimulation. A small number of these trials also included clomiphene therapy. The general trend within the data is toward a doubling of fecundity associated with intrauterine insemination, compared with timed intercourse. hMG—human menopausal gonadotropin.

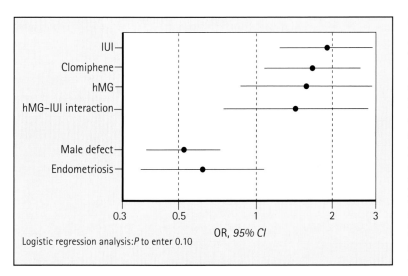

Logistic regression analysis: *P* to enter 0.10

FIGURE 12-19.

Meta-analysis of 13 randomized controlled trials. This figure shows the initial assessment of the treatment effect associated with intrauterine insemination (IUI) and clomiphene, which suggests a significant effect for both. To determine whether the effect of IUI was modified within gonadotropin induction cycles, an hMG–IUI interaction term was entered. A trend toward an effect of IUI within cycles of gonadotropin induction was present, but not significant. The presence of a World Health Organization–defined male defect was associated with a significant reduction in pregnancy rate, and the presence of endometriosis was associated with a not significant reduction in pregnancy rate. Because logistic regression analysis has expressed these treatment effects while taking into account the impact of diagnosis, the odds ratios for treatment derived from the analysis may be considered to be applicable among couples with unexplained infertility.

OVULATION INDUCTION AND INTRAUTERINE INSEMINATION

Factor	Odds Ratio (95% CI)
Clomiphene	1.7 (1.1–2.7)
hMG	2.0 (1.5–2.8)
IUI	2.1 (1.5–2.9)
Male factor	0.6 (0.4–0.8)

FIGURE 12-20.

Ovulation induction versus intrauterine insemination (IUI). The results from the logistic regression meta-analysis have been further simplified in this table. When the interaction term (hMG–IUI interaction) is removed from the analysis, the effects of both hMG and IUI are significant. Consider a typical couple with unexplained infertility (*see* Fig. 12-11); the 1-month prognosis is 2.3% (one third of the 3-month prognosis [7%]); the prognosis for a single cycle of hMG ovulation induction and IUI would be approximately 8% to 9% per cycle (2.3 × 2.0 × 2.1).

EFFECTIVENESS, SIDE EFFECTS, AND COST OF VARIOUS TREATMENTS FOR UNEXPLAINED FERTILITY

Treatment	Cost per Cycle, $	Adverse Effects	Pregnancy Rate per Cycle, %
None	0	0	2
Clomiphene	50	Minimal	4
IUI	200	Minimal	4
hMG–IUI	1200	Moderate	8
IVF	7000	Moderate	18

FIGURE 12-21.

Effectiveness, side effects, and cost of various treatments for unexplained infertility. Unexplained infertility is an especially frustrating form of infertility, and given the uncertainty about the efficacy of treatment, the options may bewilder an infertile couple. This figure summarizes the medical care evidence that may be incorporated into decision making. The costs shown are approximate, but nevertheless there is a dramatic rise in costs from the most simple to the most complex treatment. Adverse medical consequences cannot be dismissed, but are not commonly severe even with *in vitro* fertilization (IVF). The approximate pregnancy rates, drawn from the previous figures, provide the final piece of information that is required for the formulation of a plan for each couple. In many respects, infertility is similar to a chronic disease. The intensity of the disorder may alter with time; spontaneous cure may occur; cure cannot be guaranteed; and those suffering from the condition can educate themselves and become partners in their health care. hMG—human menopausal gonadotropin; IUI—intrauterine insemination.

REFERENCES

1. Collins JA, Burrows EA, Willan AR: The prognosis for live birth among untreated infertile couples. *Fertil Steril* 1995, 64:22–28.

2. Griffith CS, Grimes DA: The validity of the postcoital test. *Am J Obstet Gynecol* 1990, 162:616–620.

3. Hull *et al.*: *BMJ 1985, 291:1693–1697.*

4. Harrison RF, O'Moore RR, McSweeney J: Idiopathic infertility: a trial of bromocriptine versus placebo. *J Ir Med Assoc* 1979, 72:479–482.

5. McBain JC, Pepperell RJ: Use of bromocriptine in unexplained infertility. *Clin Reprod Fertil* 1982, 1:145–150.

6. Wright CS, Steele SJ, Jacobs HS: Value of bromocriptine in unexplained primary infertility: a double-blind controlled trial. *BMJ* 1979, 1:1037–1039.

7. Deaton JL, Gibson M, Blackmer KM, *et al.*: A randomized, controlled trial of clomiphene citrate and intrauterine insemination in couples with unexplained infertility or surgically corrected endometriosis. *Fertil Steril* 1990, 54:1083–1088.

8. Fisch H, Goluboff ET, Olson JH, *et al.*: Semen analyses in 1,283 men from the United States over a 25-year period: no decline in quality. *Fertil Steril* 1996, 65:1009–1014.

9. Glazener CMA, Coulson C, Lambert PA, *et al.*: Clomiphene treatment for women with unexplained infertility: placebo-controlled study of hormonal responses and conception rates. *Gynecol Endocrinol* 1990, 4:75–83.

10. Harrison RF, O'Moore RR: The use of clomiphene citrate with and without human chorionic gonadotropin. *Ir Med J* 1983, 76:273–274.

11. Kirby CA, Flaherty SP, Godfrey BM, *et al.*: A prospective trial of intrauterine insemination of motile spermatozoa versus timed intercourse. *Fertil Steril* 1991, 56:102–107.

12. Martinez AR, Bernardus RE, Voorhorst FJ, *et al.*: Intrauterine insemination does and clomiphene citrate does not improve fecundity in couples with infertility due to male or idiopathic factors: a prospective, randomized, controlled study. *Fertil Steril* 1990, 53:847–853.

13. Arici A, Byrd W, Bradshaw K, *et al.*: Evaluation of clomiphene citrate and human chorionic gonadotropin treatment: a prospective, randomized, crossover study during intrauterine insemination cycles. *Fertil Steril* 1994, 61:314–318.

14. Crosignani PG, Walters DE, Soliani A: The ESHRE multicentre trial on the treatment of unexplained infertility: a preliminary report. *Hum Reprod* 1991, 6:953–958.

15. Evans JH, Wells C, Gregory L, Walker S: A comparison of intrauterine insemination, intraperitoneal insemination, and natural intercourse in superovulated women. *Fertil Steril* 1991, 56:1183–1187.

16. Ho P-C, Poon IML, Chan SYW, Wang C: Intrauterine insemination is not useful in oligoasthenospermia. *Fertil Steril* 1989, 51:682–684.

17. Ho PC, So WK, Chan YF, Yeung WS: Intrauterine insemination is not useful in oligoasthenospermia. *Fertil Steril* 1992, 58:995–999.

18. Karlstrom PO, Bergh T, Lundkvist O: A prospective randomized trial of artificial insemination versus intercourse in cycles stimulated with human menopausal gonadotropin or clomiphene citrate. *Fertil Steril* 1993, 59:554–559.

19. Martinez AR, Bernardus RE, Voorhorst FJ, *et al.*: Pregnancy rates after timed intercourse or intrauterine insemination after human menopausal gonadotropin stimulation of normal ovulatory cycles: a controlled study. *Fertil Steril* 1991, 55:258–265.

20. Nulsen JC, Walsh S, Dumez S, Metzger DA: A randomized and longitudinal study of human menopausal gonadotropin with intrauterine insemination in the treatment of infertility. *Obstet Gynecol* 1993, 82:780–786.

21. teVelde ER, van Kooy RJ, Waterreus JJH: Intrauterine insemination of washed husband's spermatozoa: a controlled study. *Fertil Steril* 1989, 51:182–185.

22. Zikopoulos K, West CP, Thong PW, *et al.*: Homologous intra-uterine insemination has no advantage over timed natural intercourse when used in combination with ovulation induction for the treatment of unexplained infertility. *Hum Reprod* 1993, 8:563–567.

23. Collins JA, Hughes EG: Pharmacological interventions for the induction of ovulation. *Drugs* 1995, 50:480–494.

Assisted Reproductive Techniques

Peter L. Chang and Mark V. Sauer

Since the successful introduction 20 years ago of *in vitro* fertilization (IVF) by Steptoe and Edwards [1] for the treatment of human infertility, an explosion of medical, reproductive, and technologic research has forever changed the face of reproductive medicine. Assisted reproduction was once considered experimental, rarely successful, and of limited clinical utility. Today it is readily available in most metropolitan areas throughout the world. The story of IVF is one of unparalleled rapid growth and development.

Tens of thousands of cases of successful IVF occur annually throughout the world as the number of women undertaking IVF continues to rise. Success rates have risen over time with refinements in ovulation-induction therapy, improvements in the surveillance of recruited and growing follicles by transvaginal ultrasound, advances in nonsurgical approaches for oocyte retrieval, improvement of embryo culture techniques, and embryo cryopreservation. Over 150,000 babies have been born throughout the world as a result of assisted reproductive technology. Further breakthroughs in treating patients with gonadal failure offer options for couples who in the past were advised to adopt. Micromanipulation for severe male gamete abnormalities and oocyte donation for women with hypergonadotropic hypogonadism has radically altered the approach to these types of individuals.

Assisted reproductive techniques are now being used to address the needs of patients seeking more than traditional "fertility" care. Applications include preimplantation diagnosis of genetic disorders, sex selection, gamete and embryo banking for sick and terminally ill patients, and asexual reproduction for female homosexual and HIV-discordant couples. These latter uses represent today's biggest controversies and present complex ethical challenges. The field of IVF has always drawn the fascination of the public. Reproductive medicine has been scrutinized, criticized, condemned, and heralded. Through it all, however, assisted reproduction has stood the test of time, and is largely accepted as a tenable method of treatment for infertility. The public's preoccupation with IVF will undoubtedly remain undeterred as long as issues of sexuality, family, religion, and medicine are so intricately entwined. This chapter reviews the significant advances in assisted reproduction and documents the evolution of a technique that has become an entire field of medicine.

𝒜DVANCES

ADVANCES IN IN VITRO FERTILIZATION

Ovulation induction
   Purified or synthetic menotropins
   GnRh agonists
Monitoring
   Rapid hormone assays
   Transvaginal ultrasound measurement of follicular size
Oocyte harvesting
   Transvaginal oocyte aspiration under ultrasound guidance
   Isolettes or mobile table laboratory
Fertilization
   ICSI (micromanipulation)
   Oil overlay microdrop culture system
Laboratory techniques
   Embryo selection
   Extended growth media
   Cryopreservation
   Preimplantation genetic diagnosis

FIGURE 13-1.

Advances in *in vitro* fertilization (IVF). Since the birth of Louise Brown resulting from IVF–embryo transfer in 1978 [1], several advances have been made in ovulation induction, monitoring, oocyte harvesting, fertilization, and laboratory techniques. GnRH—gonadotropin-releasing hormone; ICSI—intracytoplasmic sperm injection.

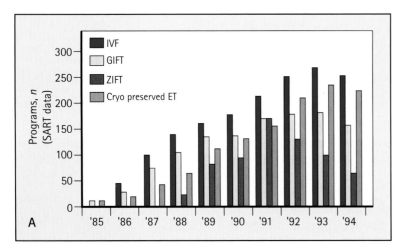

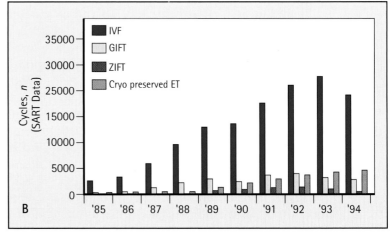

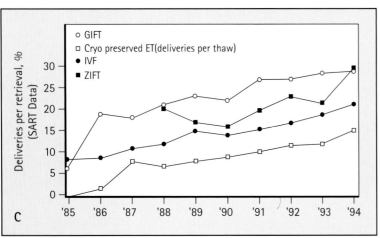

FIGURE 13-2.

Programs, cycles, and success rates of various assisted reproductive techniques. Since the first report of assisted reproductive technique activities prepared by the Society for Assisted Reproductive Technology (SART) and The American Society for Reproductive Medicine (ASRM) in 1985, the number of programs (**A**), the number of cycles (**B**), and the success of various assisted reproductive techniques (**C**) have increased considerably in the United States [2–10]. CryoET—cryopreserved embryo transfer; GIFT—gamete intrafallopian transfer; ZIFT—zygote intrafallopian transfer.

*S*UCCESS RATES AND PATIENT SCREENING

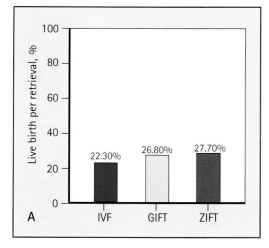

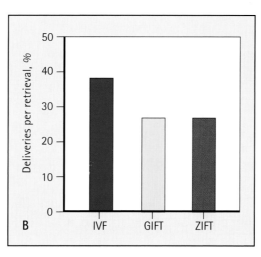

may account for the differences in success. These factors include patient age, diagnosis, length of infertility, male factor, and number of previous failed assisted reproductive technique attempts. **B**, In 1990, Tanbo *et al*. [12] randomly assigned 150 infertile patients with patent fallopian tubes to either *in vitro* fertilization (IVF), GIFT, or ZIFT. Patient characteristics (age, primary vs secondary infertility, length of infertility, and ovulatory status) and indications (unexplained, moderate male factor, and minimal endometriosis) for assisted reproductive techniques were similar in all three groups. Although there were no significant differences in pregnancy rates between the groups, the study had a power of only 24%. Studies with larger numbers are needed before concluding that there is no benefit of GIFT and ZIFT given that they involve greater costs, surgical intervention, and general anesthesia.

FIGURE 13-3.

Success rates of different types of ART. **A**, Traditionally, tubal transfers (gamete intrafallopian transfer [GIFT], and zygote intrafallopian transfer [ZIFT]) appear to have better success rates as seen in the latest Centers for Disease Control and Prevention (CDC) data 1995 [11].However, these rates are not derived from randomized groups of patients; therefore, they do not take into account the patient and diagnostic factors that

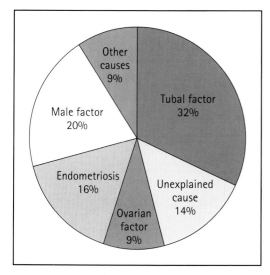

FIGURE 13-4.

Primary diagnoses for US and Canadian women undergoing assisted reproductive techniques as reported by the Centers for Disease Control and Prevention in 1995. Although essentially unchanged, these indications, since then, have extended to include others, *eg*, premature ovarian failure, postmenopausal women, homosexual couples, and postradiation and postchemotherapy cancer patients [11].

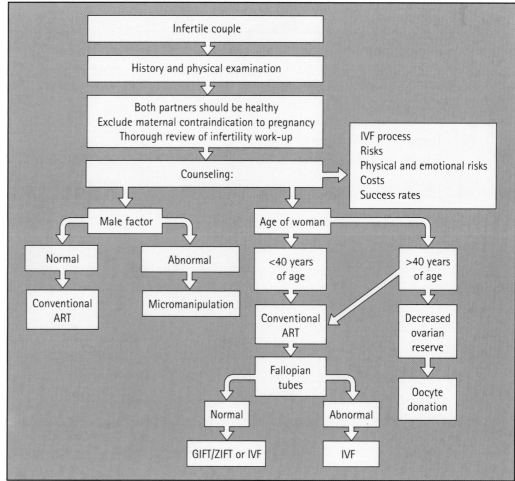

FIGURE 13-5.

Patient screening and selection process. Screening and selection are important components of the assisted reproductive technique process. Because success rates vary with different treatment options, the goal is to determine the appropriate treatment regimen to each particular couple's needs. GIFT—gamete intrafallopian transfer; IVF—*in vitro* fertilization; ZIFT—zygote intrafallopian transfer.

FACTORS ASSOCIATED WITH POOR ASSISTED REPRODUCTIVE TECHNIQUE OUTCOME

Increased maternal age

Presence of male factor

Elevated cycle day 3 FSH >15 mIU/mL or estradiol >75 pg/mL

Presence of hydrosalpinges

Severe endometriosis

Previous failed assisted reproductive technique cycles

FIGURE 13-6.

Factors associated with poor assisted reproductive technique outcome. FSH—follicle-stimulating hormone.

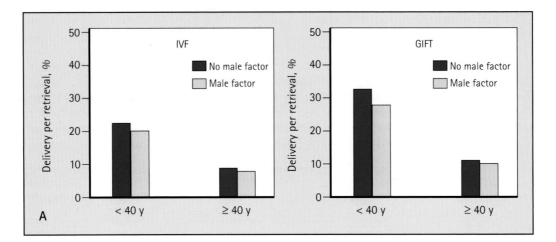

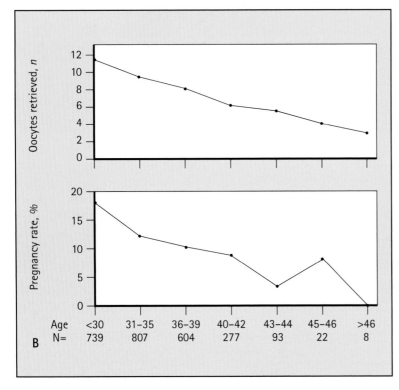

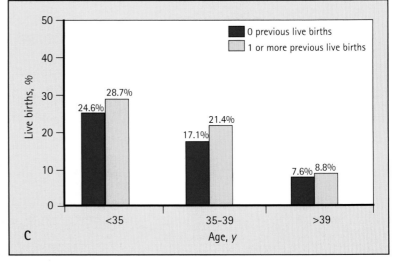

FIGURE 13-7.

Influences on success rates. **A**, Effects of female age and male factor. The dominant negative effects of maternal age on oocyte production and male factor on assisted reproductive technique (ART) success rate has long been known [10,13]. **B**, Effects of female age on *in vitro* fertilization (IVF) as reported in the 1990 Israel National Survey (*n*=2500). Note that no delivery was reported in women over 46 years of age (*n* = 8). **C**, ART live birth rates by female age and number of previous live births. (Fresh nondonor oocytes) These most recent Centers for Disease Control and Prevention (CDC) data also show a dramatic fall in live birth rates after age 39. However, ART was more likely to succeed in women of all age groups who had had a previous live birth [11].

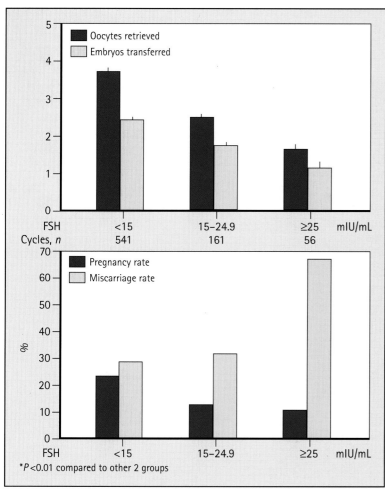

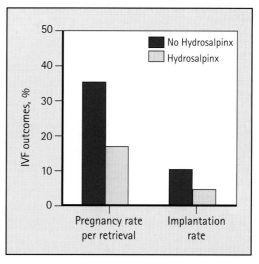

FIGURE 13-9.

Aggregate data on the effect of hydrosalpinx on *in vitro* fertilization (IVF) outcome. Although there are no randomized studies, evidence from retrospective case-control studies show a strong negative effect of hydrosalpinges on IVF outcomes such as pregnancy rate per transfer and implantation rate [15]. Although speculative, the cause may be impaired receptivity of the endometrium or detrimental effects on the developing embryo from the toxic fluid.

FIGURE 13-8.

Negative effect of elevated cycle day 3 follicle-stimulating hormone (FSH) on *in vitro* fertilization outcome [14]. All three groups had similar mean age, ampules of gonadotropin, and duration of stimulation

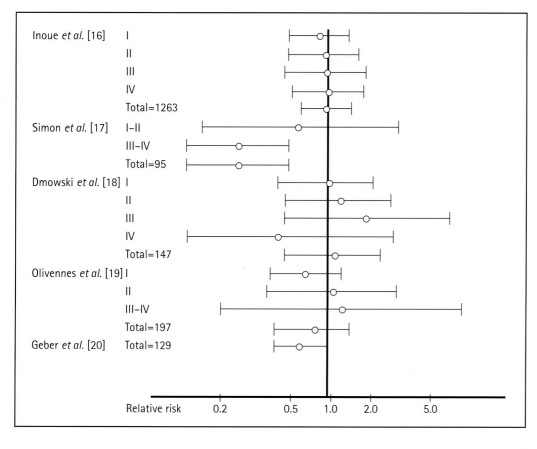

FIGURE 13-10.

The impact of endometriosis on *in vitro* fertilization (IVF)–embryo transfer outcome. Some controlled studies of patients with endometriosis treated with IVF-ET showed that severe disease (stage III and IV) is associated with poor outcome [16–20].

STEPS IN ART

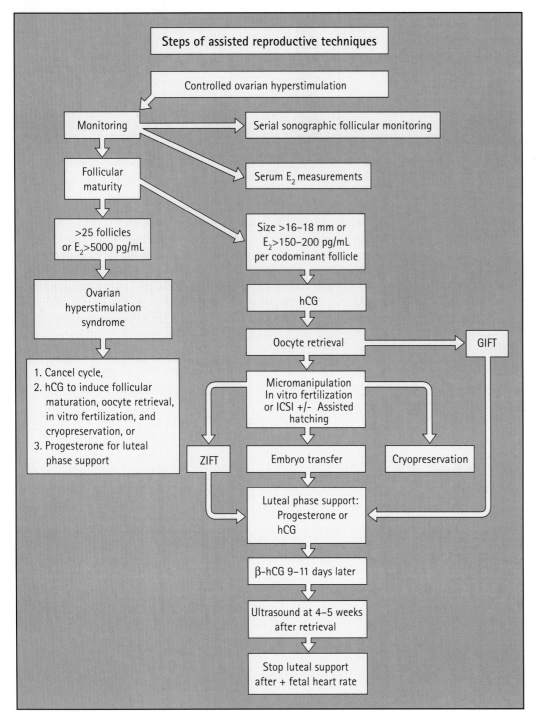

FIGURE 13-11.
Steps of assisted reproductive techniques. hCG—human chorionic gonadotropin; GIFT—gamete intrafallopian transfer; ICSI—intracytoplasmic sperm injection.

FIGURE 13-12.
Various gonadotropin preparations now available for controlled ovarian hyperstimulation: FSH—follicle-stimulating hormone; IM—intramuscular; LH—luteinizing hormone; SQ—subcutaneous.

VARIOUS GONADOTROPIN PREPARATIONS NOW AVAILABLE FOR CONTROLLED OVARIAN HYPERSTIMULATION

Gonadotropin	Route	FSH, IU	LU, IU
Menotropin	IM	75	75
Purified FSH	IM	75	<1
Recombinant FSH	SQ	75	0

DOSE, ROUTE OF ADMINISTRATION, POTENCY, AND STRUCTURE OF GONADOTROPIN-RELEASING HORMONE AGONISTS AVAILABLE WORLDWIDE

Agonist	Structure	Route	Dose, mg	Potency (GnRH=1)
Leuprorelin	D-Leu, Pro-NHEt	SQ	0.5–1.0	15–100
		IM, depot	3.75–7.5 monthly	
Buserelin	D-Ser(Bu), Pro-NHEt	SQ	0.2	100
		IN	0.9–1.2	
Histrelin	D-His(BZ), Pro-NHEt	SQ	0.1	100
Nafarelin	D-[Na(2)]	IN	0.4–0.8	200
Triptorelin	D-Trp	IN, polymer	2–4 monthly	100
Goserelin	D-Ser(tBu).aza-Gly	SQ, implant	3.6 monthly	230

FIGURE 13-13.
Dose, route of administration, potency, and structure of gonadotropin-releasing hormone agonists (GnRH-a) available worldwide [21]. Continuous high-dose GnRH infusion induces a biphasic response in pituitary gonadotropin release. Luteinizing hormone (LH) and follicle-stimulating hormone (FSH) levels increase initially followed by a progressive and sustained decline. GnRH–agonists, introduced in the late 1980s, allowed downregulation of the pituitary to prevent premature ovulation, which resulted in 15% to 30% of assisted reproductive technique cycle cancellations. IM—intramuscular; IN—intranasal; SQ—subcutaneous.

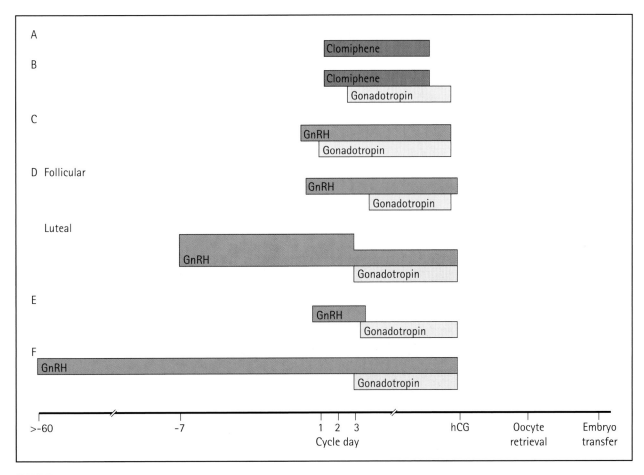

FIGURE 13-14.

Various stimulation protocols for *in vitro* fertilization (IVF) using gonadotropin-releasing hormone (GnRH) agonists and gonadotropin. A.) Clomiphene citrate. The use of clomiphene citrate as single agent for assisted reproductive techniques (ARTs) is now infrequent because of the low number of oocytes recovered (one to three oocytes per cycle) as well as high cancellation rate (25% to 50%) secondary to premature luteinizing hormone (LH) surges.

B.) The combination of clomiphene citrate with gonadotropins can be used either concurrently or sequentially.

C.) Flare or short protocol. The advantage of this protocol is a lower human menopausal gonadotropin (hMG) requirement and shorter duration of stimulation.

D.) Long protocol. The pituitary and ovaries are suppressed before starting hMG. Follicular phase downregulation has the advantage that it does not require confirmation of the luteal phase and is preferable in oligo-ovulatory patients. The luteal regimen produces a faster and more consistent ovarian suppression with fewer residual cysts.

E.) Ultrashort protocol: further reduction in cost.

F.) Ultralong protocol: for use in women with endometriosis undergoing IVF–embryo transfer.

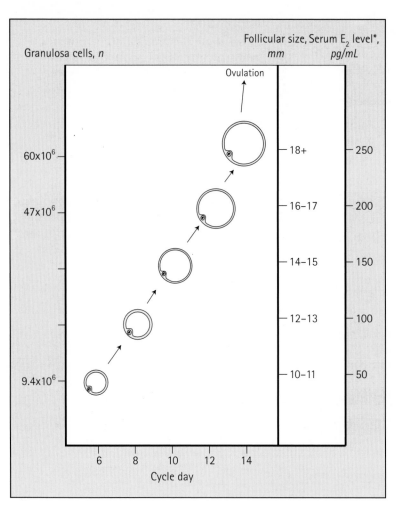

FIGURE 13-15.

Rates of follicular growth in the human ovary. Most programs use a combination of sonographic measurement of ovarian follicles and serum levels of estradiol in order to determine follicular development. Once the goal of stimulation is achieved, a single intramuscular injection of human chorionic gonadotropin (5,000 to 10,000 IU) is given to induce the final follicular maturation. *Asterisk* indicates approximate contribution of E_z per follicle size with hMGr only stimulated cycles

$\mathcal{O}$OCYTE RETRIEVAL, EVALUATION, AND FERTILIZATION

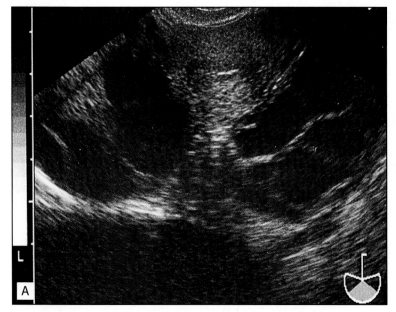 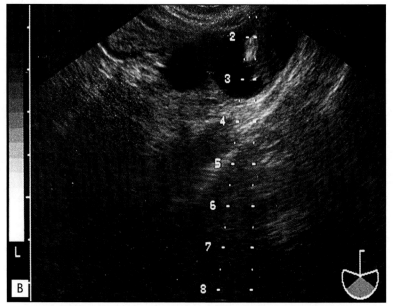

FIGURE 13-16.

Oocyte retrieval. Oocyte retrieval is usually performed approximately 34 to 36 hours after human chorionic gonadotropin injection. Most programs use the transvaginal route under ultrasound guidance. For analgesia, intravenous conscious sedation is adequate. Using a sterile needle guide attached to the vaginal ultrasound transducer and a needle path on the monitor screen, a 16- to 17-gauge needle is advanced through the vagina and the abdominal cavity into the ovary. Although a single puncture of each ovary would allow sequential aspiration of all the follicles, two or more punctures may be necessary. **A**, A stimulated ovary with needle path delineating the puncture site on the ultrasound monitor screen. **B**, An actual aspiration of a follicle with the bevel of the needle in between the 2- and 3-cm mark.

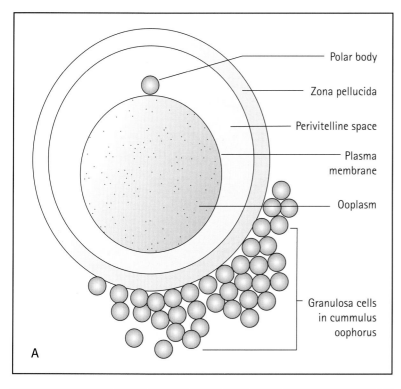

A

- Polar body
- Zona pellucida
- Perivitelline space
- Plasma membrane
- Ooplasm
- Granulosa cells in cummulus oophorus

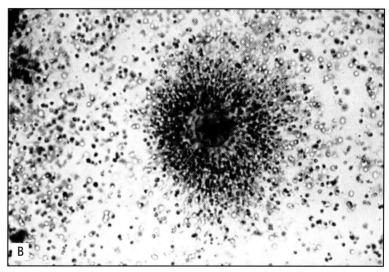

B

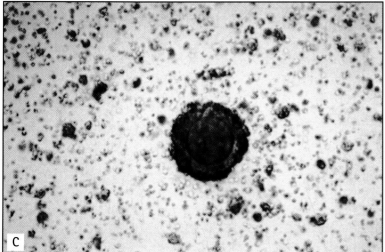

C

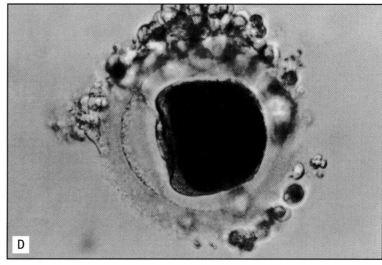

D

FIGURE 13-17.

Oocyte evaluation. At the time of retrieval, oocytes are evaluated under a light microscope and graded in order to ensure proper timing of insemination [22,23]. **A,** Structure of human oocyte. **B,** Mature oocyte with an expanded and luteinized cumulus matrix and a radiant corona radiata. **C,** Immature oocyte with a less or absent expanded cumulus or corona radiata. **D,** Postmature or atretic oocyte. Note the presence of dark and irregular ooplasm. **E,** Metaphase I: no first polar body; no germinal vesicle.

(Continued on next page)

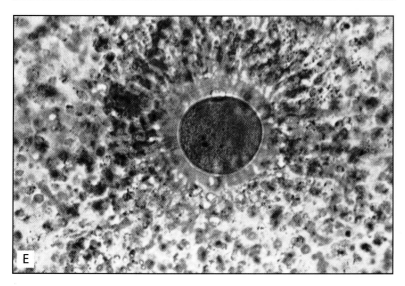

E

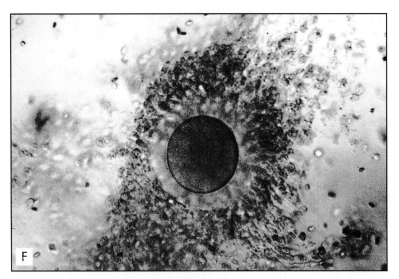

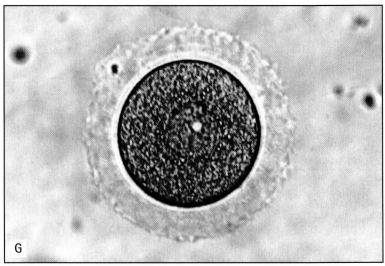

FIGURE 13-17. (*Continued*)
F, Metaphase II: first polar body present; no germinal vesicle.

G, Prophase I: germinal vesicle present. (*Panels B–G from* Veeck [22]; with permission.)

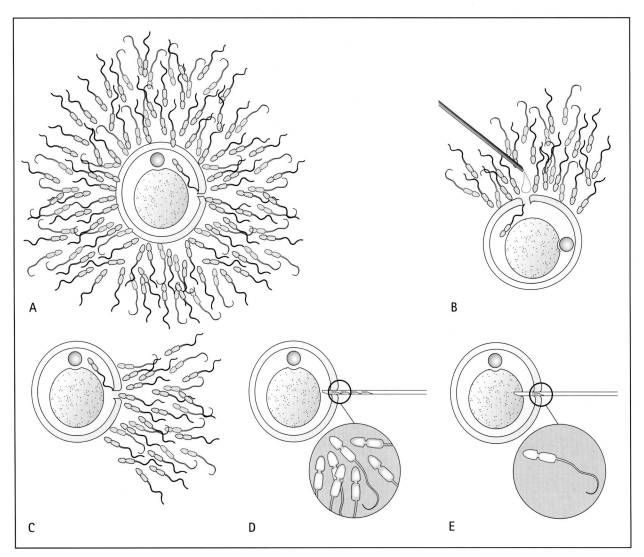

FIGURE 13-18.

Fertilization of the oocyte. Once the oocyte is deemed ready for insemination, several options are available depending on the presence of a male factor. The sperm is prepared appropriately for the procedure of choice. Note for comparison: intercourse involves 10 to 10,000 sperms. **A**, Conventional *in vitro* fertilization (IVF). The oocyte receives 50,000 to 5,000,000 washed sperm per milliliter per oocyte (if no male factor).

B, Zona drilling. The oocyte is chemically opened with acidified Tyrode's solution. **C**, Partial zona dissection. The oocyte received 5000 to 100,000 capacitated and acrosome-reacted sperms per milliliter; opened with mechanical force. **D**, Subzonal sperm insertion with one to 15 sperms introduced into the perivitelline space. **E**, Intracytoplasmic sperm injection with one sperm.

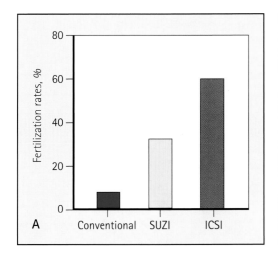

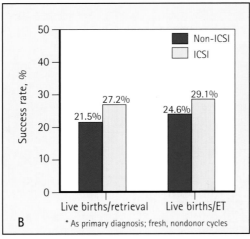

FIGURE 13-19.
Successful fertilization rates among couples with male factor infertility. **A**, Improved fertilization rates after micromanipulation in severe male factor infertility. Micromanipulation techniques for couples with severe male factor have improved considerably the fertilization rates [24,25]. **B**, Success rates for assisted reproductive technique (ART) procedures among couples with male factor infertility. In 1995, approximately 11% of ART procedures used intracytoplasmic sperm injection (ICSI) with higher success rates among couples with male factor infertility [11]. CDC—Centers for Disease Control and Prevention; ET—embryo transfer; ICSI—intracytoplasmic sperm injection; SUZI—subzonal sperm insertion.

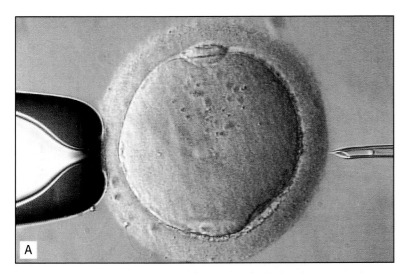

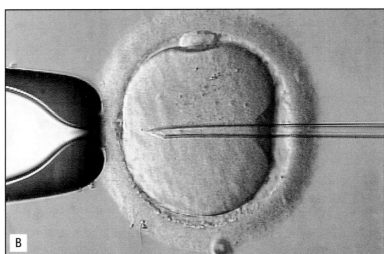

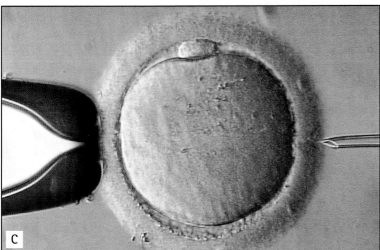

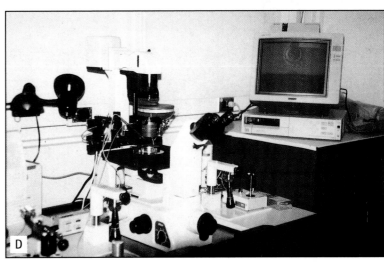

FIGURE 13-20.

Intracytoplasmic sperm injection. Oocytes are first prepared by a combination of mechanical and chemical (hyaluronidase) processes to remove the corona-cumulus complex. This removal allows visualization of the polar body and direct manipulation of the oocyte. The technique involves several steps. **A**, Immobilization of oocyte and correct placement of microinjection pipette with the sperm at a 90° angle from the polar body. **B**, Insertion of microinjection pipette into the oolemma and aspiration of the ooplasm followed by injection of sperm. **C** The microinjection pipette is then withdrawn with the sperm visualized in the oolemma. **D**, Inverted microscope with micromanipulators for intracytoplasmic sperm injection.

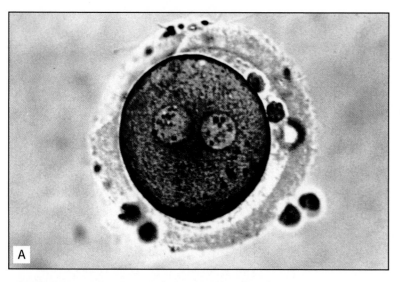

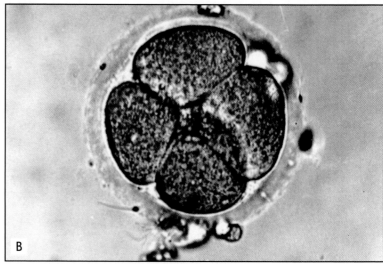

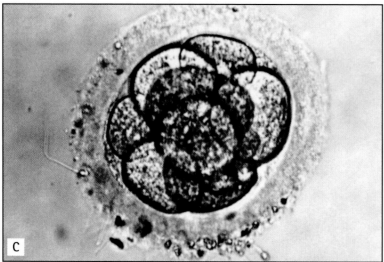

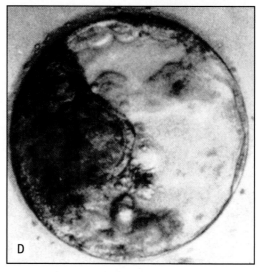

FIGURE 13–21.

Normal development of embryo *in vitro* [22,23]. **A**, Day 1 normal two pronucleus embryo. **B**, Day 2 normal four-cell embryo. **C**, Day 3 normal eight-cell embryo. Note the sperm imbedded in the zona pellucida. **D**, Day 5 normal blastocyst. **E**, Hatching blastocyst (≥ 24 hours after blastocyst formation). (*From* Veeck [23]; with permission.)

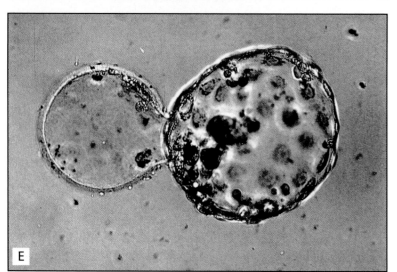

EMBRYO TRANSFER AND CRYOPRESERVATION

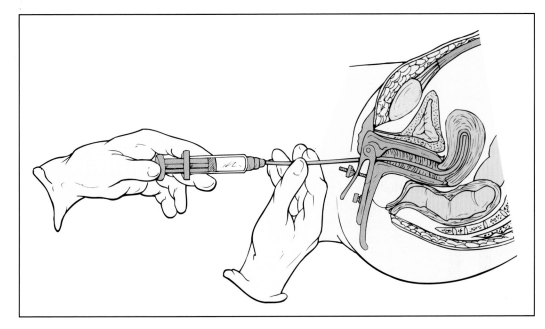

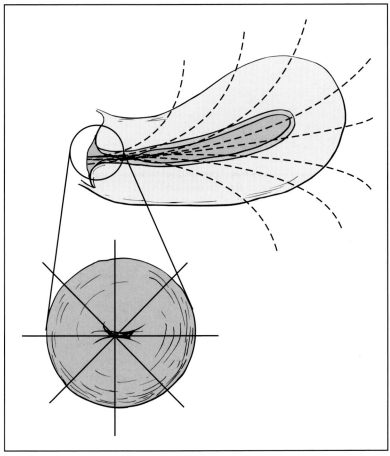

FIGURE 13-22.
Embryo transfer. **A**, Embryos in 10 to 50 μL of media are placed through the catheter at 0.5 cm from the upper fundus. The catheter is then checked for absence of embryos. **B**, A mock transfer is usually done prior to embryo transfer for measurements of the length and direction of the uterine cavity as well as for the selection of the most suitable catheter. Although embryos transferred at any stage have resulted in pregnancy, they are often transferred at four-cell through blastocyst stage (approximately 48 to 80 hours after retrieval).

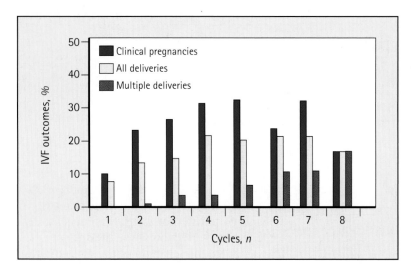

FIGURE 13-23.

The relationship between the number of fresh embryos replaced during *in vitro* fertilization (IVF) and selected outcome [5]. Maximum delivery rates occur when four to five embryos are transferred, but at the cost of a triple increase in multiple gestation rates. Therefore, there is no clear advantage in transferring more than four to five embryos. Clinical pregnancy rates are expressed as a percentage of embryo transfer (ET) cycles, all (live) delivery rates are expressed as a percentage of ET cycles, and multiple delivery rates are expressed as a percentage of ET cycles.

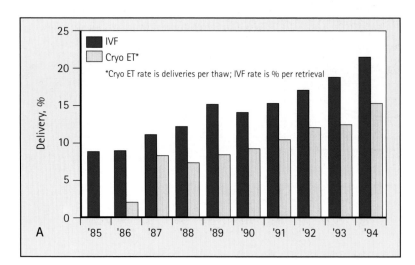

FIGURE 13-24.

Success of fresh embryo transfer (ET) versus cryogenic ET in the United States. Extra embryos can be cryopreserved at the two-pronuclei through the blastocyst stage and stored in cryostraws in liquid nitrogen storage tanks attached to an alarm system. Although rates vary with embryo stage, approximately two thirds of embryos survive the freeze–thaw process. **A,** Despite a lower pregnancy rate compared with fresh embryos [2–10], the transfer of cryopreserved embryos adds significantly to the success of an assisted reproductive technique cycle and lowers the costs considerably. **B,** The cryopreservation process.

B. CRYOPRESERVATION OF PRE-EMBRYOS AT THE PRONUCLEAR–TO EIGHT-CELL STAGE (24–50 HOURS POSTRETRIEVAL)

Equipment

Planar biomedical freezing unit

Liquid N_2 tank

Liquid N_2 storage refrigerator

Dissecting microscope

4-well Nunc dish, sterile

Pulled Pasteur micropipet, sterile

Freezing straws

0.22 μm filter and syringe

Media and Reagents

Freezing medium: phosphate-buffered saline + 10% sterile saline soak

1.5 M propanediol: 8.85 mL freezing medium + 1.15 mL propanediol

1.0 M propanediol: 1 mL freezing medium + 2 mL of 1.5 M propanediol

0.5 M propanediol: 1 mL freezing medium + 1 mL of 1.0 M propanediol

0.2 M sucrose/propanediol: 0.342 g sucrose + 5 mL of 1.5 M propanediol

Procedure

1. Sterile filter solutions with 0.22-μm filter attached to 10-mL syringe, in the following order. 0.5M, 1.0M, 1.5M, and 0.2M sucrose

2. Place 1 mL of freezing medium in an organ culture dish and warm to 37°C.

3. Place each of the solutions in one well of the Nunc dish, using 1 mL of solution per well.

4. Place the pre-embryos in the organ culture dish and allow to cool slowly to room temperature (6 min).

5. Place the pre-embryos in increasing propanediol solutions at room temperature as follows: 0.5M for 5 min, 1.0M for 5 min, 1.5M for 10 min.

6. Place pre-embryos in 1.5 M propanediol + 0.2 M sucrose for 5 min.

7. During this 5 min, load the embryos into straws, seal and label.

8. Cool from room temperature to -7° C at 2°C/min.

9. Hold at -7°C for 5 min, seed the straw manually during the 5 min, and check that seeding has occurred.

10. Cool at 0.3°C/min to -30°C.

11. Cool rapidly to -140°C and place in liquid N_2 for storage.

COMPLICATIONS OF ART

FIGURE 13-25.
Complications of assisted reproductive techniques.

COMPLICATIONS OF ASSISTED REPRODUCTIVE TECHNIQUES

Ovarian hyperstimulation syndrome: a risk if the ovaries are hyperstimulated (>25 follicles) or the estradiol level is higher than 5000 pg/mL; *this risk can be reduced* by lowering the gonadotropin dose, using progesterone instead of hCG injections for luteal support, canceling the cycle, and avoiding hCG administration

Possible ovarian neoplasm association with use of fertility drugs [26,27]

Multiple gestations: approximately 37% of births resulting from ART [11], whereas 2% of such births occur in the general population

Adverse outcome of pregnancy (22% of clinical pregnancies) [11]; ectopic pregnancy, spontaneous abortion, induced abortion, or stillbirth

Bleeding: rare; includes vaginal blood loss and intraperitoneal bleeding resulting from inadvertent laceration of vessels with the retrieval needle [28,29]

Bowel or ureteral injury with the aspiration needle

Infection: although tubo-ovarian abscess formation has been reported following transvaginal oocyte aspiration [28,29] and transcervical embryo transfer [30], infection is now rare with the use of prophylactic antibiotics

Anesthetic complications: resulting from conscious intravenous sedation; includes drug reaction, apnea, cardiac arrest, and need for intubation

OOCYTE DONATION AND ALTERNATIVE USES FOR ART

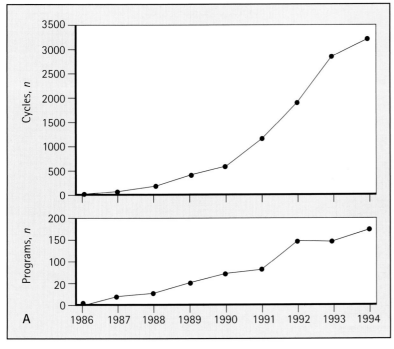

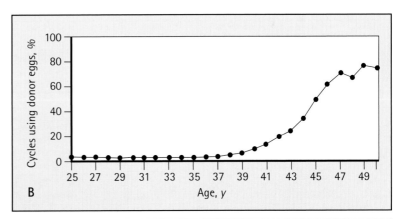

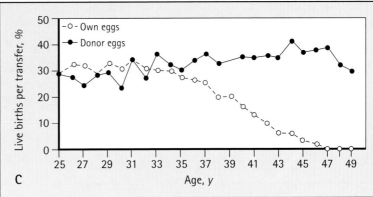

FIGURE 13-26.

The extent of the growth of oocyte donation cycles and programs in the United States [2–10]. **A**, A review of the clinic-specific data submitted to the Society for Assisted Reproductive Technology (SART) and The American Society for Reproductive Medicine (ASRM). These data may be a reflection of the increasing number of women who delay their childbearing for later years. **B**, The 1995 Centers of Disease Control data [11]. As women age, they are more likely to undergo oocyte donation. **C**, The efficacy of oocyte donation in women of advanced reproductive age remains around 40%.

GENERAL GUIDELINES FOR GAMETE DONATION ENDORSED BY THE AMERICAN SOCIETY FOR REPRODUCTIVE MEDICINE [31]

Indications
    Premature ovarian failure or gonadal dysgenesis
    Avoidance of genetic disease transmission
    Declining or absent ovarian function
    Persistent poor oocyte quality during assisted reproductive procedures
Donor selection (anonymous or known)
    Legal age
    Previous fertility desirable but not required
    Conforms with genetic screening for gamete donors
Donor screening
    Disqualify individuals at risk for HIV
    Serologic tests for syphilis, hepatitis B and C, and HIV I, II
    Match Rh-compatible couples
    Medically and psychologically
Donor payment
    Compensation for direct and indirect expenses
    Agreements executed prior to initiation of cycle
    Payments not to be excessive
    Payments not predicated on the number of oocytes obtained
Recipient age
    If over 40 years of age, thorough medical screening is required
    Treatment through the age of natural reproductive life span (50 years)

FIGURE 13-27.

General guidelines for gamete donation endorsed by The American Society for Reproductive Medicine [31].

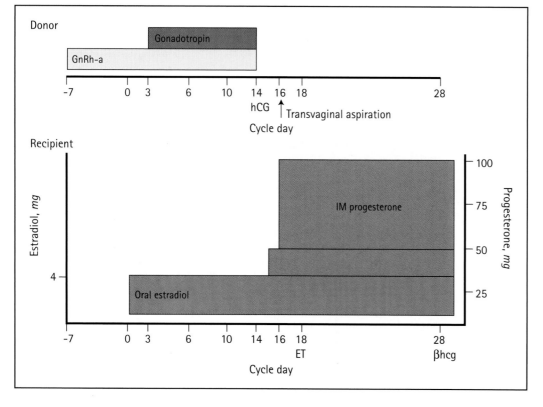

FIGURE 13-28.

Protocol for synchronizing oocyte donors and recipients. βhcg—serum levels; GnRH-a— gonadotropin-releasing hormone agonist; hCG—human chorionic gonadotropin; IM—intramuscular.

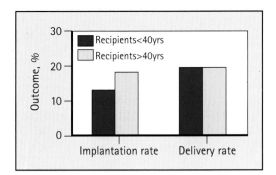

FIGURE 13-29.

Oocytes from young age donors into younger versus older recipients. The procreative capacity in women of advanced reproductive age is independent of uterine age, as demonstrated elegantly by Navot *et al.* [32]. Evenly distributed same-cohort oocytes from young donors (mean age, 30.2 years) to younger and older recipients (mean ages, 35.8 and 44.0 years, respectively) revealed no significant differences in implantation or delivery rates. The number of oocytes received, number of embryos transferred, and number of favorable embryos were similar between groups.

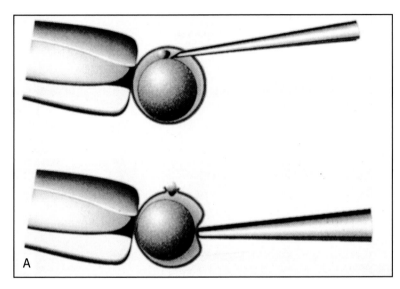

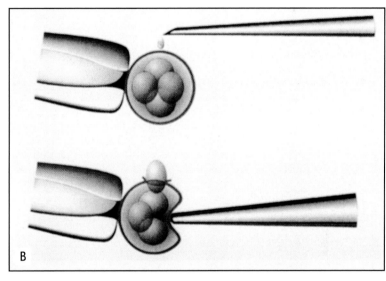

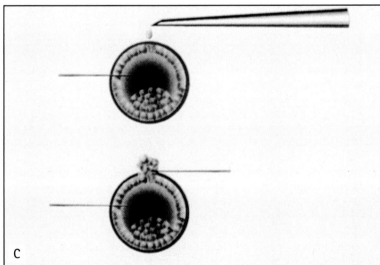

FIGURE 13-30.

Preimplantation genetic diagnosis. Preimplantation genetic diagnosis can now be accomplished successfully with polar body or embryo biopsy followed by DNA amplification using the polymerase chain reaction. **A**, Polar biopsy from a preovulatory oocyte. A beveled micropipette is inserted at 12 o'clock through the zona and the polar body is aspirated. Conversely, the polar body can also be extruded through a single slit in the zona made over the polar body. **B**, Biopsy of blastomeres at four- to eight-cell stage can be accomplished using several described techniques. Shown is the "push" variation of the extrusion technique, in which a slit is made at 12 o'clock with acid Tyrode's solution and the blastomere is extruded by pushing at the zona. The optimal stage for biopsy appears to be eight-cell stage, when one to three blastomeres can be safely removed for genetic studies. **C**, Trophectoderm biopsy at the blastocyst stage allows for removal of 10 to 30 cells for genetic studies without developmental impairment [33].

FIGURE 13-31.

Alternative uses for assisted reproduction techniques beyond conventional fertility treatment. ICSI—intracytoplasmic sperm injection; IVF—*in vitro* fertilization.

ALTERNATIVE USES FOR ASSISTED REPRODUCTIVE TECHNIQUES BEYOND CONVENTIONAL FERTILITY TREATMENT

Radiation or chemtherapy cancer patients: gamete or embryo harvest and cryopreservation prior to treatment

Homosexual female couples: asexual reproduction with use of sperm donor

Human immune-deficient virus discordant couples in whom the male partner is infected and the female is not: minimizing disease transmission with IVF-ICSI

Posthumous reproduction: posthumous retrieval of sperm for IVF-ICSI or use of frozen eggs or embryos in established surrogate

Embryo banking: surplus cryopreserved embryos for preimplantation adoption

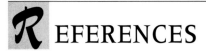

REFERENCES

1. Steptoe P, Edwards R: Birth after reimplantation of a human embryo. *Lancet* 1978, 2:366.

2. Medical Research International and the American Fertility Society Special Interest Group: In vitro fertilization/embryo transfer in the United States: 1985 and 1986 results from the National IVF/ET registry. *Fertil Steril* 1988, 49:212–215.

3. Medical Research International, the Society of Assisted Reproductive Technology, and the American Fertility Society: In vitro fertilization/embryo transfer in the United States: 1987 results from the National IVF/ET registry. *Fertil Steril* 1989, 51:13–19.

4. Medical Research International, the Society of Assisted Reproductive Technology, and the American Fertility Society: In vitro fertilization-embryo transfer in the United States: 1988 results from the IVF-ET registry. *Fertil Steril* 1990, 53:13–20.

5. Medical Research International, the Society of Assisted Reproductive Technology, and the American Fertility Society: In vitro fertilization-embryo transfer (IVF-ET) in the United States: 1989 results from the IVF-ET registry. *Fertil Steril* 1991, 55:14–23.

6. Medical Research International, the Society of Assisted Reproductive Technology (SART), and the American Fertility Society: In vitro fertilization-embryo transfer (IVF-ET) in the United States: 1990 results from the IVF-ET registry. *Fertil Steril* 1992, 57:15–24.

7. Society of Assisted Reproductive Technology and the American Fertility Society: Assisted reproductive technology in the United States and Canada: 1991 results from the Society for Assisted Reproductive Technology generated from The American Fertility Society Registry. *Fertil Steril* 1993, 59:956–962.

8. The American Fertility Society and the Society of Assisted Reproductive Technology: Assisted reproductive technology in the United States and Canada: 1992 results from The American Fertility Society/Society for Assisted Reproductive Technology Registry. *Fertil Steril* 1994, 62:1121–1128.

9. Society of Assisted Reproductive Technology and the American Society for Reproductive Medicine: Assisted reproductive technology in the United States and Canada: 1993 results from the American Society for Reproductive Medicine /Society for Assisted Reproductive Technology Registry. *Fertil Steril* 1995, 64:13–21.

10. Society of Assisted Reproductive Technology and the American Society for Reproductive Medicine: Assisted reproductive technology in the United States and Canada: 1994 results from the American Society for Reproductive Medicine /Society for Assisted Reproductive Technology Registry. *Fertil Steril* 1996, 66:697–705.

11. 1995 Assisted Reproductive Technology Success Rates. Atlanta: US Department of Health and Human Services, Centers for Disease Control and Prevention, and National Center for Chronic Disease Prevention and Health Promotion; 1997.

12. Tanbo T, Dale PO, Abyholm T: Assisted fertilization in infertile women with patent fallopian tubes: a comparison of in-vitro fertilization, gamete intra-fallopian transfer and tubal embryo stage transfer. *Hum Reprod* 1990, 5:266–270.

13. Seidman D, Lotan Y: In vitro fertilization and embryo transfer in Israel:1990 results from a national survey. *J Assist Reprod Genet* 1994, 11:1–4.

14. Scott R, Toner JP, Muasher SJ, *et al.*: Follicle-stimulating hormone levels on cycle day 3 are predictive of in vitro fertilization outcome. *Fertil Steril* 1989, 51:651–654.

15. Katz E, Akman MA, Damewood MD, Garcia JE: Deleterious effect of the presence of hydrosalpinx on implantation and pregnancy rates with in vitro fertilization. *Fertil Steril* 1996, 66:122–125.

16. Inoue M, Kobayashi Y, Honda I, *et al.*: The impact of endometriosis on the reproductive outcome of infertile patients. *Am J Obstet Gynecol* 1992, 167:278–282.

17. Simon C, Gutierrez A, Vidal A, *et al.*: Outcome of patients with endometriosis in assisted reproduction: results from in-vitro fertilization and oocyte donation. *Hum Reprod* 1994, 9:725–729.

18. Dmowski W, Rana N, Michalowska J, *et al.*: The effect of endometriosis, its stage and activity, and of autoantibodies on in vitro fertilization and oocyte donation. *Hum Reprod* 1995, 9:725–729.

19. Olivennes F, Feldberg D, Liu HC, *et al.*: Endometriosis: a stage by stage analysis—the role of in vitro fertilization. *Fertil Steril* 1995, 64:392–398.

20. Geber S, Paraschos T, Atkinson G, Margara R, Winston RML: Results of IVF in patients with endometriosis: the severity of the disease does not affect outcome, or the incidence of miscarriage. *Hum Reprod* 1995, 10:1507–1511.

21. Dawood M: Impact of medical treatment of endometriosis on bone mass. *Am J Obstet Gynecol* 1993, 168:674–684.

22. Veeck L: *Atlas of the Human Oocyte and Early Conceptus*. Baltimore: Williams & Wilkins; 1986.

23. Veeck L: *Atlas of Human Oocyte and Early Conceptus*, vol 2. Baltimore: Williams & Wilkins; 1991.

24. Gordts S, Garcia G, Vercruyssen M, *et al.*: Subzonal insemination: a prospective randomized study in patients with abnormal sperm morphology. *Fertil Steril* 1993, 60:307–313.

25. Palermo G, Cohen J, Alikani M, *et al.*: Intracytoplasmic sperm injection: a novel treatment for all forms of male factor infertility. *Fertil Steril* 1995, 63:1231–1240.

26. Whittemore AS, Harris R, Itnyre J: Characteristics relating to ovarian cancer risk: collaborative analysis of 12 U.S. case-control studies. II. Invasive epithelial ovarian cancers in white women. Collaborative Ovarian Cancer Group. *Am J. Epithelial* 1992, 136:1184-1203.

27. Shushan A, Paltiel O, Iscovich J, *et al.*: Human menopausal gonadotropin and the risk of epithelial ovarian cancer. *Fertil Steril* 1996, 65:13–18.

28. Bennett S, Waterstone JJ, Cheng WC, Parsons J: Complications of transvaginal ultrasound-directed follicle aspiration: a review of 2670 consecutive procedures. *J Assist Reprod Genet* 1993, 10:72–77.

29. Dicker D, Ashkenazi J, Feldberg D, *et al.*: Severe abdominal complications after transvaginal ultrasonographically guided retrieval of oocytes for in vitro fertilization and embryo transfer. *Fertil Steril* 1993, 59:1313–1315.

30. Sauer M, Paulson RJ: Pelvic abscess complicating transcervical embryo transfer. *Am J Obstet Gynecol* 1992, 166:148–149.

31. The American Fertility Society: Guidelines for gamete donation: 1993. *Fertil Steril* 1993, 59:1S–9S.

32. Navot D, Drews MR, Bergh PA, *et al.*: Age related decline in female fertility is not due to diminished capacity of the uterus to sustain embryo implantation. *Fertil Steril* 1994, 61:97–101.

33. Carson SA, Buster JE: Biopsy of gametes and preimplantation embryos in genetic diagnosis. *Semin Reprod Endocrinol* 1994, 12:N3:184-195.

Endometriosis

Melvin H. Thornton, Sandra M. Bello,
and Robert Israel

Endometriosis is defined as the presence of endometrial tissue, glands, and stroma outside the uterine cavity. It is estimated that the prevalence of endometriosis in the general US population is about 7% to 10%. The pathogenesis and pathophysiology still remain an enigma. The incidence varies between the populations studied. In low-risk groups, such as women undergoing laparoscopic sterilization, a prevalence of 2% to 5% has been reported. Conversely, in high-risk groups such as infertility patients, the prevalence ranges between 30% and 50%. Evidence of a genetic or familial tendency of endometriosis has been described. A recent report showed that of patients with endometriosis, approximately 7% of all first-degree relatives were affected with the disease. A polygenic, multifactorial pattern of inheritance is most likely.

Retrograde menstruation has been the longest held theory regarding the cause of endometriosis. This widely accepted transplantation theory, originally proposed by Sampson [1], suggests that viable endometrial cells reflux through the fallopian tubes during menstruation and implant on surrounding pelvic structures. The anatomic distribution of endometriosis noted at laparoscopy is consistent with this pattern of development. However, there are other theories regarding the pathogenesis of endometriosis that have merit. Coelomic metaplasia and hematogenous or lymphatic spread may account for endo-

metriosis found in unusual and distant locations. It is likely that endometriosis is a multifactorial disorder that involves the interplay of different physiologic systems. Evidence is accumulating that implicates the immune system competency, or lack thereof, along with local peritoneal factors in the propagation of this disorder. The role of macrophages and their secretory products in the pathophysiology of this condition seems to be gaining support.

Prior to the advent of ambulatory endoscopy, the diagnosis of endometriosis was almost always associated with severe symptoms of pelvic pain, dysmenorrhea, dyspareunia, and nodular pelvic masses. Today, pelvic pain, infertility, or both are the most frequent conditions found when endometriosis is diagnosed. However, the pathophysiology explaining the association of endometriosis with pain and infertility remains poorly understood. The treatment of endometriosis is based on a combination of scientific observation and clinical experience. Our lack of fundamental knowledge regarding the biology and natural history of endometriosis prevents us from treating the condition in the most effective, specific manner.

Endometriosis should be considered a chronic disease that can have variable symptoms during an affected individual's lifetime. After the diagnosis of endometriosis is established, other factors, such as the stage of the disease, the age of the patient, and the symptoms, need to be considered in developing a treatment plan. In cases of moderate to severe endometriosis associated with infertility, surgery is indicated and improves the conception rate. When infertility is present along with milder degrees of endometriosis, various therapeutic options are available to achieve pregnancy, including expectant management, controlled ovarian hyperstimulation in combination with intrauterine insemination, and assisted reproductive technologies. When pain is the main problem, medical therapy with hormonal suppression becomes the treatment of choice. In women past their childbearing years with severe pelvic pain and significant endometriosis, hysterectomy can be performed with or without ovarian conservation. It is hoped that time will give more insight into the pathophysiology of endometriosis, thus leading to a more individualized, rational approach to the treatment of women with endometriosis.

𝒫ATHOGENESIS

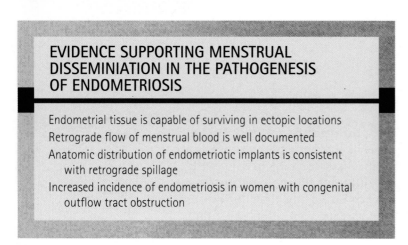

EVIDENCE SUPPORTING MENSTRUAL DISSEMINIATION IN THE PATHOGENESIS OF ENDOMETRIOSIS

Endometrial tissue is capable of surviving in ectopic locations

Retrograde flow of menstrual blood is well documented

Anatomic distribution of endometriotic implants is consistent with retrograde spillage

Increased incidence of endometriosis in women with congenital outflow tract obstruction

FIGURE 14–1.

Evidence supporting menstrual dissemination in the pathogenesis of endometriosis. In the mid-1920s, Sampson theorized that the retrograde flow of menstrual blood from the uterine cavity through the fallopian tubes could result in endometriosis. This theory remains a popular explanation for the initiation of endometriosis. The ability of endometriotic tissue to survive in an ectopic location, such as the peritoneal cavity, has been well documented. The presence of blood in the peritoneal fluid of all menstruating women, including those with endometriosis, is common. The increased incidence of endometriosis in women with menorrhagia and congenital or acquired outflow obstruction constitutes further evidence that retrograde dissemination could initiate or propagate the disease.

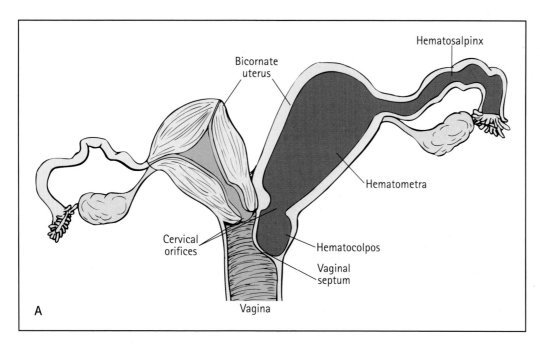

FIGURE 14–2.

Müllerian tract anomalies. **A**, Double uterus with unilateral, complete vaginal obstruction and ipsilateral renal agenesis.

(*Continued on next page*)

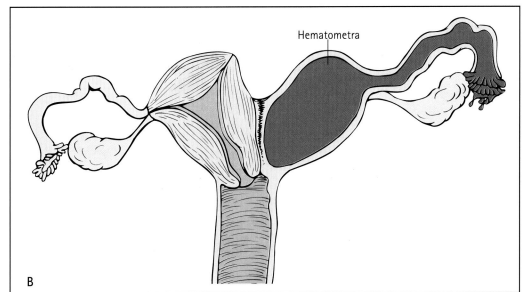

FIGURE 14-2. *(Continued)*
B, Double uterus with a noncommuni-
cating horn and hematometra. Women
with müllerian tract anomalies leading to
outflow tract obstruction have a twofold
greater incidence of endometriosis.
(*Adapted from* Thompson and Rock [2].)

SITES OF ENDOMETRIAL IMPLANTS

Most common
    Ovary
    60%–75% of patients
    Approximately 50% are bilateral
Common
    Peritoneum of posterior cul-de-sac
    Uterosacral ligaments, round ligaments, oviducts and mesosalpinx
    Peritoneum of uterus and leiomyomata
    Peritoneum of anterior cul-de-sac, rectosigmoid
Less common
    Cecum, appendix, bladder, vagina, small bowel, lymph nodes,
        omentum
Unusual
    Umbilicus, laparotomy, or episiotomy scars, inguinal canal,
        vulva, Gartner's duct, ureter
Rare
    Spinal canal, kidney, breast, pleura, lung bronchus, arm, hand,
        thigh, spleen, heart, bladder

FIGURE 14-3.
Sites of endometrial implants. The anatomic distribution of
endometrial implants lends further support to the theory of retrograde menstruation. Implants are most commonly found in the
dependent portions of the ovarian fossa or cul-de-sac.

ROLE OF THE IMMUNE SYSTEM IN ENDOMETRIOSIS

Autoantibodies against endometrium
Immunoglobulin G, IgA, complement component 3
    concentrations increase
Decreased reactivity to autologous endometrial antigens
Pelvic macrophage concentration and activity increased

FIGURE 14-4.
Role of the immune system in the pathogenesis of endometriosis.
Several investigations point toward some immune system role in
the pathogenesis of endometriosis. Amounts of T and B cells are
increased in the peritoneal fluid from women with endometriosis.
IgG and IgA autoantibodies against endometrial tissue have been
identified in the sera, peritoneal fluid, and cervical and vaginal
secretions of women with endometriosis. Alterations in cell-mediated immunity against autologous endometrial antigens have
been described in animals. In women with severe endometriosis,
cytotoxicity assays have demonstrated decreased target cell lysis
compared with control subjects.

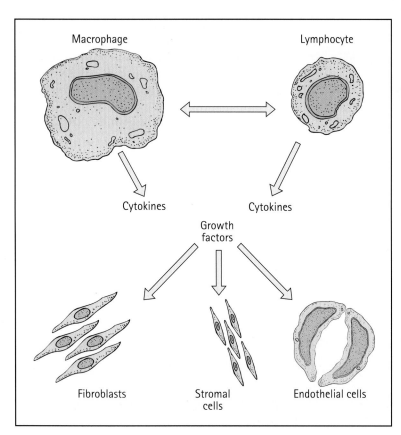

FIGURE 14–5.

Role of macrophage and lymphocyte mediators in endometriosis. In patients with endometriosis, peritoneal macrophages are increased both in numbers and activity. Macrophages are capable of secreting various substances such as growth factors, cytokines, prostanoids, and complement that may play a role in facilitating implantation and growth of endometrial cells.

THE ROLE OF CYTOKINES AND GROWTH FACTORS IN ENDOMETRIOSIS

Rantes (T-cell–specific) cytokine

    Chemoattractant for blood monocytes and T lymphocytes

    Stimulates macrophage activity

    Increase in moderate-to-severe endometriosis

IL-1

    Specific receptor antagonist (IL-1ra) absent in endometriotic implants (present in normal endometrium)

    IL-1 controls all inflammatory responses without opposition

FIGURE 14–6.

The role of cytokines and growth factors in the pathophysiology of endometriosis. These mediators are gaining increasing significance. One such cytokine, interleukin-1 (IL-1), is a mediator of the host inflammatory response. It induces prostaglandin synthesis, T-cell proliferation, and stimulation of B-lymphocyte immunoglobulin production. The increased level of these cytokines in the peritoneal fluid of patients with endometriosis suggests a role for these peptides in the pathophysiology of endometriosis. (*Data from* Khorram and coworkers [3] and Sahakian and coworkers [4].)

THE PATHOGENESIS OF ENDOMETRIOSIS

Transplantation–dissemination

    Direct extension

    Mechanical (oviducts, vascular, lymphatics)

    Iatrogenic

Coelomic metaplasia

Induction theory (combination of above)

FIGURE 14–7.

The pathogenesis of endometriosis. The literature is full of speculation and scientifically poorly supported theories. A multifactorial cause may be the reason for such a diversity of postulates. Some combination of mechanisms involving transplantation–dissemination and coelomic metaplasia probably exists. Endometrial cells and debris are transported outside the uterine cavity. An unknown host factor exists in women who will develop endometriosis. This host factor is stimulated by the transported endometrial tissue and results in the formation of endometriosis.

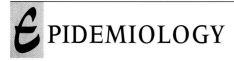# EPIDEMIOLOGY

GYNECOLOGIC HOSPITAL DISCHARGE DIAGNOSES IN THE UNITED STATES BETWEEN 1988 AND 1990

Diagnosis	Discharge, n(%)	Annual discharge rate per 10,000 women
Pelvic inflammatory disease	862,000 (17)	49.3
Ovarian cysts	571,600 (11.3)	32.7
Endometriosis	566,400 (11.2)	32.4
Menstrual disorders	549,000 (10.8)	31.4
Myomata uteri	531,200 (10.5)	30.4

FIGURE 14-8.

Gynecologic hospital discharge diagnoses in the United States between 1988 and 1990. The diagnosis of endometriosis can be made accurately only by direct visualization along with judicious histologic sampling; however, the true incidence of endometriosis is difficult to measure. Although it is estimated that the prevalence of endometriosis in the general US population is approximately 10%, the disease does comprise a large number of gynecologic hospital discharge diagnoses. (*Adapted from* Velebil *et al.* [5].)

FAMILIAL RISK OF ENDOMETRIOSIS

Endometriosis present	Cases, n/n(%)	Controls, n/n(%)	Odds ratio (95%)
In mothers (P > 0.05)	20/515 (3.9)	1/149 (0.7)	6.0 (1.0–35.8)
In sisters (P < 0.05)	25/523 (4.8)	1/169 (0.6)	8.4 (1.6–48.1)
First-degree relatives (P < 0.01)	45/1038 (4.3)	2/318 (0.6)	7.2 (2.1–24.5)

FIGURE 14-9.

Familial risk of endometriosis. Evidence of a genetic or familial tendency of endometriosis has been reported. Overall, about 7% of all first-degree relatives have been found to have endometriosis. The majority of these cases occur in families in whom the first-degree relative has had severe endometriosis. A polygenic, multifactorial pattern of inheritance is likely. (*Adapted from* Moen *et al.* [6].)

EPIDEMIOLOGY OF ENDOMETRIOSIS IN INFERTILE WOMEN

	Infertility with endometriosis, n(%)	Infertility without endometriosis, n(%)	Odds ratio (95% CI)	P value
Menarche ≤ 12 y	79 (45.4)	68 (39.3)	1.2 (0.8–2.0)	NS
Menses ≥ 8 d duration	3 (1.7)	5 (2.9)	0.6 (0.03–2.9)	NS
Cycles ≤ 27 d duration	46 (26.4)	29 (16.7)	1.8 (1.03–3.1)	0.03
High socioeconomic status	27 (15.5)	23 (13.2)	1.2 (0.6–2.3)	NS
Smoking	25 (14.4)	35 (20.1)	0.7 (0.4–1.2)	NS
Oral contraceptive use	43 (24.7)	35 (20.1)	1.3 (0.8–2.2)	NS
Intrauterine device	6 (3.4)	7 (4.0)	0.9 (0.2–2.9)	NS

FIGURE 14-10.

The epidemiology of endometriosis. An association between several menstrual characteristics and endometriosis has been demonstrated. There is an increased incidence of endometriosis in women with decreased cycle length (polymenorrhea). Endometriosis is less common in women who began smoking prior to age 17 and smoked greater than one pack per day. Women who exercise on a regular basis are less likely to have endometriosis. These findings are presumably secondary to decreased endogenous estrogen levels. (*Adapted from* Matorras *et al.* [7].)

DIAGNOSIS

DIAGNOSIS OF ENDOMETRIOSIS

History and physical examination

Pelvic examination

Pelvic ultrasound

Laparoscopy and biopsy of lesions for histologic examination

FIGURE 14–11.

Symptomatology of endometriosis. Although many women with endometriosis can be asymptomatic, symptomatology may provide the first hint toward the diagnosis of endometriosis. A constellation of symptoms, such as dysmenorrhea and dyspareunia with or without infertility, is not an uncommon finding. The finding of uterosacral nodularity or a palpable adnexal mass on bimanual examination further supports the diagnosis. Ultrasonography is a useful diagnostic modality in the presence of an ovarian mass. Computed tomographic scan and magnetic resonance imaging have a limited, if any, place in the diagnosis of endometriosis.

FIGURE 14–12.

Concentrations of CA-125, a cell-surface antigen, in 146 patients undergoing diagnostic laparoscopy or laparotomy. CA-125 has emerged as a possible noninvasive means of following therapeutic response. Because many other common conditions such as infectious or cancerous lesions are associated with elevated levels of CA-125, it cannot be used as a diagnostic marker; however, it is more likely to be elevated in severe endometriosis. Additionally, it is hoped that, in the future, another cell-surface antigen will be identified that will be diagnostic of endometriosis only. Normal controls were patients with visually normal pelvic organs at the time of diagnostic laparoscopy. *Closed circles* indicate point estimates. *T bars* indicate 95% CI. PID—pelvic inflammatory disease. *(Adapted from Barbieri et al. [8].)*

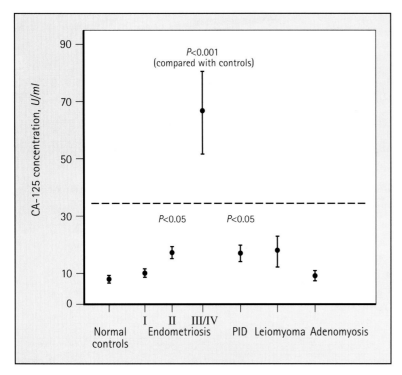

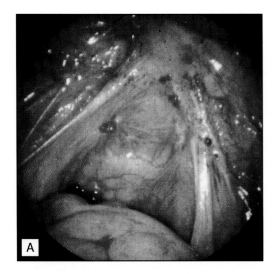

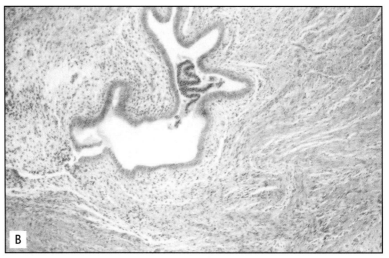

FIGURE 14–13.
Diagnosis of endometriosis. The gold standard for the diagnosis is to first visually identify endometriosis implants by laparoscopy (**A**) and then confirm the diagnosis by histologic findings (**B**) of endometrial glands and stroma outside the uterine cavity.

THE MOST COMMON LESIONS OBSERVED IN WOMEN WITH HISTOLOGICALLY CONFIRMED ENDOMETRIOSIS

Type of lesion	Incidence, %
Adhesions	91
Scarred white lesions	59
Peritoneal pockets	47
Scarred black lesions	46
Clear vesicles	30
Polypoid red lesions	26
White vesicles	25
Brown vesicles	24
Raised or flat red lesions	24
Fibrotic brown lesions	16
Black vesicles	7

FIGURE 14-14.

The most common lesions observed in women with histologically confirmed endometriosis. The morphologic appearance of endometriotic implants varies greatly and can be confused with other nonendometriotic lesions. The spectrum ranges from the classic nodular implant, varying in color from white to blue, brown, black, or red, to vesicular implants, which also have varied colors. Nonpigmented lesions have also been described. The different morphologic appearances of these lesions may represent different stages of the disease process. A significant association between deep, infiltrating lesions and pelvic pain has been demonstrated [12]. If any question exists, laparoscopic biopsy should be used liberally.

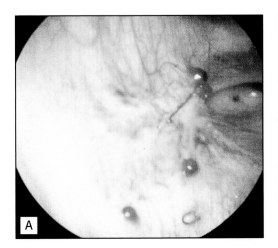
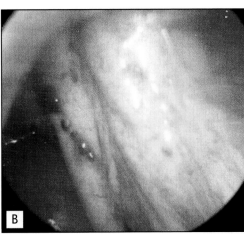

FIGURE 14-15.

Diagnostic laparoscopy. Diagnostic laparoscopy provides an excellent means to both diagnose and treat endometriosis. The visualization and search for both pigmented (**A**) and nonpigmented (**B**) lesions should be performed in a systematic manner using magnification provided by "near contact" laparoscopy.

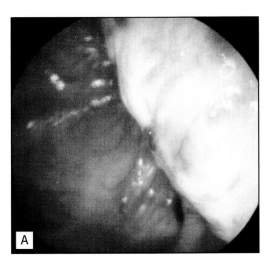
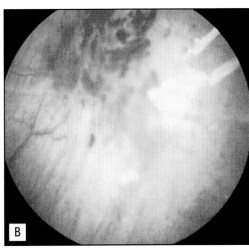
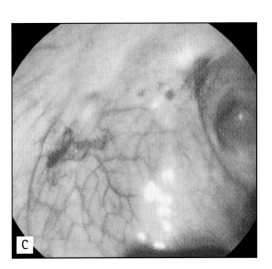

FIGURE 14-16.

Various lesions in endometriosis. **A**, Adhesions from the ovarian fossa to an implant on the surface of the ovary. **B**, Superficial pigmented lesions. **C**, Peritoneal pockets.

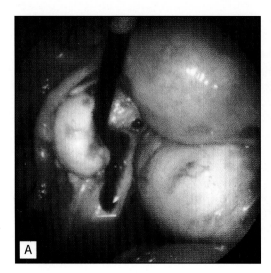
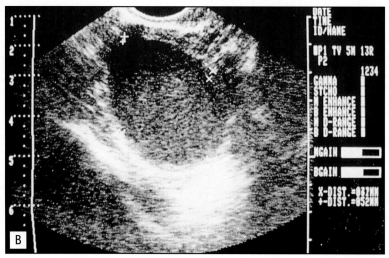

FIGURE 14-17.

Endometriomas. Ovarian endometriosis can be superficial or present as cystic masses called endometriomas. **A**, "Chocolate cyst." This term is applied to these ovarian masses because of the characteristic thick, dark brown fluid content (similar to chocolate syrup). **B**, Preoperative typical ultrasound appearance, with a concentric, half-moon layering effect of the fluid.

THE AMERICAN FERTILITY SOCIETY REVISED CLASSIFICATION OF ENDOMETRIOSIS

		< 1 cm	1–3 cm	> 3 cm
Peritoneum	Endometriosis			
	Superficial	1	2	4
	Deep	2	4	6
Ovary	R Superficial	1	2	4
	Deep	4	16	20
	L Superficial	1	2	4
	Deep	4	16	20

Posterior cul-de-sac obliteration	Partial	Complete
	4	40

		<1/3 Enclosure	1/3–2/3 Enclosure	> 2/3 Enclosure
	Adhesions			
Ovary	R Filmy	1	2	4
	Dense	4	8	16
	L Filmy	1	2	4
	Dense	4	8	16
Tube	R Filmy	1	2	4
	Dense	*	8*	16
	L Filmy	1	2	4
	Dense	4*	*	16

If the fimbriated end of the fallopian tube is completely enclosed, change the point assignment to 16.

FIGURE 14-18.

The American Fertility Society Revised Classification of Endometriosis. To encourage the careful recording of operative findings and to standardize documentation of the extent of disease, the American Fertility Society (now the American Society of Reproductive Medicine) devised a staging form in 1979 that was updated in 1985. So that therapeutic results can be interpreted in light of standardized data, use of this form in the operating room is encouraged strongly. All studies on endometriosis now refer to this classification. Although the classification does cover the superficial dimensions of endometriotic lesions and adhesions, it does not classify the depth of invasion, which is extremely important in relating topography to symptomatology. *Asterisk* indicates those point assignments that should be changed to 16 if the fimbriated end of the fallopian tube is completely enclosed. Stage I Marginal 1–5; Stage II Mild 6–15; Stage III Moderate 16–40; Stage IV Severe >40.

$\mathcal{T}$REATMENT

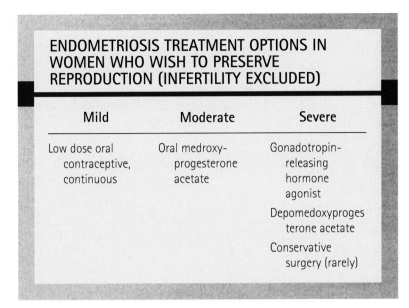

ENDOMETRIOSIS TREATMENT OPTIONS IN WOMEN WHO WISH TO PRESERVE REPRODUCTION (INFERTILITY EXCLUDED)

Mild	Moderate	Severe
Low dose oral contraceptive, continuous	Oral medroxy-progesterone acetate	Gonadotropin-releasing hormone agonist
		Depomedoxyprogesterone acetate
		Conservative surgery (rarely)

FIGURE 14-19.

Treatment of endometriosis in women during their reproductive years, excluding those with infertility. Following laparoscopic diagnosis and treatment, women with recurrent, symptomatic endometriosis who wish to preserve reproductive function should be treated medically with hormonal suppression. Unless a large endometrioma occurs requiring a surgical approach, it is best to avoid repetitive pelvic surgery, which can create adhesions and thus compromise future fertility. Because no one method of steroidal suppression may be acceptable (*eg*, patient choice, medical contraindication), many forms of medical therapy exist, all of which suppress rather than cure endometriosis. Therefore, multiple courses may be required with breaks in between while the patient is asymptomatic. It is best to start with the simplest, least expensive therapy.

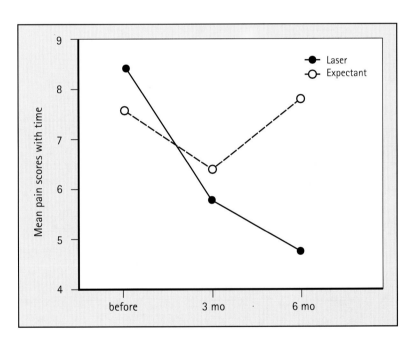

FIGURE 14-20.

Carbon dioxide laser ablation of endometriotic lesions. In women with symptomatic endometriosis, eliminating the lesions at the initial lapararoscopic procedure will provide pain relief for an extended period of time. In this computer randomized study, patients who underwent CO_2 laser ablation of their endometriotic lesions were pain-free longer than a comparable group of patients who had diagnostic laparoscopy only. In subsequent follow-up, this pain relief lasted 1 year in most patients. When symptoms recur, hormonal suppression (*see* Fig. 14-19) should be used. (*Adapted from* Sutton *et al.* [10].)

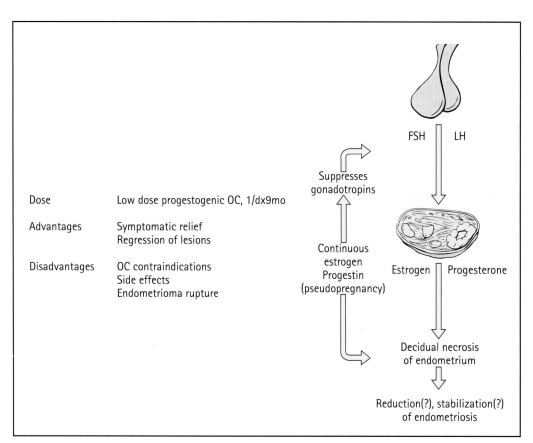

Dose	Low dose progestogenic OC, 1/dx9mo
Advantages	Symptomatic relief
	Regression of lesions
Disadvantages	OC contraindications
	Side effects
	Endometrioma rupture

FSH   LH

Suppresses gonadotropins

Continuous estrogen Progestin (pseudopregnancy)

Estrogen   Progesterone

Decidual necrosis of endometrium

Reduction(?), stabilization(?) of endometriosis

FIGURE 14–21.

Induction of pseudopregnancy for treatment of symptomatic endometriosis. A continuous, low-dose, progestogenic oral contraceptive (OC) provides a useful first-line drug for the woman with symptomatic endometriosis. It should be taken every day with no breaks. Breakthrough bleeding can be controlled with an added oral estrogen used for a short time when bleeding first occurs. FSH—follicle-stimulating hormone; LH—luteinizing hormone.

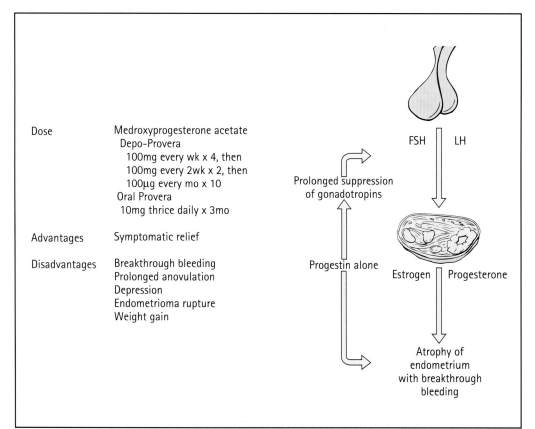

Dose	Medroxyprogesterone acetate
	Depo-Provera
	100mg every wk x 4, then
	100mg every 2wk x 2, then
	100μg every mo x 10
	Oral Provera
	10mg thrice daily x 3mo
Advantages	Symptomatic relief
Disadvantages	Breakthrough bleeding
	Prolonged anovulation
	Depression
	Endometrioma rupture
	Weight gain

FSH   LH

Prolonged suppression of gonadotropins

Progestin alone

Estrogen   Progesterone

Atrophy of endometrium with breakthrough bleeding

FIGURE 14–22.

Oral progestins for pain relief. With the availability of gonadotropin-releasing hormone agonist, the use of depomedroxyprogesterone acetate has become less useful. However, it is cheaper and can be used for a longer time. In a woman who wishes immediate fertility on cessation of therapy, depomedroxyprogesterone acetate may be a concern because of the prolonged period of anovulation after injection. FSH—follicle-stimulating hormone; LH—luteinizing hormone.

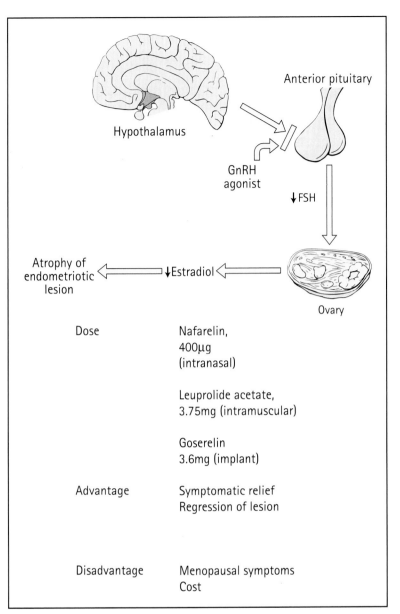

Dose | Nafarelin, 400μg (intranasal)
Leuprolide acetate, 3.75mg (intramuscular)
Goserelin 3.6mg (implant)

Advantage | Symptomatic relief
Regression of lesion

Disadvantage | Menopausal symptoms
Cost

FIGURE 14-23.

Suppression of ovarian function using gonadotropin-releasing hormone (GnRH) agonist. GnRH agonist lowers estradial levels to those of ovariectomized women, suggesting that suppression of ovarian function using a GnRH agonist may have effects on endometriosis similar to those of castration. However, GnRH agonist therapy may cause rupture of endometriomas larger than 5 cm. The main negative aspects of this form of treatment are hot flushes (in 95% of women) and a decrease in bone mass during the normal 6-month course of therapy. However, with cessation of therapy, bone mass is recovered during the next 12 to 24 months. FSH—follicle-stimulating hormone.

INDICATIONS FOR TREATMENT OF PATIENT WITH INTRACTABLE PAIN WHO DOES NOT DESIRE FUTURE FERTILITY

Mild-to-moderate pain	Moderate-to-severe pain
Medical therapy	Surgery
Low-dose OC	TAH
Oral MPA	TAH ± BSO if involved or significant disease left
GnRHa	After BSO postoperative estrogen replacement therapy if pelvic wall disease left, HRT or progestin for 3-6 mo before starting ERT

FIGURE 14-24.

Treatment of the patient with intractable pain who does not desire future fertility. When pelvic pain can be directly attributed to endometriosis and its accompanying adhesions, hysterectomy is the most successful treatment for the appropriately selected women who do not desire future fertility. With ovarian involvement, or if significant endometriosis is left behind, consideration should be given to performing a bilateral salpingo-oophorectomy (BSO) as well. Obviously, the patient's age and desires will ultimately decide for or against undergoing BSO. Following a BSO, estrogen replacement therapy (ERT) can begin. Caution is necessary when residual endometriosis or ovarian tissue is left along the pelvic side wall; in such cases, it would be prudent to use 3 to 6 months of hormonal replacement therapy (HRT)—(ie, estrogen and progestin), or progestin alone to further reduce the chance of endometriosis recurrence. GnRHa—gonadotropin-releasing hormone agonist; MPA—medroxyprogesterone acetate; OC—oral contraceptive; TAH—total abdominal hysterectomy.

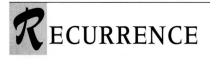

TOTAL ABDOMINAL HYSTERECTOMY WITH AND WITHOUT OVARIAN CONSERVATION: SIGNIFICANTLY DIFFERENT PATIENT CHARACTERISTICS

	Ovarian conservation (n = 29)	Bilateral oophorectomy (n = 109)	P value
Mean age at TAH	33 (range, 24–45)	35 (range, 22–44)	0.03
Mean parity	1.3 (range, 0–2)	0.8 (range, 0–4)	0.004
Mean stage at TAH			0.0002
I, II (%)	51.8	18.3	
III (%)	20.7	13.8	
IV (%)	27.5	67.8	

FIGURE 14–25.

Characteristics of patients undergoing total abdominal hysterectomy (TAH) with and without ovarian preservation at the time of hysterectomy for endometriosis. This treatment remains controversial. In this historical, prospective study from Johns Hopkins Hospital, bilateral oophorectomy had been performed in 109 women and the ovaries left in the other 29 women. Patient characteristics differed only in the areas noted. TAH—total abdominal hysterectomy. (*Adapted from* Namnoum *et al.* [11].)

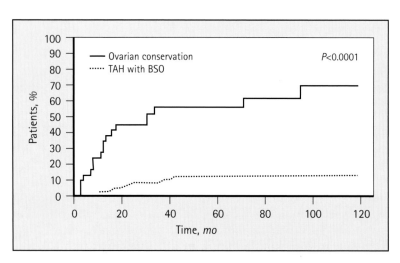

FIGURE 14–26.

Cumulative incidence of symptom recurrence. All patients were contacted in the prospective part of the study by Namnoum and colleagues [11]. In those women who had ovarian preservation, 62% (18 of 29) had recurrence of symptoms, most within a year of surgery. In the group who had undergone total abdominal hysterectomy (TAH) with bilateral salpingo-oophorectomy (BSO), 10.1% (11 of 109) had symptom recurrence and all eleven had received postoperative hormone replacement therapy. (*Adapted from* Namnoum *et al.* [11].)

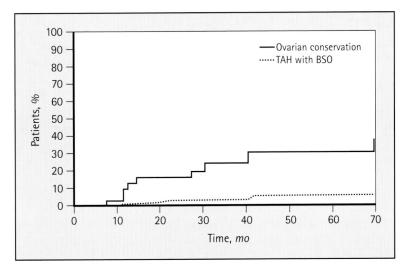

FIGURE 14-27.

Cumulative incidence of reoperation. In the women who had ovarian conservation studied by Namnoum and colleagues [11], 31% (nine of 29) required pelvic reoperation, and five of nine still have persistent pain. In the group who had undergone total abdominal hysterectomy (TAH) with bilateral salpingo-oophorectomy (BSO), 3.7% (four of 109) required pelvic reoperation; no ovarian remnants were found. P<0.0001 (*Adapted from* Namnoum *et al.* [11].)

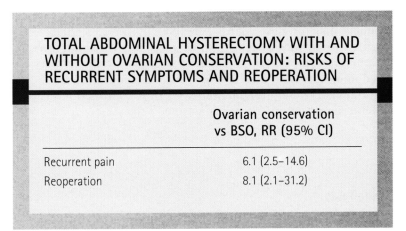

TOTAL ABDOMINAL HYSTERECTOMY WITH AND WITHOUT OVARIAN CONSERVATION: RISKS OF RECURRENT SYMPTOMS AND REOPERATION	
	Ovarian conservation vs BSO, RR (95% CI)
Recurrent pain	6.1 (2.5–14.6)
Reoperation	8.1 (2.1–31.2)

FIGURE 14-28.

Risks of recurrent symptoms and reoperation in women with total abdominal hysterectomy (TAH) with and without ovarian conservation. The relative risk (RR) of recurrent pain or reoperation after ovarian conservation rather than BSO are 6.1 and 8.1 respectively. RR values were adjusted for age, stage, and prior medical or surgical therapy. (*Adapted from* Namnoum *et al.* [11].)

*E*FFECTS ON FERTILITY

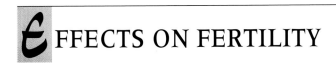

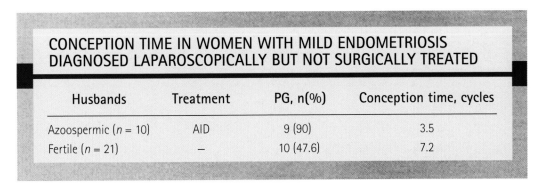

CONCEPTION TIME IN WOMEN WITH MILD ENDOMETRIOSIS DIAGNOSED LAPAROSCOPICALLY BUT NOT SURGICALLY TREATED			
Husbands	Treatment	PG, n(%)	Conception time, cycles
Azoospermic (*n* = 10)	AID	9 (90)	3.5
Fertile (*n* = 21)	—	10 (47.6)	7.2

FIGURE 14-29.

Conception time in women with mild endometriosis diagnosed laparoscopically but not surgically treated. It is uncertain whether the infertility in women with endometriosis is caused by the endometriosis or whether the endometriosis develops secondary to the infertility. Numerous studies have shown that infertility associated with mild endometriosis diagnosed surgically does not need active therapy for fertility to occur. After laparoscopic diagnosis only of mild endometriosis, 10 of 31 patients had azoospermic husbands and postoperative donor insemination produced a high conception rate over a short time period. The other 21 patients, where husbands had a normal semen analysis, who postoperatively used well-timed, midcycle intercourse only, also had a reasonable pregnancy rate. However, because endometriosis is a progressive gynecologic process, surgical eradication of obvious lesions at the time of diagnosis seems prudent. (*Adapted from* Portunado *et al.* [9].)

PATHOPHYSIOLOGY OF INFERTILITY IN ENDOMETRIOSIS

Mechanical obstruction

Impaired implantation and embryogenesis

Defects in fertilization

Sperm dysfunction

FIGURE 14-30.

The pathophysiology of infertility in endometriosis. It is easy to understand how severe endometriosis affects fertility. Obviously, the presence of dense adhesions can interfere with ovum pick-up and tubal transport. However, infertility in patients with minimal and mild endometriosis without adhesions cannot be explained easily. Prostaglandins have been implicated as possibly interfering with implantation. A deleterious effect of certain cytokines (*eg*, interleukin-1) on the developing embryo in culture has been shown. Studies have demonstrated more sperm in the peritoneal fluid of women without endometriosis compared with those with endometriosis. This finding suggests that sperm phagocytosis by macrophages may be a cause of infertility in women with endometriosis. Numerous other theories have tried to explain why, or if, mild endometriosis causes infertility. The answer remains unknown.

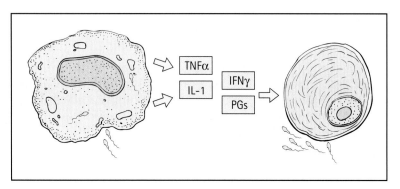

FIGURE 14-31.

Possible mechanisms by which macrophages, or their secretory products, may interfere with the reproductive process. These mechanisms include phagocytosis of sperm by macrophages and the interference of sperm function by secretory products of activated monocytes and macrophages, such as tumor necrosis factor-alpha (TNF-alpha), interleukin-1 (IL-1), prostanoids (PGs), and interferon gamma (IFN-gamma).

CLASSIFICATION AND TREATMENT OF MINIMAL-TO-MODERATE ENDOMETRIOSIS

Classification	Treatment
Minimal	
Mild	
Moderate	Laparoscopic fulguration, ablation, excision
Accessible adhesions	
Endometriomas (<5 cm)	

FIGURE 14-32.

Classification and treatment of minimal-to-moderate endometriosis. The stage of endometriosis is diagnosed at laparoscopy. The disease is fulgurated, ablated, and excised, and adhesions are lysed and excised. Although surgical therapy may not improve fertility, eradication of the lesions is indicated because endometriosis can be a progressive gynecologic disorder. Postoperatively, the use of ovarian stimulation and intrauterine insemination will improve cycle fecundity compared with timed intercourse alone.

CLASSIFICATION AND TREATMENT OF INFERTILITY WITH MODERATE-TO-SEVERE ENDOMETRIOSIS

Classification	Treatment
Moderate	
Extensive adhesions	GnRH agonist
Endometriomas (> 5cm)	Laparoscopy or laparotomy
Severe	

FIGURE 14-33.

Classification and treatment of late-stage or moderate-to-severe endometriosis. The stage of endometriosis is determined at the time of laparoscopy and all visible endometriotic lesions and adhesions are resected. The selection of laparoscopy or laparotomy depends on the surgeon's skills with either technique. If a prior diagnostic laparoscopy has revealed extensive, active endometriosis, a short (3 month) course of gonadotropin-releasing hormone (GnRH) agonist might be considered preoperatively. Postoperatively, ovarian stimulation and intrauterine insemination are performed.

REFERENCES

1. Sampson JA. Peritoneal endometriosis due to dissemination of endometrial tissue into the peritoneal cavity. *Am J Obstet Gynecol* 1927, 14: 422–469

2. Thompson JD, Rock JA, eds.: *Te Linde's Operative Gynecology*, edn 7. Philadelphia: JB Lippincott; 1992.

3. Khorran O, *et al.*: Peritoneal fluid concentrations of the cytokine RANTES correlate with the severity of endometriosis. *Am J Obstet Gynecol* 1993, 169:1545–1549.

4. Sahakian V, *et al.*: Selective localization of interleukin-1 receptor antagonist in eutopic endometrium and endometriotic implants. *Fertil Steril* 1993, 60:276–279.

5. Velebil P, *et al.*: Rate of hospitalization for gynecologic disorders among reproductive-age women in the United States. *Obstet Gynecol* 1995, 86:764–769.

6. Moen MH, *et al.*: The familial risk of endometriosis. *Acta Obstet Gynecol Scand* 1993, 72:560–564.

7. Matorra R, *et al.*: Epidemiology of endometriosis in infertile women. *Fertil Steril* 1995, 63:34–38.

8. Barbieri RL, *et al.*: Elevated serum concentrations of CA-125 in patients with advanced endometriosis. *Fertil Steril* 1986, 45:630.

9. Portunado JA, Echanojauregui AD, Herran C, Alijarte I: Early conception in patients with untreated mild endometriosis. *Fertil Steril* 1983, 39:22.

10. Sutton CJG, *et al.*: Prospective, randomized, double-blind, controlled trial of laser laparoscopy in the treatment of pelvic pain associated with minimal, mild, and moderate endometriosis. *Fertil Steril* 1994, 62:696–700.

11. Namnoum AB, Hickman TN, Goodman SB, *et al.*: Incidence of symptom recurrence after hysterectomy for endometriosis. *Fertil Steril* 1995, 64:898–902.

12. Stovall DW, Bowser LM, Archer DF, Guzick DS: Endometriosis-associated pelvic pain: evidence for an association between the stage of disease and a history of chronic pelvic pain. *Fertil Steril* 1997, 68:13–18.

SELECTED BIBLIOGRAPHY

Adamson GD, Hurd SJ, Pasta DJ, Rodriguez BD. Laparoscopic endometriosis treatment: is it better? *Fertil Steril* 1993, 59:35–44.

Adamson GD, Pasta DJ: Surgical treatment of endometriosis-associated infertility: meta-analysis compared with survival analysis. *Am J Obstet Gynecol* 1994, 171:1488–1505.

American Fertility Society: Revised AFS classification of endometriosis. *Fertil Steril* 1985, 43:351–352.

American Fertility Society: Management of endometriosis in the presence of pelvic pain. *Fertil Steril* 1993, 60:952–955.

American Society for Reproductive Medicine: Revised ASRM classification of endometriosis: 1996. *Fertil Steril* 1997, 67:817–821.

Barbieri RL: Hormone treatment of endometriosis: the estrogen threshold hypothesis. *Am J Obstet Gynecol* 1992, 166:740.

Berga SL: A skeleton in the closet? Bone health and therapy for endometriosis revisited. *Fertil Steril* 1996, 65:702–703.

Bergquist A, Fernö M, Mattson S: A comparison of cathepsin D levels in endometriotic tissue and in uterine endometrium. *Fertil Steril* 1996, 65:1130–1134.

Braun DP, Gebel H, House R, *et al.*: Spontaneous and induced synthesis of cytokines by peripheral blood monocytes in patients with endometriosis. *Fertil Steril* 1996, 65:1125–1129.

Cornillie FJ, Oosterlynck D, Lauweryns JM, *et al.*: Deeply infiltrating pelvic endometriosis: histology and clinical significance. *Fertil Steril* 1990, 53:978.

Dawood MY, Ramos J, Khan-Dawood FS: Depot leuprolide acetate versus danazol for treatment of pelvic endometriosis: changes in vertebral bone mass and serum estradiol and calcitonin. *Fertil Steril* 1995, 63:1177–1183.

Donnez J, Nisolle M, Gillerot S, *et al.*: Ovarian endometrial cysts: the role of gonadotropin-releasing hormone agonist and/or drainage. *Fertil Steril* 1994, 62:63–66.

Friedman AJ, Juneau-Norcross M, Rein MS: Adverse effects of leuprolide acetate depot treatment. *Fertil Steril* 1993, 59:448–450.

Friedman AJ, Hornstein MD: Gonadotropin-releasing hormone agonist plus estrogen-progestin "add-back" therapy for endometriosis-related pelvic pain. *Fertil Steril* 1993, 60:236–241.

Guzick DS, Yao YAS, Berga SL, *et al.*: Endometriosis impairs the efficacy of gamete intrafallopian transfer: results of a case-control study. *Fertil Steril* 1994, 62:1186–1191.

Hornstein MD, Yuzpe AA, Burry KA, *et al.*: Prospective randomized double-blind trial of 3 versus 6 months of nafarelin therapy for endometriosis associated with pelvic pain. *Fertil Steril* 1995, 63:955–962.

Israel R: Pelvic endometriosis. In *Infertility, Contraception and Reproductive Endocrinology*, edn 3. Edited by Mishell DR Jr., Davajan V, Lobo RA. Cambridge, MA: Blackwell Scientific Publications; 1991:723–753.

Jansen RPS, Russell P: Nonpigmented endometriosis: clinical, laparoscopic, and pathologic definition. *Am J Obstet Gynecol* 1986, 155:1154.

Kettel LM, Murphy AA, Morales AJ, *et al.*: Treatment of endometriosis with the antiprogesterone mifepristone (RU486). *Fertil Steril* 1996, 65:23–28.

Koninckx PR, Meuleman C, Demeyere S, *et al.*: Suggestive evidence that pelvic endometriosis is a progressive disease, whereas deeply infiltrating endometriosis is associated with pelvic pain. *Fertil Steril* 1991, 55:759.

Koninckx PR, Martin DC: Deep endometriosis: a consequence of infiltration or retraction or possibly adenomyosis externa? *Fertil Steril* 1992, 58:924–928.

Leather AT, Studd JWW, Watson NR, Holland EFN: The prevention of bone loss in young women treated with GnRH analogues with "add-back" estrogen therapy. *Obstet Gynecol* 1993, 81:104–107.

Letterie GS, Stevenson D, Shah A: Recurrent anaphylaxis to a depot form of GnRH analogue. *Obstet Gynecol* 1991, 78:943.

Mäkäräinen L, Rönnberg L, Kauppila A: Medroxyprogesterone acetate supplementation diminishes the hypoestrogenic side effects of gonadotropin-releasing hormone agonist without changing its efficacy in endometriosis. *Fertil Steril* 1996, 65:29–34.

Morcos RN, Gibbons WE, Findley WE: Effect of peritoneal fluid on in vitro cleavage of 2-cell mouse embryos: possible role in infertility associated with endometriosis. *Fertil Steril* 1985, 44:678.

Mukherjee T, Barad D, Turk R, Freeman R: A randomized, placebo-controlled study on the effect of cyclic intermittent etidronate therapy on the bone mineral density changes associated with six months of gonadotropin-releasing hormone agonist treatment. *Am J Obstet Gynecol* 1996, 175:105–109.

Muse KN, Wilson EA: How does mild endometriosis cause infertility? *Fertil Steril* 1982, 38:145.

Olivennes F, Feldberg D, Liu H-C, *et al.*: A stage by stage analysis: the role of in vitro fertilization. *Fertil Steril* 1995, 64:392–398.

Parazzini F, Fedele L, Busacca M, *et al.*: Postsurgical medical treatment of advanced endometriosis: results of a randomized clinical trial. *Am J Obstet Gynecol* 1994, 171:1205–1207.

Paoletti AM, Serra GG, Cagnacci A, *et al.*: Spontaneous reversibility of bone loss induced by gonadotropin-releasing hormone analog treatment. *Fertil Steril* 1996, 65:707–710.

Pittaway DE, Maxon W, Daniell J, *et al.*: Luteal phase defects in infertility patients with endometriosis. *Fertil Steril* 1983, 39:712.

Punnonen J, Teisala K, Ranta H, *et al.*: Increased levels of interleukin-6 and interleukin-10 in the peritoneal fluid of patients with endometriosis. *Am J Obstet Gynecol* 1996, 174:1522–1526.

Rana N, Braun DP, House R, *et al.*: Basal and stimulated secretion of cytokines by peritoneal macrophages in women with endometriosis. *Fertil Steril* 1996, 65:925–930.

Rock JA, Truglia JA, Caplan RJ, the Zoladex Endometriosis Study Group: Zoladex (goserelin acetate implant) in the treatment of endometriosis: a randomized comparison with danazol. *Obstet Gynecol* 1993, 82:198–205.

Rock JA: The revised American Fertility Society classification of endometriosis: reproducibility of scoring. *Fertil Steril* 1995, 63:1108–1110.

Rock JA: Endometriosis and pelvic pain. *Fertil Steril* 1993, 60:950–951.

Ryan IP, Tseng JF, Schriock ED, *et al.*: Interleukin-8 concentrations are elevated in peritoneal fluid of women with endometriosis. *Fertil Steril* 1995, 63:929–932.

Schenken RS: *Endometriosis: Contemporary Concepts in Clinical Management.* Philadelphia: JB Lippincott; 1989.

Schenken RS, Malinak RL: Conservative surgery versus expectant management for the infertile patient with mild endometriosis. *Fertil Steril* 1982, 37:183.

Schmidt CL: Endometriosis: a reappraisal of pathogenesis and treatment. *Fertil Steril* 1985, 44:157.

Suginami H, Yano K, Watanabe K, Matsuura S: A factor inhibiting ovum capture by the oviductal fimbriae present in endometriosis peritoneal fluid. *Fertil Steril* 1986, 46:1140.

Suginami H, Yano K: An ovum capture inhibitor (OCI) in endometriosis peritoneal fluid: an OCI-related membrane responsible for fimbrial failure of ovum capture. *Fertil Steril* 1988, 50:648.

Surrey ES, Voigt B, Fournet N, Judd HL: Prolonged gonadotropin-releasing hormone agonist treatment of symptomatic endometriosis: the role of cyclic sodium etidronate and low-dose norethindrone "add-back" therapy. *Fertil Steril* 1995, 63:747–755.

Taylor BA, Frizelle FA, Dozois RR, Williams TJ: Intestinal endometriosis: clinicopathologic characteristics and surgical management. *Journal of Pelvic Surgery* 1996, 2:122–127.

Thomas EJ: Endometriosis 1995: confusion or sense? *Int J Gynecol Obstet* 1995, 48:149–155.

Tummon IS, Asher LJ, Martin JSB, Tulandi T: Randomized controlled trial of superovulation and insemination for infertility associated with minimal or mild endometriosis. *Fertil Steril* 1997, 68:8–12.

Vercellini P, Vendola N, Bocciolone L, *et al.*: Laparoscopic aspiration of ovarian endometriomas: effect with postoperative gonadotropin releasing hormone agonist treatment. *J Reprod Med* 1992, 37:577–580.

Vercellini P, Trespidi L, Colombo A, *et al.*: A gonadotropin-releasing hormone agonist versus a low-dose oral contraceptive for pelvic pain associated with endometriosis. *Fertil Steril* 1993, 60:75–79.

Waller KG, Shaw RW: Endometriosis, pelvic pain, and psychological functioning. *Fertil Steril* 1995, 63:796–800.

Waller KG, Shaw RW: Gonadotropin-releasing hormone analogues for the treatment of endometriosis: long-term follow-up. *Fertil Steril* 1993, 59:511–515.

CHAPTER 15

Recurrent Abortion

Bruce R. Carr

Recurrent abortion is a serious personal tragedy that can lead to depression in a couple seeking parenthood. Likewise it is a formidable clinical challenge for any physician who tries to diagnose and treat this disorder.

Recurrent abortion is usually defined as three or more consecutive losses. In couples with one live-born infant, the outcome is significantly better than in women with no live-born births.

This chapter discusses the prevalence and risks that predispose to recurrent abortion. Potential treatments and evaluation of pregnancy loss also are discussed. The causes of recurrent pregnancy loss that can be defined clinically or by laboratory tests include genetic, anatomic, endocrine, immunologic, infectious, and environmental factors. Spontaneous and recurrent abortion occur most commonly in the first trimester and usually the cause is unknown.

$\mathcal{P}$REVALENCE AND RISKS

REPRODUCTIVE SUCCESS AND FAILURE IN THE HUMAN OVUM

Survivors, n	Outcome	Week After Ovulation
100 Ova	13 (not fertilized)	–
87 Fertile	15 (not implanted)	0
72 Implant	18 (preclinical loss)	1–8
54	6 (early clinical loss)	8–14
48	2 (late clinical loss)	15–22
46	1 (perinatal demise)	23–44
45 Viable Infants	–	–

FIGURE 15-1.

The reproductive success and failure of the human ovum. In this model it is assumed that the couple is young and healthy and without fertility problems. The data for this figure show frequency of early pregnancy loss based on human chorionic gonadotropin testing starting 3 weeks after the last menstrual period. The maximum fecundability is approximately 45%, which is similar to previous studies by Hertig and coworkers [1]. (*Adapted from* Leridon [2].)

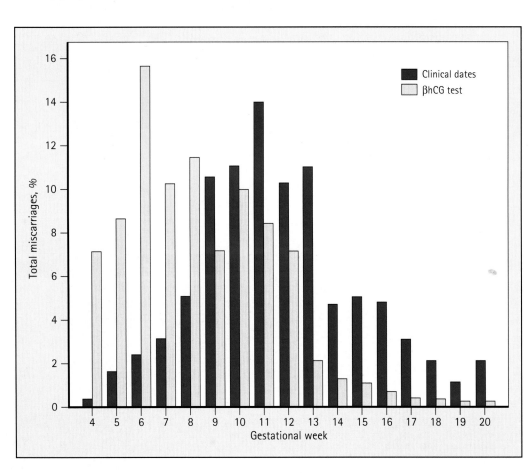

FIGURE 15-2.

The occurrence of spontaneous miscarriages during the first 20 weeks of pregnancy. These data were determined clinically by dates in 610 women (*solid blue bars*) or by sensitive human chorionic gonadotropin (hCG) assay in 707 menstrual cycles (*yellow bars*). The mean gestational age at the time of clinically recognized pregnancy loss was 11 weeks based on clinical dates. However, a sensitive β-hCG assay found that the mean age of pregnancy loss was 7 weeks. When the results of sensitive β-hCG tests are combined with ultrasound data, the mean age of pregnancy loss is 8 weeks [3]; thus, in most cases of early spontaneous abortion, fetal viability ceases several weeks before clinical signs such as bleeding or cramping are present. (*Data from* Kallen [3], Mills and coworkers [4], and Kutteh and Carr [5].)

RELATION OF ABORTION FREQUENCY TO MATERNAL AND PATERNAL AGE AT CONCEPTION

Maternal age, y	Abortion, %	Paternal age, y	Abortion, %
<20	12.2	<20	12.0
20–24	14.3	20–24	11.8
25–29	13.7	25–29	15.7
30–34	15.5	30–34	13.1
35–39	18.7	35–39	15.8
40–44	33.8	40–44	19.5
>44	53.2	–	–

FIGURE 15-3.

The relationship of maternal and paternal age at the time of conception. Advanced maternal age is known to be a risk factor for spontaneous abortion. The rate of abortion in women older than 40 years of age is almost three times that of women younger than 20 years of age. Likewise, paternal age is also important, but to a lesser extent. (*Data from* Kutteh and Carr [5] and Warburton and Fraser [6].)

RECURRENCE RISK RELATIVE TO PRIOR GESTATIONAL EVENTS

Prior Outcome	Prior Losses, n	Recurrence, %
Live born	0	12
	1	24
	2	26
	3	32
	4	26
Miscarriage		
	1	19
	2	35
	3	47
	4	54

FIGURE 15-4.

The risk of recurrent abortion related to prior pregnancy outcome. The outcome of a previous pregnancy is also an important factor in predicting subsequent pregnancy outcome. In a study of over 2000 pregnancies, it was determined that in couples with at least one full-term live birth, the recurrence of pregnancy loss increased from 12% with no previous loss to 24 to 32% after one to four losses. In other words, the chance of successful outcome in subsequent pregnancy remained relatively constant at 70% to 76% with a history of one to four losses. In contrast, in couples without a live birth, the risk of recurrent pregnancy loss progressively increased. Couples with three or four consecutive losses without a prior liveborn infant face a risk of 50% pregnancy loss in subsequent pregnancies. (*Data from* Poland and coworkers [7], Warburton and Fraser [6], and Kutteh and Carr [5].)

PREVALENCE OF RECURRENT PREGNANT LOSS

Year	RPL, n*	Deliveries†	RPL, %
1991	153	15,183	1.00
1992	212	15,035	1.41
1993	198	14,888	1.33
1994	203	13,929	1.46
1995	219	13,585	1.61
Total	985	72,620	1.36

* New cases of RPL identified
† Total women delivered of infants ≥ 500 g is an approximation of the women at risk.

FIGURE 15-5.

Prevalence rate of recurrent pregnancy loss (RPL). Based on approximately 1000 new cases of recurrent spontaneous abortion at one hospital, the risk of a couple experiencing RPL was between 1% and 2% per year. This estimate is based on 72,620 deliveries occur ring at Parkland Memorial Hospital in Dallas, Texas, during a 5-year period. *Asterisk* indicates new cases identified; *dagger* indicates that the total women delivered of infants ≥ 500 g is an approximation of the number of women at risk. (*Adapted from Kutteh and Carr [5].*)

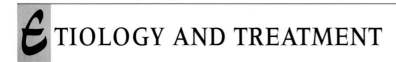

*E*TIOLOGY AND TREATMENT

ABNORMALITIES IN WOMEN WITH VIABLE PREGNANCIES AND THOSE WITH SINGLE AND RECURRENT PREGNANCY LOSS

Abnormalities	Viable Pregnancies, %	Single Loss, %	Recurrent Loss, %
Müllerian anomalies	1–3	2–5	10–15
Cervical incompetence	1–2	6–10	8–15
Leiomyomata	15	15	15–20
Asherman's syndrome	<1	<1	5
Luteal phase defect	8	8–12	10–15
Autoimmune	0.5	2	10
Chromosomal			
Parental	0.2	NA	3–5
Fetal	0.5	55	20

FIGURE 15–6.

The percentage of women diagnosed with various clinical disorders related to pregnancy outcome. The data in this table are based on literature reports of the pregnancy outcome with müllerian anomalies, cervical incompetence, leiomyomas, Asherman's syndrome, luteal phase defects, and chromosomal abnormalities. Thus, müllerian anomalies are only found in 1% to 3% of fertile women but 10% to 15% in women with recurrent pregnancy loss. The percentages refer to estimated frequencies of abnormalities that are found in couples who have had a viable pregnancy, single pregnancy loss, or recurrent pregnancy loss. NA—data not available. (*Adapted from* Kutteh and Carr [5].)

GENETIC FACTORS

FREQUENCY OF CHROMOSOMAL COMPLEMENTS DETECTED IN FIRST TRIMESTER SPONTANEOUS ABORTIONS

Complement		Frequency, %	Complement		Frequency, %
Normal (46,XX or 46,XY)		54.1	Autosomal trisomy		22.3
Triploidy		7.7	Chromosome 5	0.04	
69,XXX	2.7		Chromosome 6	0.14	
69,XYY	0.2		Chromosome 7	0.89	
69,XXY	4.0		Chromosome 8	0.79	
Other	0.8		Chromosome 9	0.72	
Tetraploidy		2.6	Chromosome 10	0.36	
92,XXX	1.5		Chromosome 11	0.04	
92,XXYY	0.55		Chromosome 12	0.18	
Not stated	0.55		Chromosome 13	1.07	
Monosomy X (45,X)		8.6	Chromosome 14	0.82	
Structural abnormalities		1.5	Chromosome 15	1.68	
Sex chromosomal polysomy		0.2	Chromosome 16	7.27	
47,XXX	0.05		Chromosome 17	0.18	
47,XXY	0.15		Chromosome 18	1.15	
Autosomal monosomy (G)		0.1	Chromosome 19	0.01	
Autosomal trisomy		22.3	Chromosome 20	0.61	
Chromosome 1	0		Chromosome 21	2.11	
Chromosome 2	1.11		Chromosome 22	2.26	
Chromosome 3	0.25		Double trisomy		0.7
Chromosome 4	0.64		Mosaic trisomy		1.3
			Abnormality not specified		0.9

FIGURE 15–7.

Frequency of chromosome complements detected in first trimester pregnancy loss. Autosomal trisomies are the most frequent chromosomal anomalies in first trimester pregnancy loss. Of these, trisomy 16 occurs most frequently. Monosomal anomalies are the second most common abnormality, followed closely by triploidy. However, the majority of first trimester pregnancy losses (*ie*, 50%) have a normal karyotype. (*Adapted from* Simpson [8].)

FIGURE 15-8.

The percentage of chromosomal anomalies related to gestational age. The frequency of an abnormal karyotype at 12 weeks gestation is approximately 60%, 45% by 16 weeks, 12% by 20 weeks, and in full-term infants is less than 1%. Thus, the frequency of an abnormal chromosome analysis is much greater in early versus late pregnancy. These differences may be explained by the fact that the majority of chromosomally abnormal fetuses are aborted in early gestation. (*Data from* Scott [9].)

DISTRIBUTION OF CHROMOSOME ABNORMALITIES ACCORDING TO THE SEX OF THE CARRIER

Abnormality	Male carriers, n	Female carriers, n	Both, n
Reciprocal translocations	150	265	415
Robertsonian translocations	58	133	191
Inversions	25	35	60
Sex chromosome aneuploidy	7	19	26
Supernumerary chromosome	2	9	11
Total abnormalities, n	242	461	703

FIGURE 15-9.

The distribution of the chromosome abnormalities in the sex of the carrier (mother, father, or both). Overall abnormalities are more frequent in the mother. The most common abnormalities are reciprocal followed by robertsonian translocations. In couples with recurrent pregnancy loss, a chromosomal anomaly in either parent occurs in 2% to 6%. Thus, in couples with recurrent spontaneous abortion (more than three), a chromosomal analysis should be obtained. (*Adapted from* DeBraekeleer and Dao [10].)

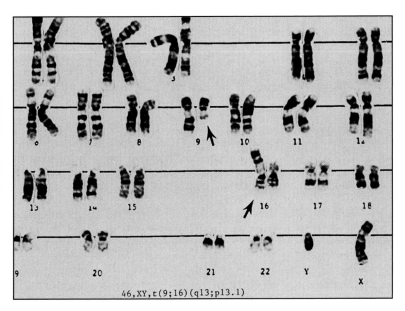

46,XY,t(9;16)(q13;p13.1)

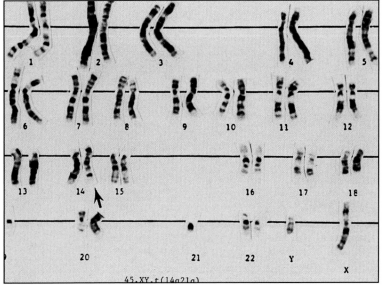

45,XY,t(14q21q)

FIGURE 15-10.

Reciprocal translocation. The father has 46 chromosomes and a balanced translocation between 16 and 9 (*arrows*). Although the subject was phenotypically normal, his offspring have an increased risk of an abnormal karyotype. The risk of spontaneous abortions is estimated to be as high as 50% [11]. Donor sperm may be offered as therapy.

FIGURE 15-11.

Robertsonian translocation. The father has 45 chromosomes and a balanced translocation involving chromosomes 14 (*arrow*) and 21. The outcome of normal conception with this disorder is unlikely. In this case, only a trisomy 14 or 21 or a monosomy 14 or 21 may result in the conceptus. The father should consider sterilization and request donor sperm for treatment [11].)

ANATOMIC FACTORS CAUSING RECURRENT ABORTION

Cervix	Uterus
Cervical incompetence	Leiomyomas
	Polyps
	Intrauterine adhesions (Asherman's syndrome)
	Developmental anomalies
	Unicornuate
	Didelphys
	Bicornuate
	Septate
	Diethylstilbesterol (DES) exposure

FIGURE 15–12.

Anatomic risk factors for recurrent abortion. Several uterine abnormalities have been reported to be associated with recurrent abortion. Cervical incompetence usually involves second trimester loss. Disorders of the uterine corpus include pathologic conditions such as leiomyoma, polyps, and intrauterine adhesions. Developmental müllerian anomalies are associated with reduced or constricted uterine volume, which is often associated with poor pregnancy outcome.

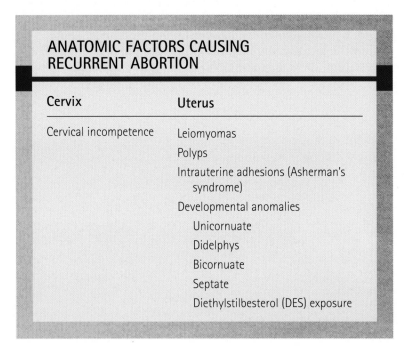

Patient's Name _____ Date _____ Chart # _____

Age _____ G _____ P _____ Sp Ab _____ VTP _____ Ectopic _____ Infertile Yes _____ No _____

Other Significant History (i.e. surgery, infection, etc.)_____

HSG _____ Sonography _____ Photography _____ Laparoscopy _____ Laparotomy _____

EXAMPLES

I. Hypoplasis/Agenesis
A. Vaginal   B. Cervical
C. Fundal   E. Combined
D. Tubal

II. Unicornuate
A. Communicating   B. Non-communicating
C. No cavity   D. No horn

III. Didelphus

IV. Bicornuate
A. Complete   B. Partial

V. Septate
A. Complete   B. Partial

VI. Arcuate

VII. DES Drug related

*Uterus may be normal or take a variety of abnormal forms
**May have two distinct cervices

FIGURE 15–13.

The American Fertility Society (now known as the American Society for Reproductive Medicine) classification of müllerian anomalies. A number of classifications have been proposed for müllerian anomalies. Currently, evaluation of clinical studies to confirm the relevance of this classification are ongoing. (Courtesy of the American Society for Reproductive Medicine, Birmingham, AL.)

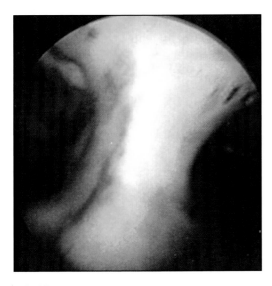

FIGURE 15–14.

Uterine septum. This figure demonstrates a uterine septum as seen at the time of hysteroscopy. A concomitant laparoscopy is also required to differentiate this disorder from a bicornuate uterus. Not only do these procedures performed concomitantly provide an accurate diagnosis, they simultaneously allow outpatient surgical correction. The hysteroscopy surgery can be performed using Hyskon, saline, or 3% glycerine as a distending medium. The septum can be incised with microscissors, or removed by an electrodessicator with a wire loop, or treated with various laser modalities [12].

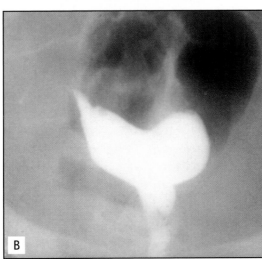

FIGURE 15–15.

A hysterosalpingogram (HSG) demonstrating a uterine septum before and after hysteroscopic surgery. **A,** A uterine septum is suggested by the typical findings at the time of HSG. The patient had experienced three prior consecutive pregnancy losses. A uterine septum was confirmed and incised at the time of hysteroscopic surgery. **B,** The postoperative view reveals a more unified cavity with absence of the septum.

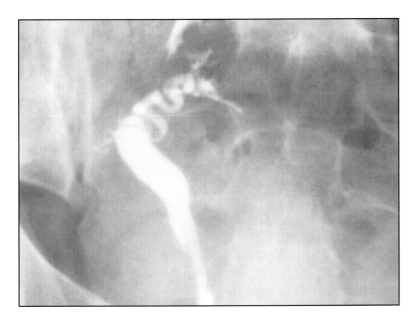

FIGURE 15–16.

Unicornuate uterus. This figure demonstrates a unicornuate uterus on hysterosalpingogram (HSG) in a patient with recurrent abortion. The uterine cavity volume is reduced in size and the chance of a term pregnancy is predicted to be only about 60%. No surgical therapy is available [12].

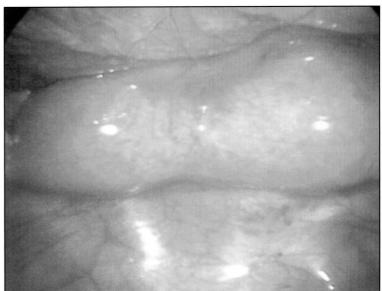

FIGURE 15–17.

Uterus didelphys. This laparoscopic view of uterus didelphys, with two vaginas, two cervices, and two uterine fundi, is shown in a woman with 1 year of infertility. Surgery is not recommended unless recurrent abortion occurs, because a successful pregnancy outcome without treatment is about 70%.

RESULTS OF SURGICAL CORRECTION OF PARTIAL OR COMPLETE UTERINE DUPLICATION

Study	Metroplasty technique	Patients, *n*	Type of uterine defect	Successful pregnancy rate, % Preoperative	Successful pregnancy rate, % Postoperative
Musich and Behman	Tompkins	11	Didelphys	57	–
	Jones	28	Septate/bicornuate	7	75
	Strassmann				
Mercer *et al.*	Jones	15	Septate/bicornuate	73	
	Strassmann	2			
Rock and Jones	Jones	76	Double uterus (didelphys, bicornuate, septate)	0–59	1–81
Strassmann	Strassmann	128	Double uterus	19	86
Daly *et al.*	Hysteroscopic; sharp incision	25	Septate uterus	10	73
Perino *et al.*	Hysteroscopic; sharp incision	24	Septate	11	78.6
DeCherney *et al.*	Hysteroscopy	72	Septate		80.5
DeCherney and Polan	Hysteroscopy	11	Septate		81

FIGURE 15–18.

Results of surgical correction of partial or complete uterine duplication. The outcome of surgical procedures for uterine anomalies differs greatly depending on the disorder, surgeon, and other causes of recurrent abortion. As seen in this figure, the majority of procedures for septate uteri increase gestational outcome. However, none of the studies included a control or untreated group. (*Adapted from Winkel [12].*)

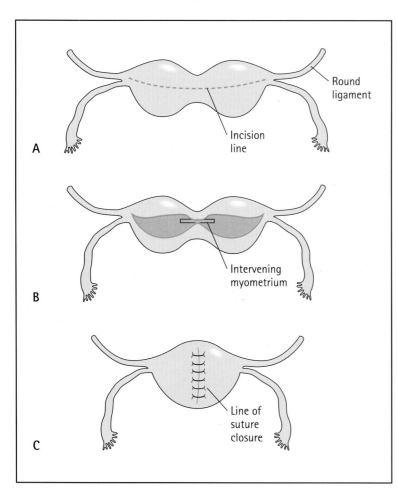

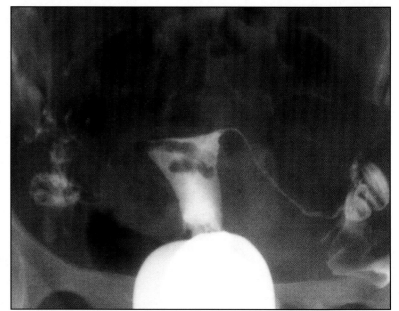

FIGURE 15–20.

Hysterosalpingogram demonstrating an endometrial polyp. Endometrial polyps develop as a hyperplastic growth of a segment of endometrium and might be quite long, as shown. The polyp itself may or may not demonstrate atypical hyperplastic changes, whereas the adjacent endometrium can be histologically normal. Polyps can be present in women with infertility, recurrent pregnancy loss, or menorrhagia.

FIGURE 15–19.

Surgical technique for treatment of the bicornuate uterus. The procedure of choice is the Strassman technique, which requires a transverse surgical incision (**A** and **B**) and a vertical closure (**C**). (*Adapted from Winkel [12].*)

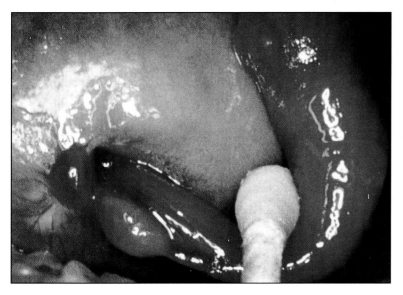

FIGURE 15–21.

Endometrial polyp extending through external cervical os. The patient had a history of recurrent pregnancy loss, infertility, and postcoital bleeding. The base of this polyp extended high into the uterine cavity and was removed at the time of hysteroscopy.

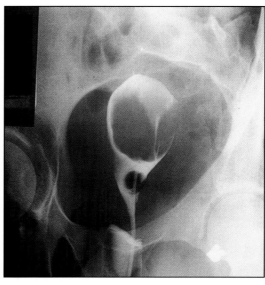

FIGURE 15–22.

A hysterosalpingogram demonstrating a large uterine leiomyoma-induced filling defect. An intramural–submucous leiomyoma was 9 cm in diameter and grossly distorted the endometrial cavity and occluded the left fallopian tube. The patient was a 34-year-old black woman with two pregnancy losses and 2 years of infertility. A myomectomy was performed by laparotomy. The patient conceived 3 months following surgery and delivered at term by cesarean section 12 months later.

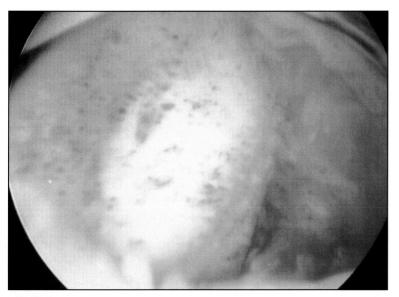

FIGURE 15–23.

Hysteroscopic appearance of a cervical leiomyoma. This patient presented with recurrent pregnancy loss and menorrhagia. A sonogram revealed a lower uterine mass suggestive of a uterine leiomyoma. At the time of hysteroscopy a 2.5-cm leiomyoma was identified and removed.

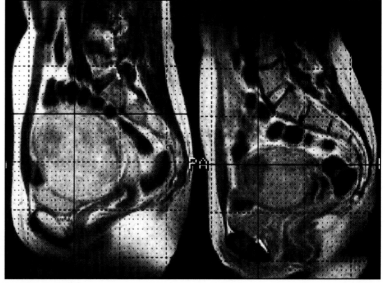

FIGURE 15–24.

Pelvic magnetic resonance imaging (MRI) scan of a 24-year-old woman with recurrent pregnancy loss. The scan confirmed the presence of a large uterine leiomyoma. *Left,* A single uterine leiomyoma. *Right,* The leiomyoma and uterine volume were reduced after 3 months of treatment with a gonadotropin-releasing hormone agonist. The leiomyoma was then removed by an abdominal myomectomy.

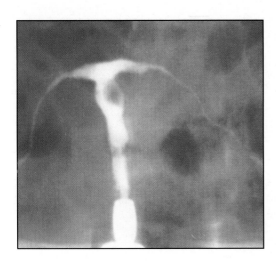

FIGURE 15–25.

Hysterosalpingogram (HSG) of a diethylstilbesterol (DES)-induced uterine deformity. The patient was a 24-year-old woman with infertility. A cervical hood was detected on pelvic examination, and the patient's mother had taken DES during her pregnancy. HSG revealed typical findings of a T-shaped fundus and a filling defect on the left lower segment. The patient subsequently conceived but delivered prematurely at 33 weeks of gestation.

ENDOCRINE FACTORS

DEFINITIONS, ETIOLOGY, AND DIAGNOSIS OF LUTEAL PHASE ABNORMALITIES POSSIBLY ASSOCIATED WITH RECURRENT ABORTION OR INFERTILITY

Definition	Etiology	Diagnosis
Short luteal phase	Abnormal follicular development, low FSH, elevated prolactin, stress	Basal body termperature chart
Inadequate luteal phase	Abnormal or subnormal follicular development	Midluteal phase progesterone, endometrial biopsy
"Normal" luteal phase	Reduced progesterone receptors	Endometrial steroid receptor determination
	Abetalipoproteinemia	Low cholesterol and low density lipoprotein levels
Polycystic ovarian syndrome	Unknown	High LH:FSH ratio

FIGURE 15–26.

Disease states, etiology, and diagnosis of luteal phase abnormalities possibly associated with recurrent abortion and infertility. These disorders vary as defined in the figure. A short luteal phase may result from problems that alter or affect follicular growth such as stress, exercise, elevated prolactin, or ovarian hyperstimulation.

An inadequate luteal phase is associated with abnormal follicular development. A "normal" luteal phase may be associated with reduced endometrial steroid receptors or abetalipoproteinemia. Polycystic ovarian syndrome is associated with high luteinizing hormone (LH) to follicle-stimulating hormone (FSH) ratios.

DIAGNOSTIC METHODS FOR LUTEAL PHASE DEFECT

Methods	Diagnostic criteria	Advantages	Disadvantages
BBT recording	Luteal phase <11 days	Simplicity	Lacks both sensitivity and specificity
Progesterone determinations	Midluteal concentration <10 ng/mL	Objective	Misinterpretation due to short-term fluctuations in serum levels
Endometrial biopsy	Histology >2 days out of phase with known day of sampling as judged by onset of subsequent menses during at least 2 cycles	Identifies abnormalities resulting from both deficient corpus luteum, steroid production and endometrial response	Discomfort; requires expertise in histopathology; expense

FIGURE 15–27.

Diagnostic methods used for luteal phase defects. Tests that are useful in confirming the diagnosis of luteal phase defect include the basal body temperature chart (BBT), progesterone levels, and endometrial biopsy. All of these tests have advantages and disadvantages. The least useful is the BBT chart. A day 21 progesterone level of greater than 10 ng/mL is usually consistent with a normal luteal phase. (*Adapted from Rein [13].*)

TREATMENT OPTIONS FOR LUTEAL PHASE ABNORMALITIES

Abnormality	Treatment
Short luteal phase	Clomiphene citrate
	Bromocriptine (if prolactin level is elevated)
Inadequate luteal phase	Clomiphene citrate
	Bromocriptine (if prolactin level is elevated)
	Progesterone suppositories or injections
	Gonadotropins
"Normal" luteal phase	
Reduced progesterone receptors	Possibly clomiphene citrate, gonadotropins
Abetalipoproteinemia	Progesterone suppositories or injections
Polycystic ovarian syndrome	Ovarian drilling (laparascopic ovarian wedge)

FIGURE 15-28.

Treatment options for luteal phase abnormalities. Clomiphene citrate is the treatment of choice. Clomiphene citrate increases follicular recruitment, development, and subsequent luteal phase quality. Bromocriptine is only indicated when the luteal phase deficiency is associated with elevated prolactin levels. Progesterone suppositories or injections are used as indicated. Occasionally, gonadotropin may be beneficial.

IMMUNE FACTORS

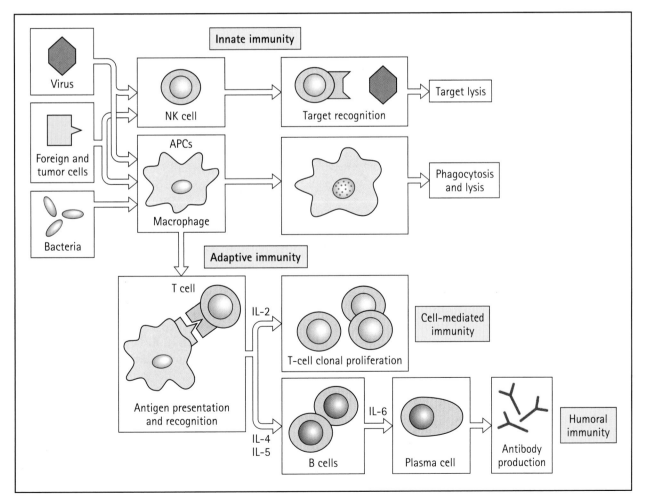

FIGURE 15-29.

Function of antigen-presenting cells (APCs). Two interactive systems make up the immune system. The innate system (*top*) is a more basic. The APCs of the innate system include macrophages, neutrophils, monocytes, and natural killer (NK) cells. There is nonspecificity of this system, *ie,* the APCs recognize most nonself antigens. The innate systems do not increase resistance of the host to repeated exposure of antigen. In contrast, the adaptive system (*bottom*) does provide increased resistance after repeated exposures. This system includes T cells derived from the thymus. The T-cell clones provide cell-mediated immunity. The B cells derived from the marrow provide humoral immunity. IL—interleukin. (*Adapted from* Hatasaka and Scott [14].)

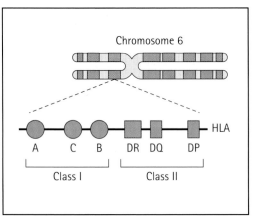

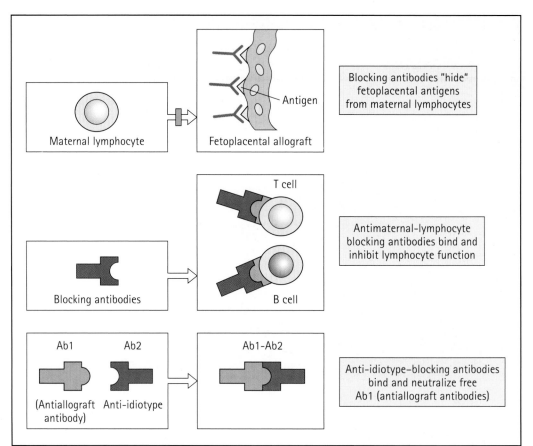

FIGURE 15–30.

The histocompatability locus antigene (HLA) loci of the major histocompatibility complex (MHC). The MHC is located on the short arm of chromosome 6. In humans, the MHC complex is also known as human leukocyte antigen (HLA). Six major antigens are encoded by this locus: class I (HLA-A, -B, and -C), and class II (HLA-DR, -OP, and -DQ).

FIGURE 15–31.

Proposed mechanisms whereby blocking antibodies may contribute to the maintenance of a fetal–placental allograph. *Top,* The fetal-trophoblast antigens are hidden by blocking antibodies from maternal lymphocytes. *Middle,* Antimaternal-lymphocyte blocking antibodies bind and inhibit lymphocyte function (see figure 15-16). *Bottom,* Anti-idiotype–blocking antibodies bind and neutralize free antiallograft antibodies. (*Adapted from Hatasaka and Scott [14].*)

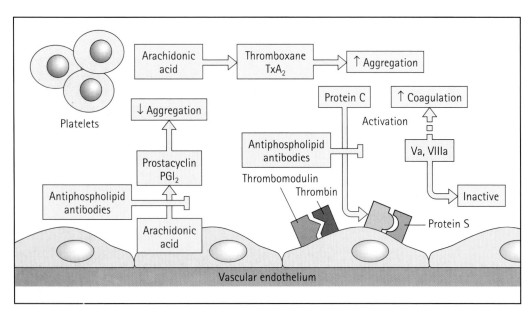

FIGURE 15–32.

Possible mechanisms of antiphospholipid antibody (APA)-induced thrombosis. Three potential mechanisms are shown: decreased prostacyclin production by endothelial cells, increased thromboxane production by platelets, and decreased protein C activation. Endothelial cells normally convert plasma membrane arachidonic acid into prostacyclin, which is released into the circulation and prevents platelet aggregation.

Antiphospholipid antibodies may predispose to thrombosis by inhibiting endothelial cells from producing prostacyclin. Platelets normally convert plasma membrane arachidonic acid into thromboxane, which is released and induces platelet aggregation. Antiphospholipid antibodies may increase thrombosis by enhancing thromboxane release. During clotting, thrombin (a product of the clotting cascade) forms a complex on the surface of endothelial cells with its receptor, thrombomodulin. The thrombin–thrombomodulin complex is enzymatically active and can activate circulating protein C. The activated protein C binds with protein S on the surface of endothelial cells (and platelets). The protein C–protein S complex degrades circulating activated components of the clotting cascade (factors Va and VIIIa). If factors Va and VIIIa were allowed to remain in the circulation, they would increase coagulation activity of the blood. PG—prostaglandin. (*Adapted from* Rote [15].)

SUGGESTED CLINICAL AND LABORATORY CRITERIA FOR THE ANTIPHOSPHOLIPID SYNDROME

Clinical features	Laboratory features
Pregnancy loss	Lupus anticoagulant
Fetal death	
Recurrent pregnancy loss	IgG anticardiolipin antibodies
	(≥ 20 IGG phospholipid units)
Thrombosis	
Venous	
Arterial, including stroke	
Autoimmune thrombocytopenia	
Other	IgM anticardiolipin antibodies
Coombs' positive hemolytic	(≥ 20 IGM phospholipid units)
anemia	
Livedo reticularis	

FIGURE 15-33.

Suggested clinical and laboratory criteria for the antiphospholipid (APA) syndrome. There are a number of clinical features of APA syndrome. Fetal death and recurrent pregnancy loss are characterized by an abnormal lupus anticoagulant level. A history of thrombosis may be associated with elevated IgG anticardiolipin antibodies. Other disorders, *ie*, Coombs' positive hemolytic anemia or levido reticularis, may demonstrate IgM anticardiolipin antibodies. Patients with APA syndrome should have at least one clinical and one laboratory test during the course of their illness. Laboratory tests should be positive on at least two occasions more than 8 weeks apart. GPL—IGG phospholipid units; MPL—IGM phospholipid units.) (*Adapted from* Kutteh [16].)

LABORATORY TESTS USED TO DETECT THE PRESENCE OF LUPUS ANTICOAGULANT

Test	Advantages	Disadvantages
APTT	Inexpensive, automated	Reduced sensitivity
dRVVT	No significant effect during pregnancy, readily available	Manual technique, altered by anticoagulants
PCT	Readily available	Manual technique, fresh plasma required
KCT	No significant effect during pregnancy, not altered by anticoagulants, very sensitive	Manual technique, expensive

FIGURE 15-34.

Laboratory screening tests available to detect the presence of lupus anticoagulant (LAC). The most sensitive test is the kaolin clotting time (KCT) test, but it is expensive and must be done manually. Other tests include the plasma clotting time (PCT) and dilute Russell viper venom time (dRVVT). The activated partial thromboplastin time (APTT) is automated but is the least sensitive. Tests shown are listed in order of least to most sensitive.

FIGURE 15-35.

Treatment protocol. Proposed treatment regimen and protocol used for women with recurrent abortion caused by antiphospholipid antibodies (APAs) at the University of Texas Southwestern Medical Center at Dallas. CBC—complete blood count; FHT—fetal heart tone; LA—lupus anticoagulant; PT—prothrombin time; PTT—partial thromboplastin time.

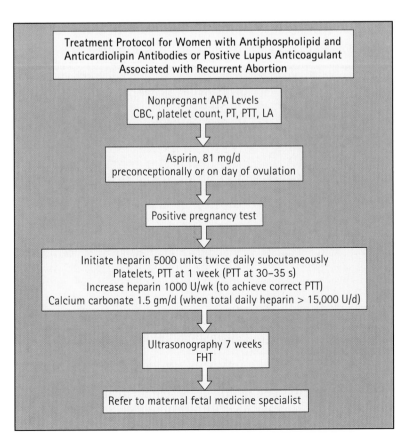

Treatment Protocol for Women with Antiphospholipid and Anticardiolipin Antibodies or Positive Lupus Anticoagulant Associated with Recurrent Abortion

Nonpregnant APA Levels
CBC, platelet count, PT, PTT, LA

↓

Aspirin, 81 mg/d
preconceptionally or on day of ovulation

↓

Positive pregnancy test

↓

Initiate heparin 5000 units twice daily subcutaneously
Platelets, PTT at 1 week (PTT at 30–35 s)
Increase heparin 1000 U/wk (to achieve correct PTT)
Calcium carbonate 1.5 gm/d (when total daily heparin > 15,000 U/d)

↓

Ultrasonography 7 weeks
FHT

↓

Refer to maternal fetal medicine specialist

COMPARISON OF TREATMENTS AND PREGNANCY OUTCOME IN PATIENTS WITH REPEATED PREGNANCY LOSS AND ANTIPHOSPHOLIPID ANTIBODIES

Study	Inclusion criteria	Treatments compared*	Live birth rate, n/n (%)	P value
Laskin (1996)	≥ 2 Fetal losses LA or aCL>20 GPL	Prednisone 0.5–0.8 mg/kg + aspirin 100 mg Placebo	25/42(47.8) 24/46(52.4)	0.57
Hasegawa (1992)	≥ 2 Fetal losses LA or aCL>33 GPL	Prednisone 40 mg + aspirin 81 mg No treatment	13/17(76.5) 1/12(8.3)	0.01
Passaleva (1992)	≥ 2 Fetal losses/SAB LA or aCL	Prednisone 20 mg + aspirin 100 mg No treatment Aspirin 100 mg	5/5(100.0) 1/6(17.0) 9/11(81.8)	
Kutteh (1996)	≥ 3 Pregnancy losses aCL>20 GPL	Heparin 10,000–30,000 U + aspirin 81 mg Aspirin 81 mg	20/25(80.0) 11/25(44.0)	0.02
Cowcheck (1992)	≥ 2 Fetal losses LA or aCL	Heparin 20,000 U + aspirin 81 mg Predisone 40 mg + aspirin 81 mg	9/12(75.0) 6/8(75.0)	1.00
Branch (1992)	≥ 2 Fetal losses LA or aCL>20 GPL[†]	Heparin 15,000–20,000 U + aspirin 81 mg Predisone 40 mg + aspirin 81 mg	14/19(73.7) 21/39(53.8)	0.17
Ketteh (1996)	≥ 3 Pregnancy losses aCL>20 GPL	Low-dose heparin + aspirin 81 mg High-dose heparin + aspirin 81 mg	19/25(76.0) 20/25(80.0)	0.50
Rai (1997)	≥ 3 Pregnancy losses LA or aCL	Heparin 10,000 U + aspirin 81 mg Aspirin 81 mg	32/45(71.0) 19/45(42.0)	0.01

*Converted to equivalent prednisone dose

FIGURE 15–36.

Comparison of treatments and pregnancy outcome in women with recurrent abortions and antiphospholipid antibodies (APAs). In these studies, treatment included aspirin, prednisone, or heparin. All the treatments appeared to improve the pregnancy outcome, but heparin and aspirin appear to be superior to trials with prednisone when one considers maternal and fetal complications. Concomitant use of prednisone and heparin is not better than either alone and may increase the risk of fractures. *Asterisk* indicates converted to equivalent prednisone dose; *dagger* indicates that some patients had previous thromboembolic events but no prior pregnancy loss. aCL—anticardiolipin; GPL—IGG phospholipid units; LA—lupus anticoagulant; SAB—spontaneous abortion. (*Adapted from* Kutteh [16].)

PUBLISHED AND UPDATED TRIALS OF LEUKOCYTE THERAPY FOR RECURRENT SPONTANEOUS ABORTION

Study	Treatments and subjects (n)	Route	Doses, n	Live birth rate, %	P value	Power to detect 50% increase over baseline	Updated RR (95% CI)
Mowbray (1985)	Paternal leukocytes (22) vs maternal leukocytes (27)	3/5 IV 1/5 SC 1/5 ID	1	77 37	0.01	0.26	1.45 (0.95–2.21)
Ho (1991)	Paternal and donor leukocytes (50) vs maternal leukocytes (49)	ID	>1	78 65	0.16	0.48	1.20 (0.93–1.56)
Cauchi (1991)	Paternal leukocytes (21) vs saline (25)	1/2 IV 1/4 C 1/4 ID	1	62 76	0.31	0.23	0.89 (0.59–1.35)
Gatenby (1993)	Paternal leukocytes (19) vs maternal leukocytes	3/5 IV 1/5 SC 1/5 ID	1	68 47	0.14	0.19	1.14 (0.71–1.82)

FIGURE 15–37.

Published controlled trials of leukocyte therapy for recurrent spontaneous abortion. Although the live-birth rate was high, controlled treatment resulted in similar rates in three of four studies. Only one reached statistical significance. Because of the expense of this procedure and potential morbidity, full disclosure of benefits and risks and informed consent are required. ID—intradermal; IV—intravenous; RR—relative risk; SC—subcutaneous. (*Adapted from* Kutteh [16].)

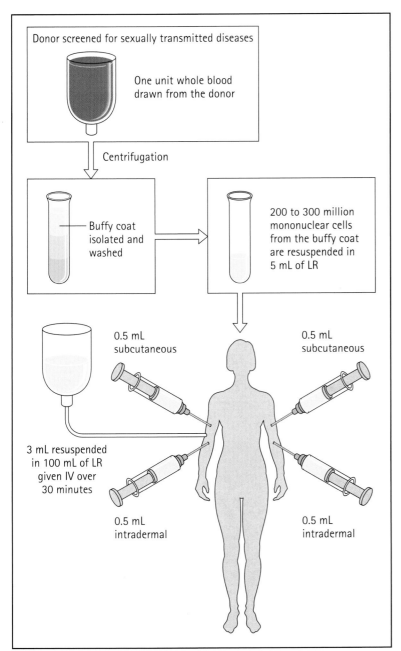

FIGURE 15-38.

Protocol for use of leukocyte immunization for recurrent pregnancy loss as proposed by the American Society for Immunology of Reproduction. Originally, couples with shared HLA of two or more were selected for treatment with donor leukocytes. However, HLA sharing has not been shown to predict pregnancy outcome in couples treated with immunotherapy [17]. Recently, this protocol has been used—with strict inclusion and exclusion criteria—in couples with unexplained recurrent abortion and three losses [18]. In this protocol, enriched lymphocyte and monocyte populations are prepared and infused over 30 minutes. The remaining preparation is injected into two intradermal and two subcutaneous sites in the upper arm. The immunization is performed on a single occurrence confirmation of pregnancy, but before 6 weeks gestation. IV—intravenously; LR—lactated ringers. (*Adapted from* Hataska and Scott [14].)

IMMUNOGLOBULIN THERAPY FOR RECURRENT SPONTANEOUS ABORTION

Study	Treatments compared and subjects (*n*)	Dose frequency, *d*	Therapy interval, *wk*	Live birth rate, %	*P* value
German recurrent spontaneous abortion/Intravenous Immunoglobulin (1994)	Immunoglobulin 20g (33) vs Albumin (31)	every 21	8–25 gestation	60.6 67.7	0.173
Coulam (1995) Christiansen (1995)	Immunoglobulin 500 mg/kg (29) vs Albumin (32)	every 28	0–32 gestation	62 38	0.04
	Immunoglobulin 30–35g (17) vs Albumin (17)	every 7–14	5–34 gestation	52.9 29.4	0.16

FIGURE 15-39.

Controlled studies of immunoglobulin therapy for recurrent abortion. Recently, investigators initiated studies using intravenous gamma globulin (IVIGG) as an alternative for leukocyte therapy for the treatment of unexplained recurrent abortion. However, it should be noted that the mechanism whereby IVIGG affects immune function is unknown. Only one of the three studies demonstrate statistical significance. Further studies are needed to confirm the clinical usefulness of this form of therapy. GRSA/IVIGG—German Recurrent Spontaneous Abortion/Intravenous Immunoglobulin Group. (*Adapted from* Kutteh [16].)

ORGANISMS POTENTIALLY CAUSING RECURRENT ABORTION

Type	Infecting agent	Route of infection	Cause of recurrent abortion
Parasites	*Toxoplasma gondii*	Hematogenous	Uncertain
Bacteria	*Treponema pallidum*	Hematogenous	Yes
	Mycoplasma spp	Ascending	Uncertain
	Chlamydia trachomatis	Ascending	Uncertain
	Listeria monocytogenes	Hematogenous	No
Viruses	HSV	Ascending	Uncertain
	CMV	Ascending	Uncertain

FIGURE 15-40.

Organisms potentially causing recurrent abortion. A number of infectious agents including bacteria, yeast, virus, and parasites have been associated with infections and sporadic abortion. In addition, some agents have been reported to cause recurrent abortion. Those agents and the most likely route of infection are shown in this table. *Treponema pallidum* is the only agent listed as certain. HSV—herpes simplex virus; CMV—cytomegalovirus. (*Adapted from* Hegone and Gibbs [19].)

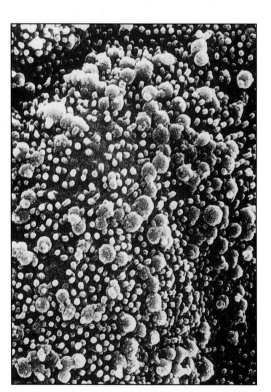

FIGURE 15-41.

A scanning electron micrograph demonstrating *Ureaplasma urealyticum* attached to the endometrium. Both *U. urealyticum* and *Mycoplasma hominis* can be isolated from the endometrium with or without evidence of inflammation. The presence of these organisms can also be demonstrated by culture of the endometrium and by immunofluorescence. In general, *Mycoplasma* organisms, including *M. hominis* and *U. urealyticum*, have received extensive attention as potential causes of pregnancy loss. These organisms are characterized by small size and lack of a cell wall, which renders them resistant to antibiotics. However, bacteriostatic antibiotics such as doxycycline and tetracycline are the treatments of choice for these organisms. *Mycoplasma* organisms require special culture techniques and may be found in 35% of sexually active women, and are possibly transmitted from their sexual partners. Some but not all investigators have demonstrated causal links between *Mycoplasma* organisms and recurrent abortion. Although this cannot be clarified completely, it is prudent to perform cultures from patients and, if positive, to treat the husband and wife appropriately. (*From* Cassell [20]; with permission.)

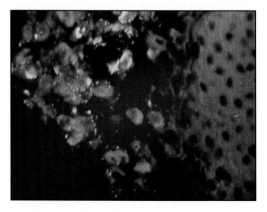

FIGURE 15-42.

Immunofluorescence study demonstrating *Mycoplasma* organisms attached to the surface of inflammatory cells in the cervix. (*From* Barnes [21]; with permission.)

DIAGNOSIS AND MANAGEMENT OF RECURRENT PREGNANCY LOSS

Etiology	Diagnostic evaluation	Therapy
Genetic	Karyotype partners	Genetic counseling
		Donor gametes
Anatomic	Hysterosalpingography	Septum transection
	Hysteroscopy	Remove polyp
	Sonohysterography	Resect synechiae
Endocrinologic	Endometrial biopsy	Progesterone
	Midluteal progesterone	Clomiphene citrate
	Thyrotropin	Thyroxine
	Prolactin	Bromocriptine
Immunologic	Lupus anticoagulant	Prednisone
	Antiphospholipid antibodies	Heparin
	(? Antithyroid antibodies)	Aspirin
	(? Embryotoxic factors)	(? Intravenous immunoglobulin)
Microbiologic	Cervical cultures	Antibiotics
Psychologic	Interview	Support group, counseling
Environmental	Exposure to tobacco, ethanol, toxins	Eliminate consumption
		Eliminate exposure

FIGURE 15-43.

Diagnosis and management of recurrent pregnancy loss. This table summarizes the previously discussed causes of recurrent pregnancy loss, the appropriate diagnostic tests to confirm the diagnosis, and the variety of therapies available. (*Adapted from Kutteh and Carr [5].*)

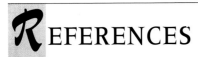EFERENCES

1. Hertig AT, Rock J, Adams EC, Menkin MC: Thirty-four fertilized human ova, good, bad, and indifferent, recovered from 210 women of known fertility. *Pediatrics* 1959, 23 (suppl.):202.

2. Leridon H: Intrauterine mortality. In *Human Fertility: The Basic Components*. Edited by Leridon H. Chicago: The University of Chicago Press; 1977; and *Williams Obstetrics*, edn 18. Norwalk: Appleton & Lange; 1989.

3. Kallen B: *Epidemiology of Human Reproduction*. Boca Raton: CRC Press; 1988:1–18.

4. Mills JL, Simpson JL, Driscoll SF, *et al.*: Incidence of spontaneous abortion among normal women and insulin-dependent diabetic women whose pregnancies were identified within 21 days of conception. *N Engl J Med* 1988, 319:1617.

5. Kutteh WH, Carr BR: Recurrent Pregnancy Loss. In *Textbook of Reproductive Medicine*. Edited by Carr BR, Blackwell RE. Norwalk: Appleton & Lange; 1993:559–570.

6. Warburton D, Fraser FC: Spontaneous abortion risks in man: data from reproductivehistories collected in a medical genetics unit. *Am J Hum Genet* 1964, 16:1.

7. Poland BJ, Miller JR, Jones DC, Trimble BK: Reproductive counseling in patients who have had a spontaneous abortion. *Am J Obstet Gynecol* 1977, 127:685.

8. Simpson JL: *Genetics: CREOG Basic Science Monographs in Obstetrics and Gynecology*. Washington, DC: Council on Resident Education in Obstetrics and Gynecology; 1986.

9. Scott JR: Spontaneous abortion. In *Danforth's Obstetrics and Gynecology*, edn 6. Edited by Danforth DN, Scott JA. Philadelphia: JB Lippincott; 1990:209.

10. DeBraekeleer M, Dao TN: Cytogenetic studies in couples experiencing repeated pregnancy losses. *Hum Reprod* 1990, 5:519.

11. Neri G, Serra A, Campana M, *et al.*: Reproductive risks for translocation carriers: cytogenetic study and analysis of pregnancy outcome in 58 families. *Am J Med Genet* 1983, 16:535–561.

12. Winkel CA: Diagnosis and treatment of uterine pathology. In *Textbook of Reproductive Medicine*. Edited by Carr BR, Blackwell RE. Norwalk, CT: Appleton & Lange; 1993:481–506.

13. Rein MS: Luteal phase defect and recurrent pregnancy loss. In *Infertility and Reproductive Medicine Clinics of North America*. Edited by Diamond MP, DeCherney AH, Friedman AJ. Philadelphia: WB Saunders Co; 1991:121–136.

14. Hatasaka HH, Scott JR: The immune factor. In *Reproductive Endocrinology, Surgery and Technology*, vol 2. Edited by Adashi EY, Rock JA, Rosenwaks Z. Philadelphia: Lippincott-Raven; 1996:2287–2308.

15. Rote NS: Pregnancy-associated immunological disorders. *Curr Opin Immunol* 1989, 1:1165.

16. Kutteh WH: Recurrent pregnancy loss. In *Textbook of Reproductive Medicine*, edn 2. Edited by Carr BR, Blackwell RE. Stamford, CT: Appleton & Lange; in press.

17. Cowchok SF, Smith JB, David S, *et al.*: Paternal mononuclear cell immunization therapy for repeated miscarriage: predictive variables for pregnancy success. *Am J Reprod Immunol* 1990, 22:12–17.

18. Coulam CB: Workshop A: unification of immunotherapy protocols. The report from the tenth anniversary meeting of the American Society for the Immunology of Reproduction, Chicago, June 20–23, 1990. *Am J Reprod Immunol* 1991, 25:1–6.

19. Heyborne KD, Gibbs RS: The infectious factor. In *Reproductive Endocrinology, Surgery and Technology*, vol 2. Edited by Adashi EY, Rock JA, Rosenwaks Z. Philadelphia: Lippincott-Raven; 1996:2310–2318.

20. Cassell G, Waites K, Taylor-Robinson D: Genital mycoplasma. In *Slide Atlas of Sexually Transmitted Diseases*. Edited by Morse S, Moreland A, Thompson S. New York: Gower Medical Publishing; 1992.

21. Barnes R: Infections caused by *Chlamydia trachomatis*. In *Slide Atlas of Sexually Transmitted Diseases*. Edited by Morse S, Moreland A, Thompson S. New York: Gower Medical Publishing; 1992.

Index --- I.1

Stress *(continued)*
    prolactin secretion and, 3.7
Submucous myoma, 9.9
Superovulation, 10.1
Superovulatory cycle monitoring, 9.17–9.18
Suppressor T cells, antigen-specific, 2.15
Surgery
    for abnormal uterine bleeding, 6.24
    for anovulation, 10.3
    for endometriosis, 14.9, 14.11, 14.13
    for hyperprolactinemia, 3.14
    for premenstrual syndrome, 7.1
    prolactin secretion and, 3.7
Syndrome X, 5.11

T

Teratogenicity, 10.2
Teratoma, 9.10
Testicle, 11.3
Testicular agonadism, 1.17
Testicular determining factor genes, 1.15
Testicular sperm aspiration, 11.9
Testicular volume, measurement of, 11.5
Testis, 11.2
    biopsy of, 11.9
        for male infertility, 11.1
        normal spermatogenesis in, 11.8
    development of, 1.15
    regulation of function of, 11.2
Testosterone, 4.3
    in acne, 4.6
    analogue of for Turner syndrome, 1.8
    metabolism of, 11.2
    postmenopausal production of, 8.4
    serum levels of, 4.9
        in abnormal uterine bleeding, 6.9
        after surgery for arrhenoblastoma, 2.13
        in amenorrhea, 1.14
        in polycystic ovary syndrome, 5.7, 5.8
    target tissues of, 4.3
Testosterone replacement therapy, 11.10
    side effects of, 11.10
    transdermal, 11.10
Testosterone-secreting tumor, 2.12
Thrombosis, antiphospholipid antibody-induced, 15.14
Thyroid-stimulating hormone test, 6.9
Thyroid-stimulating hormone (TSH)
    in anovulation and polycystic ovary syndrome, 2.6
    elevated levels of in primary amenorrhea, 1.18
    measurement of in infertility evaluation, 10.2
    serum levels of in primary amenorrhea, 1.21
Thyronine, 2.6
Thyrotropin-releasing hormone, 3.3, 3.5
Thyroxine
    in anovulation and polycystic ovary syndrome, 2.6
    for recurrent abortion, 15.17
Tibolone, 8.8
Tooth loss, 8.12

Toxoplasma gondii, 15.16
Transforming growth factors, 10.19
Transvaginal sonography
    for abnormal uterine bleeding, 6.9
    advantages and disadvantages of, 6.13
    in follicle size measurement, 13.2
    for hyperandrogenism, 4.12
    indications for, 6.13
Treponema pallidum, 15.16
TRH. *See* Thyrotropin-releasing hormones
Tricyclic antidepressants, 7.7
Trisomies, 15.5
Tubal transfers, success rates of, 13.3
Tubovarian adhesions, 9.7
Tumor necrosis factor, 10.19
Turner syndrome
    fertility options in, 1.8
    Hashimoto's thyroiditis and, 2.15
    with hypergonadotropic hypogonadism, 1.6
    internal genitalia with, 1.7
    in primary amenorrhea, 1.8
    treatment of, 1.8

U

Ultrasonography. *See also* Transvaginal sonography
    for abnormal uterine bleeding, 6.9, 6.13–6.16
    pelvic, for infertility, 9.10–9.11
    in polycystic ovary syndrome, 5.1, 5.2–5.4
    vaginal, for infertility, 9.10–9.11
Ureaplasma urealyticum, 15.16
Urinary frequency, postmenopausal, 8.5
Urinary tract infections, postmenopausal, 8.5
Urinary urgency, 8.5
Uterine septum, 9.9
    in recurrent abortion, 15.7
Uterovaginal agenesis, 1.13
Uterus
    absence of, 1.4, 1.16–1.17
    agenesis of, 1.13
    in amenorrhea, 2.1, 2.14
    anomalies of in recurrent abortion, 15.6, 15.8–15.10
    in Asherman's syndrome, 2.14
    bicornuate, surgical treatment of, 15.8
    congenital absence of, 1.16
        differential diagnosis of, 1.16
    DES-induced deformity of, 15.10
    double, 14.3
    duplication of
        in recurrent abortion, 15.7
        surgical correction of, 15.7
    dysfunctional bleeding of, 6.1–6.2
        biopsy for, 6.9–6.12
        causes of, 6.4–6.7
        definition of, 6.3
        diagnostic evaluation of, 6.8–6.17
        hysteroscopy for, 6.16–6.17
        medication for, 6.20–6.23
        menstrual cycle variability and, 6.2–6.3
        surgery for, 6.24
        transvaginal sonography for, 6.13–6.16

    treatment of, 6.17–6.24
    enlargement of, 6.15
    leiomyoma of, 15.9
    leiomyoma-induced filling defect of, 15.9
    lesions of with abnormal uterine bleeding, 6.7
    myoma of, 9.7
    unicornuate, in recurrent abortion, 15.8
Uterus didelphys, 15.6

V

Vagina
    abnormalities of, 6.7
    congenital absence of, 1.13
    development of, 1.15
    layers of, 8.5
    normal versus estrogen-deficient epithelium of, 8.5
Vaginitis, atrophic postmenopausal, 8.5
Vanishing testes syndrome, 1.17
Varicocele, 11.6
    clinical aspects of, 11.6
    effects of repair on pregnancy rates, 11.11
Vas, congenital absence of, 11.8
Vas deferens, obstruction of, 11.8
Vascular endothelial growth factor (VEGF)
    definition of, 5.13
    distribution in ovary, 5.14
    serum levels in polycystic ovary syndrome, 5.14
    during *in vitro* fertilization, 5.15
Vasectomy
    azoospermia with, 11.8
    reversal of, 11.9
Venous thromboembolic disease, 8.13
Virilization, 4.7
Viruses, 15.18
Vitamin B_6, 7.9
Vitamin D, 8.8
Vitamin E, 7.9
Vitamins, 7.3

X

X chromosome
    features of, 1.9
    with hypergonadotropic hypogonadism, 1.6

Y

Y chromosome, 1.9, 11.2
    counseling for, 1.15

Z

Zona dissection, partial, 13.10
Zona drilling, 13.10
Zona-free hamster ova-*in vitro* sperm penetration assay, 11.7